Resolving Ethical Dilemmas

A GUIDE FOR CLINICIANS

Sixth Edition

Resolving Ethical Dilemmas

A GUIDE FOR CLINICIANS

Sixth Edition

Bernard Lo, M.D.
President & CEO
The Greenwall Foundation
New York, New York
Professor Emeritus of Medicine
Director Emeritus, Program in Medical Ethics
University of California
California, San Francisco

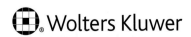
Wolters Kluwer

Philadelphia • Baltimore • New York • London
Buenos Aires • Hong Kong • Sydney • Tokyo

Director, Medical Practice: Rebecca Gaertner
Editorial Coordinator: Jeremiah Kiely
Senior Editorial Assistant: Brian Convery
Marketing Manager: Rachel Mante-Leung
Senior Production Project Manager: Alicia Jackson
Design Coordinator: Holly McLaughlin
Manufacturing Coordinator: Beth Welsh
Prepress Vendor: S4Carlisle Publishing Services

Sixth Edition

Library of Congress Cataloging-in-Publication Data

Names: Lo, Bernard, author.
Title: Resolving ethical dilemmas : a guide for clinicians / Bernard Lo.
Description: Sixth edition. | Philadelphia, PA: Wolters Kluwer Health,
   [2020] | Includes bibliographical references and index.
Identifiers: LCCN 2018054744 | ISBN 9781975103545
Subjects: | MESH: Ethics, Clinical | Clinical Decision-Making—ethics | Case
   Reports
Classification: LCC R724 | NLM WB 60 | DDC 174.2—dc23 LC record available at https://lccn.loc.gov/2018054744.

shop.lww.com

Contents

SECTION V   CONFLICTS OF INTEREST

SECTION VI   ETHICAL ISSUES IN CLINICAL SPECIALTIES

Preface to the First Edition

As a resident, I was paged by the intensive care unit late one night. I recognized the patient, a 17-year-old boy who had undergone bone marrow transplantation for leukemia and now had chronic interstitial fibrosis. The shy, bright smile I remembered from a previous admission was gone. According to the chart, he had developed progressive respiratory failure. His thin, intubated body was squirming restlessly in the bed. The patient's father grabbed my hand and pointed to the ventilator, saying, "Stop, it's enough. He doesn't want this." I phoned the attending physician, an eminent hematologist, who said that the patient was expected to die in the next few days. I asked whether we should extubate the patient, as his father had requested, and sedate him. The hematologist said that the bone marrow transplant service wanted to continue intensive care; although he did not defend their decision, he deferred to it. We did agree on a Do Not Resuscitate (DNR) order. I gave some sedation to the patient and tried to comfort him and his family. The boy died just before I went off duty the next morning, more comfortable perhaps, but by no means peaceful. The father asked me, "Why didn't they stop? Why?" Later, the attending physician told me that after my phone call, he couldn't get back to sleep. He said that he wanted to call me back to tell me to extubate the patient.

Like this boy's father, I kept asking, "Why?" Why were we so insistent on imposing our medical technology on dying patients? Why were decisions driven by physicians' personalities, hospital politics, research priorities, or staffing problems rather than by what was best for the patient? Why were we comfortable withholding cardiopulmonary resuscitation (CPR), but uneasy administering high doses of narcotics to a patient with intractable ventilatory failure? Although we spent much time on rounds talking about the use of immunosuppressive agents, antibiotics, ventilators, and a vast array of treatments, why did we avoid discussing what to do when such interventions were no longer helpful or appropriate?

My interest in medical ethics, and ultimately this book, grew from such perplexing cases as this and from the illnesses of family members and friends. From visiting my favorite aunt, who had developed multi-infarct dementia, I learned how hard it is to say that life is no longer worth living. She had become almost immobile, dependent on others for all her needs, and would often moan and shout when moved. But she would smile when I held her hands or stroked her cheek. Although mute most of the day, she laughed when I showed her pictures of my son and would ask me, "How old?" We could spend an hour looking at the same pictures over and over, with her repeating the same questions. But even as her family and I despaired over her deteriorating condition, it was not yet time to let her go. Life was still a precious gift, not yet an intolerable burden.

As I began writing and speaking about medical ethics, I learned that many colleagues shared my concerns. At professional meetings, practitioners often tell me about cases whose ethical dilemmas still bother them. I have tried to keep in mind such physicians struggling to do what was right in difficult situations. This book features realistic cases that physicians can relate to their own experience. The goal of *Resolving Ethical Dilemmas* is to help clinicians resolve the mundane ethical issues in patient care, as well as the dilemmas that keep them awake at night. In some cases, there are persuasive reasons for a course of action, but in others the countervailing arguments are equally compelling. Yet even when the philosophic debate is closely balanced, physicians must act, choosing one plan of care or another.

This book grew in several ways beyond my initial work on decisions regarding life-sustaining interventions. First, over the years I realized that physicians need help with many ethical issues. Friends and colleagues often asked me why no one has written about impaired colleagues, about patients' requests to deceive insurance companies, and about the ethical problems in managed care. Second, as the AIDS epidemic ravaged San Francisco, we grappled with new ethical dilemmas, such as the duty to provide care, access to experimental therapies, and the fear of nosocomial HIV infection. Third, a personal calamity broadened the issues of this book. On October 20, 1991, a firestorm raged through the Oakland hills. Our house and more than 2,000 others burned to the ground in a few hours. My wife and I felt sad, angry, frustrated, and overwhelmed by the task of putting our lives back together. It was hard to make any choices, much less informed or rational ones. Gradually, I realized I was struggling with the same issues in this book as in life. Issues of autonomy, informed consent, and fiduciary responsibility took on increasing prominence. How can people make informed decisions when they are emotionally overwhelmed? Why must physicians act in their patients' best interests, even to their personal financial disadvantage, when insurance companies and other businesses have no such obligation?

Colleagues sometimes ask me why I work on such "depressing" topics. Although the issues are indeed somber, it is also a special privilege when patients and their families trust us with their grief, anger, and tranquility and show us how to endure turmoil and sorrow. An elderly patient who had hidden for months the severity of her bone cancer pain was delighted when I made a home visit, saying, "I am so glad I could show you my garden. Now you know why I want to die here, looking at my flowers." Another of my patients died from breast cancer and recurrent pleural effusions. She always cried and moaned as we tapped her effusions, even though she knew that her breathing would be easier. I wondered whether we were hurting her rather than helping her. After her death, I said to her son that it must have been hard for him to care for her. He replied softly, "Doc, it made me a better man." As physicians, we see the worst and the best of people. At times, they are helpless and angry and make foolish decisions. But when confronting problems that are too large for them, people often become heroes. Ultimately, I hope this book will help patients who struggle with such problems by guiding the physicians who care for them.

Bernard Lo

Preface to the Sixth Edition

This sixth edition contains extensive new materials to keep up with significant new developments and the best recent thinking in resolving ethical dilemmas in clinical care.

Chapter 46 is a new chapter that analyzes the ethical issues in big data and artificial intelligence in health care. Although big data and artificial intelligence might provide important benefits for patients, they also raise complex ethical issues that need to be addressed.

Conscientious objection has taken on increased significance in medicine and in US society in general. Chapter 24 has a new, extended discussion of the topic. Chapter 1 contains a rewritten section on claims of conscience.

Professionalism has become more prominent in medical education. Chapter 1 discusses how clinical ethics differs from professional codes. Chapter 36 discusses the differences between clinical ethics and professionalism training, particularly how clinical ethics analyzes the reasons for a decision or action, whereas professionalism tends to focus on the physician's observable behavior and actions.

Chapter 12 contains new expanded sections on advance care planning and Physician Orders for Life-Sustaining Treatment (POLST). The emphasis is on preparing surrogates to make an actual clinical decision for a patient who no longer has decision-making capacity.

Chapter 14, entitled *Potentially Inappropriate Interventions* (formerly called Futile Interventions), discusses disputes when patients or their surrogates disagree with physician recommendations that an intervention is not medically appropriate. There is emerging agreement that institutional procedures for resolving these disputes should replace unilateral decisions by physicians to withhold the intervention.

Chapter 19 provides a new analysis of ethical issues regarding physician-assisted suicide. With several states reporting their experience with legalized physician aid-in-dying (PAD), the chapter incorporates empirical evidence relevant to concerns about legalization of PAD. In addition, there is more discussion of ethical dilemmas confronting physicians after a patient requests PAD; both supporters and opponents of legalization of PAD need to decide how they will respond to these dilemmas.

Chapter 20, entitled *Unresponsive Wakefulness And the Minimally Conscious State,* (formerly called The Persistent Vegetative State, now entitled Unresponsive Wakefulness And the Minimally Conscious State), contains up-to-date information about the minimally conscious state (MCS) and unresponsive wakefulness. There is new information on the neurobiology of the MCS, on how it differs from unresponsive wakefulness (formerly called the persistent vegetative state), and on the long-term prognosis in patients who receive intensive and extensive neurorehabilitation after severe brain injury. This revised chapter analyzes how this new knowledge impacts on how physicians should respond to the ethical dilemmas in the care of these patients.

Chapter 26 on sexual contact between physicians and patients contains a new section on physicians who sexually abuse patients. In several prominent cases, serial abusers were allowed to continue to practice medicine, putting additional patients at risk. The chapter discusses the responsibility of individual health care workers to speak out when they learn of such illegal conduct and the responsibility of health care organizations to address it.

The new Chapter 30 analyzes the dilemmas that health care policy and health economics must address in the United States. The United States per capita expenditures of health care are significantly higher than in other countries, yet health outcomes in the United States lag substantially behind outcomes in countries that have much lower expenditures for health care, with wide disparities in outcomes according to social determinants of health. Furthermore, access to health care is substantially worse than the vast majority of other countries. Political leaders do not agree on the relative importance of these problems.

Chapter 31 on payment to physicians and health care organizations is substantially rewritten.

Chapter 36 on ethical issues students and house staff face contains updated and expanded discussions of the ethical dilemmas created by house staff duty hours restrictions. Throughout, this chapter emphasizes the responsibility of the health care organization.

Chapter 38 on ethical issues in surgery contains an expanded and updated discussion of ethical issues regarding concurrent surgery.

Chapter 41 on transplantation has a revised, updated section on ethical issues concerning organ donation after cardiac determination of death.

Chapter 43 on ethical issues in caring for diverse populations contains a new section on responding to racist requests by patients, which may well have become more prominent in recent years.

Chapter 44 contains a new section on learning health systems.

Fundamentals of Clinical Ethics

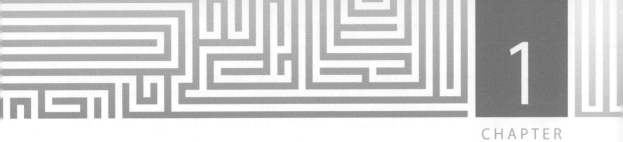

An Approach to Ethical Dilemmas in Patient Care

INTRODUCTION

"This case is really bothering me. I haven't been able to stop worrying about it. I'm just not sure what the right thing to do is." Cases that present ethical dilemmas can perplex physicians. Strong reasons for an action or decision might be balanced by strong arguments against it. Key parties in the case may disagree sharply. Being a good person and having good intentions, common sense, and clinical experience do not guarantee that a physician will respond appropriately. Ethical dilemmas often evoke powerful emotions and strong personal opinions; however, emotions and reflexive opinions alone are not a satisfactory way of addressing ethical dilemmas.

This chapter describes how clinical ethics can help physicians respond to dilemmas. Specific ethical problems are discussed in detail in subsequent chapters.

WHAT IS CLINICAL ETHICS?

We use the term *clinical* to limit our topics to the doctor–patient encounter in the office or at the hospital bedside, when a physician is caring for an individual patient. Such patient care is the essence of a physician's work. In addition to the doctor's interaction with the patient, the physician's relationships with the family, other health care workers, and medical institutions, such as insurance companies, may also present dilemmas in patient care.

We use the term *ethics* to refer to judgments about what is right or wrong and worthy of praise or blame. This refers to moral judgments about right and wrong, not biotechnical or clinical judgments about the most effective or safest test or treatment.

Clinical ethics analyzes the reasons for and against a decision or action and suggests which reasons are convincing and which are not, as well as why this is the case.

CASE 1.1	Decisions about life-sustaining interventions

Mrs. D is a 76-year-old nursing home resident with severe dementia who does not respond to questions. She develops fever, cough, shortness of breath, and purulent sputum. Her daughter, who visits her several times a week, insists that hospitalization and administration of antibiotics would be pointless and that the patient would not want such "heroics." However, Mrs. D's son, who visits infrequently, demands that her pneumonia be treated because he believes that life is sacred.

In Case 1.1, the biotechnical issue is which antibiotic would be most effective for community-acquired pneumonia. There may be medical uncertainty or controversy, for example, because of emerging patterns of antibiotic resistance. These biotechnical questions can often be resolved by referring to the medical literature, clinical experience, or expert judgment. The clinical ethics question in this case, however, is whether to administer or withhold antibiotics.

We also distinguish clinical ethics from several other closely related fields that are beyond the scope of this book. *Health policy* refers to public and private policies that set the context in which physicians deliver care to patients. It includes health insurance arrangements, access to care for the uninsured, public health policies, and relevant laws and regulations.

Bioethics refers to broader philosophical questions raised by biomedical advances, for example, whether genetically modified crops or germ-line gene therapy is acceptable.

HOW DOES CLINICAL ETHICS DIFFER FROM PROFESSIONAL CODES?

Many physicians seek ethical guidance from professional codes and the oaths that they took as students at white-coat ceremonies and at graduation. At these ceremonies, new physicians pledge to the public and to their patients that they will be guided by the oath or code. Although professional oaths and codes are important, they have several shortcomings (1, 2). First, medical schools administer a variety of different oaths; hence, neither colleagues nor patients know what an individual doctor has pledged to do.

Second, professional oaths are unilateral declarations by groups of physicians, without significant input from patients or the public. Codes of ethics and professional oaths do not acknowledge that society has granted the medical profession responsibility for self-regulation, for example, to set standards for training and certification. In return for such self-regulation, the public may expect physicians to meet certain expectations.

Third, professional codes have been criticized for falling short on respect for patients and acting in their interests. The Hippocratic tradition, for example, is highly paternalistic, granting patients little role in making decisions. It does not require physicians to disclose information to patients, to be truthful, or to allow them to make informed choices. In recent years, physician professional codes have lagged behind public views of acting in the best interests of patients. Compared with physicians, patients want more disclosure of errors and explicit apologies for them (see Chapter 34), greater public disclosure of impaired and incompetent physicians and stricter sanctions for them (*see* Chapter 35), and more detailed disclosure of information regarding proposed surgical procedures, including risks and the physician's experience (*see* Chapter 38). Critics also charge that professional codes do not adequately address problems that concern patients, such as poor access to care as well as its high cost. Professional organizations historically have served as advocacy groups for physicians in ways that arguably were not in the interests of patients (3), and their efforts to obtain favorable reimbursement for physicians may conflict with patients' desires for more affordable health care.

Fourth, oaths and codes articulate broad general precepts but often do not provide practical guidance in specific cases. Codes often do not discuss the reasons for their precepts and how to interpret them in various situations. In addition, the principles embodied in codes may be in conflict in a particular case, leaving the physician in a quandary about how to act. This book provides physicians and medical students the tools to respond to such dilemmas and how to interpret and apply broad ethical guidelines (such as those contained in professional codes) in specific situations and how to act when ethical guidelines are in conflict or do not apply.

Chapter 36 covers education in professionalism for trainees, which has increased and become more systematic in recent years. Professionalism education focuses on behaviors that can be learned, practiced, and refined over a professional career (4, 5). Professionalism training assumes that all physicians share a common view on what maxims should guide physician behaviors and what actions are appropriate in a specific clinical situation; that is, there is a shared understanding of what is right to do. However, this assumption is questionable for several reasons. First, there is no agreement on what the term *professionalism* means or requires (5). Second, individual physicians bring values to guide their actions from their personal, religious, secular, and cultural traditions, which may differ from professional values (1). Third, as noted, patients and the public may have different views from physicians on both guiding principles and specific physician actions.

Chapter 36 discusses the differences between clinical ethics and professionalism, particularly how clinical ethics analyzes the reasons for a decision or action, whereas professionalism tends to focus on the physician's observable behavior and actions.

HOW DOES CLINICAL ETHICS DIFFER FROM LAW?

Statutes, regulations, and court decisions also guide what physicians may or may not do. On many issues, the law reflects an ethical consensus in society. Appellate courts give reasons for decisions and therefore provide an analysis of pertinent issues. Physicians should be familiar with what the law requires regarding issues in clinical ethics. However, the law may not provide definitive answers to ethical dilemmas.

First, the law, particularly criminal law, sets only a minimal standard of conduct. It identifies acts that are so *wrong* that physicians will be held legally liable for committing them. In contrast, ethics may focus on the *right* or the best decision in a situation. Ethical standards may be higher than legal requirements; for example, respect for patients requires physicians to do more than the legal requirements.

CASE 1.2	Physician certification of eligibility

A 67-year-old man with chronic obstructive lung disease has dyspnea after walking one block. He is on an optimal medical regimen of inhaled bronchodilators and corticosteroids. His resting arterial O_2 level is 65 mm Hg, and it does not decrease with exercise. This exceeds the level that qualifies for Medicare coverage of home oxygen. The patient pleads, "Can't you just write that the oxygen level is 58? I need to do something about this breathing."

In Case 1.2, the Medicare criteria for coverage of home oxygen are clear: an arterial oxygen level of under 60 mm Hg. Giving false information to obtain Medicare coverage is considered fraud, a criminal violation. Physicians, like all citizens, should follow the law. Beyond that, clinical ethics may require physicians to go beyond their legal duties, for example, acting with compassion and respect and responding to the patient's distress. The law cannot compel such ideals.

Second, the law may be silent in some situations. In Case 1.1, most states do not give physicians explicit legal authority to determine when a patient lacks the decision-making capacity to identify a surrogate to make decisions on his or her behalf (*see* Chapter 11). However, this practice is widely accepted and practiced, and the option of seeking the legal appointment of a guardian in every case is impractical. In these circumstances, physicians must turn to ethical and clinical considerations, not legal ones.

Finally, law and ethics might differ. Abortion is currently legal throughout the United States, but remains controversial ethically. Many health care workers consider it morally wrong and do not participate in it. Conversely, people might consider some actions that the law prohibits to be ethical. In a few states, laws establishing who may act as a surrogate for a patient who lacks decision-making capacity do not include domestic partners, long-standing partners, or close friends as acceptable surrogates. In some cases, however, these persons meet the ethical criteria for an appropriate surrogate because they know the patient's goals, values, and preferences and care about the patient (*see* Chapter 12). In such cases, most physicians feel ethically uncomfortable simply following the letter of the law.

SOURCES OF MORAL GUIDANCE

Distinguishing Morality and Ethics

The terms *morality* and *ethics* are often used interchangeably to refer to standards of right and wrong behavior. It is helpful to draw some distinctions. Moral choices ultimately rest on values or beliefs that cannot be proved but are simply accepted. Morality usually refers to conduct that conforms "to the accepted customs or conventions of a people" (6). Children usually learn from parents and religious and community leaders what their culture or group regards as correct and commonly accept it without deliberation. Ultimately, such fundamental moral beliefs are part of a person's character. Yet ordinary moral rules, which usually provide an adequate guide for daily conduct, fail to provide clear direction for health care workers in many clinical situations.

In contrast to morality, ethics connotes deliberation and explicit arguments to justify particular actions. Ethics also refers to a branch of philosophy that deals with the "principles governing ideal human character" (6). To philosophers, ethics focuses on the reasons *why* an action is considered right or wrong. It asks people to justify their positions and beliefs by rational arguments that can persuade others who may not share their specific cultural or religious affiliation.

Personal Moral Values

Physicians, like all people, draw on many sources of moral guidance, including parental and family values, cultural traditions, and religious beliefs. However, additional guidance in clinical ethics is needed.

First, these personal moral values might not address important issues in clinical ethics. Often, doctors face an ethical dilemma for the first time during their training and clinical practice. Laypeople have little experience with such topics as life-sustaining treatment or surrogate decision-making. In addition, personal moral values might offer conflicting or ambiguous advice on a particular situation. For instance, moral precepts to respect the sanctity of life can be used in Case 1.1 to justify both continuing and withholding antibiotics.

Second, physicians have role-specific ethical obligations that go beyond their obligations as good citizens and people. Doctors have special duties to avoid misrepresentation when certifying a patient's medical condition, as in Case 1.2 (*see* Chapter 6). Personal moral values do not address these special professional roles.

Third, the physician's moral values might differ from those of the patient or other health care workers. The United States is increasingly diverse in terms of cultural heritage and religious beliefs. In such a pluralistic society, physicians cannot assume that other people directly involved in a case share their moral beliefs. Thus, physicians need to persuade other health care workers, patients, and family members of their plans to resolve ethical dilemmas in patient care, using reasons that do not depend on a particular religious or cultural perspective.

Claims of Conscience

Sometimes people explain their actions as a matter of conscience; to act otherwise would breach deeply held core values that define them as individuals, violate their sense of moral integrity, and make them feel ashamed, guilty, or lose self-respect (7).

Deeply held claims of conscience should be honored. It would be dehumanizing and disrespectful to compel people to act in ways that contradict their sense of moral integrity. In a society that respects claims of conscience, people are encouraged to engage in moral reflection and act with integrity. Having deep moral commitments and living by them is an aspect of human flourishing, which, in the US vision of a good society, should be encouraged and fostered. Of note, a person can, and should, respect the actions another person takes in accordance with his or her conscience and deeply held religious beliefs, without agreeing with the substance of the moral belief or his or her decision or action (8). Thus, respect for the conscience of other people is closely aligned with the values of religious liberty and pluralism, which are core American values dating back to colonial times (9).

Claims of conscience, however, are not absolute. In many situations, there are important countervailing interests and ethical principles that also deserve to be respected. Physicians and hospitals have an ethical and professional obligation to prevent imminent, serious harm to patients in need. Claims of conscience by a health care worker or even a health care institution should not place patients at significant harm in a medical emergency (10, 11). One party's claim to live by his or her own deeply held values should not block others from doing the same (10).

Appeals to conscience do not end discussions about what to do in a particular case; to persuade others to accept such claims, it is often necessary to provide reasons and arguments and to address countervailing interests and rights. Chapter 14 discusses physician insistence on interventions, and Chapter 24 discusses refusals to provide medical services for reasons of conscience.

Claims of Rights

To explain their positions on ethical issues, people often appeal to rights, such as a "right to die" or a "right to health care." To philosophers, rights are justified claims that a person can make on others or on society. The language of rights is widespread in US culture, yet appeals to rights are often controversial. Other people might deny that the right exists or assert conflicting rights. For example, many people believe there is a right to health care; however, such claims cannot be enforced against government agencies or private health insurers. Some general rights that are broadly acknowledged, for example, are the right to be free of unwanted medical interventions, the right to privacy, and the right not to be discriminated against. However, these rights need to be specified, particularly in terms of who needs to do what under the law or as a matter of ethics. Although claims of rights are often used to end debates, asserting a right instead should open a new discussion: are there persuasive arguments that support the claim of a right and what specifically does that right entail?

HOW CAN CLINICAL ETHICS HELP PHYSICIANS?

Certain situations commonly recur in clinical practice. Physicians learn to recognize individual cases as examples of syndromes, such as "angina" or "hyponatremia" (12). Placing cases into cognitive schemas or conceptual categories allow physicians to organize relevant data, draw on experiences with similar cases, and to help with problem solving (13). For each type of case, the physician learns to gather additional information, anticipate associated problems or complications, and develop an approach to the case. The more detailed and nuanced schema physicians have prepare them for clinical practice.

Clinical ethics can help physicians identify, understand, and resolve common ethical issues in patient care. By studying paradigmatic "teaching cases," physicians can gain vicarious experience in identifying and resolving ethical dilemmas (14). Cases help physicians learn how to interpret ethical guidelines in particular situations, how to distinguish a case from other apparently similar cases, which differences between cases should lead to a different decision or action, and when exceptions to guidelines are justified. The cases in this book are based on real cases, and information in a case is presented in chunks to pause the process of care at key junctures to allow reflection, analysis, and discussion.

Identify Ethical Issues

By studying realistic cases that illustrate common ethical problems, physicians may better recognize the ethical issues in their own cases. In some instances, physicians might have only a vague uneasiness that important ethical issues are at stake. In other situations, health care workers might be perplexed about difficult decisions but fail to identify problems as specifically ethical in nature, as opposed to issues of clinical management or interpersonal conflict.

Understand Areas of Ethical Consensus and Controversy

On many ethical issues, physicians, philosophers, and the courts agree on what should be done (15, 16). For example, it is well established that trustworthy advance directives, such as a Physician Orders for Life-Sustaining Treatment (POLST) form, should be respected. Such an agreement is often possible even when it holds different reasons for the action (17). Subsequent chapters point out areas of widespread ethical agreement as well as areas of ongoing controversy.

Clinical ethics can identify actions that are clearly right or wrong under the circumstances and those that are controversial. Philosophers also distinguish among actions that are obligatory, permissible, and prohibited. In Case 1.2, there are strong reasons why physicians should not misrepresent the patient's condition to insurers (*see* Chapter 6); not misrepresenting the patient's laboratory value is obligatory. Other actions may be optional or ethically *permissible,* but not required. The arguments for and against them may be so evenly balanced that reasonable people may disagree. Alternatively, it may be praiseworthy for the physician to perform them, but the physician should not be faulted for not doing so. For instance, it would be commendable for a busy physician in Case 1.2 to devote considerable time to explaining to the patient why he or she cannot fulfill his request. The physician should not be blamed, however, if he or she gave his or her recommendation with a brief explanation of his or her reasoning, referred the patient for more information on home oxygen, for example to the website of the Global Initiative for Chronic Obstructive Lung Disease, and continued the discussion at a later visit.

Understanding the reasons for and against a decision or action can reduce moral uncertainty and prevent or alleviate moral distress. Clinical ethics also can help the physician respond to reasons others offer for a different course of action.

AN APPROACH TO ETHICAL DILEMMAS IN CLINICAL MEDICINE

A systematic approach to ethical problems helps ensure that no important considerations are overlooked and that similar cases are resolved consistently (Table 1-1). In any particular case, an experienced physician may need to modify the general approach.

What Is the Problem or Dilemma?

As a first step, it is helpful to state the problem or dilemma in straightforward terms. In Case 1.1, should Mrs. D receive antibiotics? Should she be transferred from the nursing home to the hospital?

What Are the Medical Facts and Issues?

Sound ethical decision-making requires accurate medical facts and clinical judgment. The physician needs to clarify the patient's diagnosis and prognosis, the options for care, and the benefits and burdens of each alternative. Health outcomes need to be specified and characterized in probabilistic terms insofar as possible. In Case 1.1, how likely is it that with antibiotics, Mrs. D will be able to return to the nursing home and regain her former functional status? Furthermore, the strength of the medical evidence needs to be assessed. Uncertainty and disagreement over the interpretation of medical facts are common. Often they can be resolved by going to the medical literature or by having the various specialty services or physicians caring for the patient meet face to face.

What Are the Patient's Concerns, Values, and Preferences?

Informed consent and shared decision-making require the physician to understand the patient's perspective (*see* Chapter 3). A good first step is to ask open-ended questions about the patient's understanding of the clinical situation: "What is your understanding of your medical situation?"

TABLE 1-1.   An Approach to Ethical Dilemmas in Clinical Medicine
In plain terms, what is the problem or dilemma?
What are the medical facts and issues?
What are the concerns, values, and preferences of the patient?
What are the concerns, values, and preferences of the physicians?
What are the ethical issues?
What ethical guidelines are at stake?
What practical considerations need to be addressed?

or "What have the doctors told you about your illness?" Any misunderstandings should be discussed and corrected.

Physicians should elicit the patient's or surrogate's concerns, hopes, and fears: "As you think about your medical situation, what concerns you the most?" Addressing the patient's concerns demonstrates caring, strengthens the doctor–patient relationship, and makes patients and surrogates more open to the physician's recommendations. Next, the physician needs to understand the patient's goals for care and preferences regarding specific decisions that need to be made.

In Case 1.1, has Mrs. D previously indicated her goals for care and values? Has she given preferences for hospitalization and medical care in such a situation? Has she indicated whom she would want to make decisions for her?

If the patient lacks decision-making capacity, an appropriate surrogate needs to be identified, generally a family member (*see* Chapter 13).

What Are the Clinicians' Concerns, Values, and Preferences?

Physicians have expertise regarding diagnosis, prognosis, options for care, and their risks and benefits. They also have their own values and preferences. In Case 1.1, a physician might believe that prolonging life is beneficial and that he or she should provide effective, low-risk treatments that prolong life. The physician's personal beliefs may differ from those of the patient or family. Physicians must identify their own values and distinguish medical expertise from value judgments, where the patient's values and preferences must be taken into account, and generally should be decisive.

Physicians do not all have the same attitudes, preferences, and values regarding uncertainty, risk, and the doctor–patient relationship. They need to acknowledge that other health care workers may have quite different values and preferences. One way to assess such differences is to ask questions: Would another attending physician have different goals of care and make different recommendations?

What Are the Ethical Issues or Questions?

It is generally fruitful to frame the ethical issues and questions in specific terms, rather than as broad ethical concepts, such as autonomy and beneficence. In Case 1.1, the specific questions are: Who should serve as the surrogate for Mrs. D, who lacks decision-making capacity (*see* Chapter 11)? What should be the basis for the surrogate's decision (*see* Chapter 12)? Should antibiotics for pneumonia be considered heroic or extraordinary care in this context (*see* Chapter 15)?

The importance of specificity can be illustrated by comparing how physicians pose medical issues. In a case of diabetic ketoacidosis, it is not useful to frame the issue as "homeostasis," although that is a fundamental unifying concept in this situation. For clinical management, it is much more useful to identify specific problems, such as volume replacement, hyperglycemia, potassium disorders, acidosis, and precipitating events. Posing medical issues in such specific terms facilitates clinical reasoning and management. Each specific medical issue triggers considerations for the physician to take into account. For example, identifying serum potassium as an issue emphasizes that the potassium level should be elevated in the face of acidosis and suggests the magnitude of total body potassium loss and the rate of replacement.

What Ethical Guidelines Are at Stake, and How Can the Dilemma Be Resolved?

Once identified, specific ethical issues and guidelines should be taken into account and an approach developed to resolve the issues. Subsequent chapters analyze how to resolve these specific ethical issues. The guidelines need to be more specific than "respect for persons," "beneficence," and so on, which are too abstract and general to guide the physician's decisions and actions. In each clinical situation and case, these abstract guidelines need to be specified, interpreted, and applied. In addition, countervailing arguments and interpretations need to be considered. Moreover, the physician needs to consider how additional ethical guidelines or moral intuitions might apply to the case, and how different ethical guidelines might need to be balanced.

Although physicians should learn an approach to each common ethical issue, difficult cases cannot be resolved by mechanically applying rules. Physicians must interpret guidelines in the particular circumstances of the patient's situation. Furthermore, guidelines may conflict or be accorded different weight in various circumstances. Physicians also need to think through the reasons supporting their plan, so that they can explain them to others in a persuasive manner.

What Practical Considerations Need to Be Addressed?

What Is the Plan for Communication?

The physician should consider how to discuss the ethical issues with other health care workers, patients, and surrogates. Team meetings can clarify the clinical situation and provide additional information about the patient's or surrogate's views. Health care workers from different clinical, personal, religious, and cultural backgrounds can frequently point out hidden assumptions and value judgments, call attention to neglected issues, and suggest fresh alternatives. Health care workers caring for the patient should agree on a plan for care, or at least clarify the points of disagreement and the process for resolving them.

A series of family meetings is usually required. Chapter 13 suggests how physicians can negotiate an ethically acceptable resolution when relatives of a patient disagree. Often the key is first to listen to the patient's and family's needs, concerns, and values. Patients or families might hear mixed messages from different clinicians, so family conferences that include key consulting services enhance consistent communication.

Physicians need to try to reach a decision that is acceptable to them, the patient or surrogate, and other health care providers caring for the patient. Decisions also need to be consistent with the ethical guidelines discussed in later chapters.

What Psychosocial Issues Complicate the Case?

Emotions, misunderstandings, interpersonal conflicts, and time pressures often complicate ethical dilemmas. Although analysis of ethical issues is essential, few dilemmas in clinical ethics are resolved solely by philosophical arguments. Indeed, many ethical dilemmas are settled by addressing psychosocial issues rather than through philosophical debate. Showing respect, concern, and compassion builds patient and family trust and makes them more likely to carefully consider the physician's recommendations.

When Should Physicians Seek Assistance?

In difficult cases, the physician may seek assistance from the hospital ethics committee or an ethics consultant (*see* Chapter 16). A second opinion from another physician not directly involved in the case might also be helpful. A chaplain, social worker, or nurse who has good rapport with the patient or family can help address their concerns or facilitate discussions.

What Are the Legal Constraints?

Physicians need to understand the legal risk of the course of action they have determined to be ethically appropriate; however, decisions should not be based primarily on defensive medicine. Ethics and law may differ. Some states do not explicitly authorize surrogate decision-making by family members who have not been designated as proxies by the patient, even though this is standard clinical practice and ethically sound. Physicians can minimize legal risk by documenting in the medical record the reasons that justify the plan for care and the process by which the decision was reached.

Moral Distress

Health care providers, including residents, medical students, and nurses, may experience moral distress when they cannot carry out an ethically appropriate action because of institutional policies, decision-making hierarchies, legal barriers, limited resources, or other external constraints (18). Such situations may compromise a person's sense of moral integrity. For example, many students are distressed if asked to carry out intimate examinations of patients or to perform invasive procedures without patient consent. Moral distress can lead to anger, anxiety, frustration, helplessness, fatigue, work dissatisfaction, and burnout. Similar feelings may be experienced when a heath care worker is unsure what the morally appropriate action is in a situation (18). Moral distress is related to conscientious objection, which is a health care worker's refusal to carry out an action that violates a deeply held core moral belief (*see* Chapter 2).

To address their moral distress, health care workers should discuss complex or unfamiliar clinical situations with colleagues and seek assistance with difficult decisions. Personal ways to help relieve distress include mindfulness meditation, cognitive reappraisal, and yoga. Health care institutions have important responsibilities to prevent and mitigate moral distress by establishing a culture of open communication, speaking up, mutual respect, and flatter power hierarchies. Root causes should be addressed, such as a lack of an effective forum to discuss end-of-life decisions.

SUMMARY

1. Reading about ethical issues, thinking about them, and discussing them with colleagues can help physicians resolve ethical dilemmas.
2. As with any clinical problem, following a systematic approach helps ensure that all pertinent considerations are taken into account.
3. Physicians should gather information about the medical situation and the patient's values and preferences, identify the ethical guidelines at stake, and address practical considerations.

References

1. Veatch RM. Hippocratic, religious, and secular ethics: the points of conflict. *Theor Med Bioeth* 2012;33: 33-43.
2. Veatch RM. Assessing Pellegrino's reconstruction of medical morality. *Am J Bioeth* 2006;6:72-75.
3. Harris JM, Jr. It is time to cancel medicine's social contract metaphor. *Acad Med* 2017;92:1236-1240.
4. Levinson W, Ginsburg S, Hafferty FW, et al. *Understanding Medical Professionalism.* Columbus, OH: McGraw-Hill Education; 2014.
5. Livingston EH, Ginsburg S, Levinson W. Introducing JAMA professionalism. *JAMA* 2016;316:720-721.
6. *Webster's New Dictionary of Synonyms.* Springfield: Merriam-Webster Inc.; 1984: 547.
7. Wicclair M. Conscientious objection in healthcare and moral integrity. *Camb Q Healthc Ethics* 2017;26: 7-17.
8. Wicclair MR. *Conscientious Objection in Health Care*: Cambridge University Press; 2011.
9. Laycock D. Religious liberty and the culture wars. *U Ill L Rev* 2014;136:839-880.
10. Laycock D. Religious liberty for politically active minority groups: a response to NeJaime and Siegel. *Yale LJ F* 2016;136:369-386.
11. Stahl RY, Emanuel EJ. Physicians, not conscripts—conscientious objection in health care. *N Engl J Med* 2017;376:1380-1385.
12. Kassirer JP. Diagnostic reasoning. *Ann Intern Med* 1989;110:893-900.
13. Minter DJ, Manesh R, Cornett P, et al. Putting schemas to the test: an exercise in clinical reasoning. *J Gen Intern Med* 2018.
14. Lo B, Jonsen AR. Ethical dilemmas and the clinician. *Ann Intern Med* 1980;92:116-117.
15. Meisel A, Cerminara KL, Pope TM. *The Right to Die.* 3rd ed. New York: Wolters Kluwer; 2014.
16. Beauchamp TL, Childress JF. *Principles of Biomedical Ethics.* 7th ed. New York: Oxford University Press; 2012.
17. Jonsen AR, Toulmin S. *The Abuse of Casuistry: A History of Moral Reasoning.* Berkeley: University of California Press; 1988.
18. Campbell SM, Ulrich CM, Grady C. A broader understanding of moral distress. *Am J Bioeth* 2016;16:2-9.

ANNOTATED BIBLIOGRAPHY

1. Beauchamp TL, Childress JF. *Principles of Biomedical Ethics*. 7th ed. New York: Oxford University Press; 2012.
   Lucid exposition of philosophical foundations of clinical ethics.
2. Meisel A, Cerminara KL, Pope TM. *The Right to Die*. 3rd ed. New York: Wolters Kluwer; 2014.
   Comprehensive legal treatise of court cases and laws on care of patients near the end of life.
3. Wicclair MR. *Conscientious Objection in Health Care*. Cambridge: Cambridge University Press; 2011.
   Book on conscientious objection in health care that analyzes different ways in which term is used.
4. Laycock D. Religious Liberty and the Culture Wars. *U Ill L Rev* 2014;136:839-880.
   Thoughtful analysis of conscientious objection by an advocate of religious liberty.

Overview of Ethical Guidelines

INTRODUCTION

Ethical dilemmas arise in clinical medicine because there are often good reasons for conflicting courses of action. In resolving dilemmas, physicians need to refer to, specify, apply, and balance general ethical guidelines to inform their choices and justify their decisions. This chapter provides an overview of guidelines in clinical ethics. Subsequent chapters discuss them in detail and apply them to specific cases.

RESPECT FOR PERSONS

Treating patients with respect entails several ethical obligations. First, physicians must respect the medical decisions of persons who are autonomous (1). The term *autonomy* literally means "self-rule." Autonomous people act intentionally, are informed, and are free from interference and control by others. People should be allowed to shape their lives in accordance with their core values and goals, free from unwanted bodily intrusion or touching. The concept of autonomy includes the ideas of self-determination, independence, and liberty. Doctors should promote patient autonomy, for example, by disclosing information and helping patients deliberate.

With regard to health care, autonomy justifies the doctrine of informed consent (*see* Chapter 3). Informed consent has several specific aspects. Informed, competent patients may refuse unwanted medical interventions, such as surgery and invasive procedures, and may choose among medically feasible alternatives. Important clinical choices need not involve a major bodily invasion, for instance, choosing on whether to have an electrocardiogram or among several drugs for a condition. Competent, informed patients have the right to make choices that differ from the wishes of family members or the recommendations of their physicians.

A person's autonomy is not absolute and may be justifiably restricted for several reasons. If a person is incapable of making informed decisions, trying to respect his or her autonomy might be less important than acting in his or her best interests. Autonomy might also be constrained by the needs of other individuals or society at large. A person is not free to act in ways that violate other people's autonomy, harm others, or impose unfair claims on society's resources.

A second meaning of respect for persons concerns patients who are not autonomous because their decision-making capacity is impaired by illness or medication. Physicians should still treat them as persons with individual characteristics, preferences, and values. Decisions should reflect their preferences and values, so far as they are known. In addition, all patients, whether autonomous or not, should be treated with attention, dignity, and compassion.

Third, respect for persons requires physicians to avoid misrepresentation, maintain confidentiality, and keep promises. There are additional reasons for these other guidelines, as we will discuss.

Maintain Confidentiality

Maintaining the confidentiality of medical information respects patient privacy. It also encourages people to seek treatment and to discuss their problems frankly. In addition, confidentiality protects patients from harm that might occur if information about sensitive conditions such as psychiatric illness, sexual preference, or alcohol or drug use were widely disseminated. Patients and the public expect physicians to keep medical information confidential. However, maintaining confidentiality is not an absolute duty. In some situations, physicians need to override confidentiality to protect third parties from harm (*see* Chapter 5).

Avoid Deception and Nondisclosure

Truth telling—avoiding lies—is a cornerstone of social interaction. If people cannot depend on others to tell the truth, no one would make agreements or contracts. Physicians might mislead patients without technically lying, for example, by giving partial information that is literally true but intended to mislead. Deception violates the autonomy of people who are deceived because it causes them to make decisions on the basis of false premises. To cover these broader issues, this book uses the term *deception* rather than *lying*. In addition, physicians sometimes withhold information about their diagnosis or prognosis from patients. Doctors may do so to protect patients from bad news. However, patients cannot make informed decisions about their medical care if they do not receive all pertinent information about their condition.

Keep Promises

Promises generate expectations in other people, who, in turn, modify their plans on the assumption that promises will be kept. The very concept of promises is undermined if people are free to break them. It is unfair for someone to expect others to honor their promises, but to break his or her own. Keeping promises also enhances trust in both the individual physician and the medical profession. Furthermore, promises relieve patients' anxiety about the future by providing reassurance that doctors will not abandon them.

ACT IN THE BEST INTERESTS OF PATIENTS

The guideline of *nonmaleficence*, or *do no harm*, forbids physicians from providing ineffective therapies or from acting selfishly or maliciously (2, 3). This oft-cited precept, however, provides only limited guidance because many beneficial interventions also entail serious risks and side effects. Literally doing no harm would preclude risky treatments such as surgery and cancer chemotherapy.

The guideline of *beneficence* requires physicians to provide a net benefit to patients: the benefits of an intervention must outweigh the burdens and be proportionate (*see* Chapter 4). Because patients do not possess medical expertise and might be vulnerable because of illnesses, they rely on physicians to provide sound advice and to promote their well-being (4). Physicians encourage such trust and for these reasons have a fiduciary duty to act in the best interests of their patients and place the well-being of patients before their own self-interest or the interests of third parties.

Unwise Decisions by Patients

Acting in patients' best interests might conflict with respecting their informed choices, as when patients' refusals of care might thwart their own goals or cause them serious harm. Simply accepting such refusals, in the name of respecting autonomy, would be highly problematic. Physicians should listen to patients, educate them, and try to persuade them to accept beneficial treatment, or negotiate a mutually acceptable compromise. If disagreements persist, the patient's informed choices and judgment of his or her best interests should prevail.

Patients Who Lack Decision-Making Capacity

The choices and preferences of many patients who lack decision-making capacity are unknown or unclear. In this situation, respecting autonomy is not pertinent. Instead, physicians should be guided by the patient's best interests (*see* Chapters 4 and 12).

Conflicts of Interest

Physicians should act in the patient's best interests rather than in their own self-interest when conflicts of interest occur (*see* Chapters 29–36). Patients trust their physicians to act on their behalf and feel betrayed if that trust is abused. When considering whether or not a conflict of interest exists, physicians should consider how patients, the public, and colleagues would react if they knew about the situation. Even situations where the likelihood of bias or undue influence is low might damage trust in the individual physician and in the profession.

ALLOCATE RESOURCES JUSTLY

The term *justice* is used in a general sense to mean fairness—that is, people should get what they deserve. People who are similar in ethically relevant respects should be treated similarly, and people who differ in ethically significant ways should be treated differently. Otherwise, decisions would be arbitrary and biased. To make this formal statement of justice operational, the physician would need to specify what counts as an ethically relevant distinction and what it means to treat people similarly.

In health care settings, *justice* also refers to the allocation of health care resources. Allocation decisions are unavoidable because resources are limited and could be spent on other social goods, such as education or the environment, instead of on health care. Ideally, allocation decisions should be made as public policy and set by legislatures or government officials, according to appropriate procedures. Physicians should participate in public debates about allocation and help set policies. In general, however, rationing medical care at the bedside should be avoided because it might be inconsistent, discriminatory, and ineffective. At the bedside, physicians usually should act as patient advocates within constraints set by society and sound clinical practice (*see* Chapter 32). In some cases, however, two patients might compete for the same limited resources, such as physician time or a bed in intensive care. When this occurs, physicians should ration their time and resources according to patients' medical needs and the probability and degree of benefit.

THE USE OF ETHICAL GUIDELINES

Having summarized guidelines for clinical ethics, we next discuss how physicians should use them in specific cases. This book uses the term *guidelines* to connote that ethical generalizations cannot be mechanically or rigidly applied but need to be used with discretion and judgment in the circumstances of a particular case. Guidelines are derived from decisions made in previous cases and from moral theories (5, 6). In turn, guidelines shape decisions in similar cases in the future. Guidelines might be difficult to apply in new cases for several reasons.

Interpreting Guidelines in Specific Cases

The meaning or force of a guideline might not be clear in a particular case. Uncertainty and case-by-case variation are inherent in clinical medicine. Furthermore, patients have different priorities and goals for care. A crucial issue is whether the case at hand can be distinguished in ethically meaningful ways from previous cases to which the guideline was applied. Unforeseen or novel cases might point out the shortcomings of an existing guideline and suggest that it needs to be modified or an exception made.

Exceptions to Guidelines

Guidelines are not absolute. A particular case might have distinctive features that justify making an exception to a guideline (6). To ensure fairness, physicians who make an exception to a guideline should justify their decisions. The exception and its justification should apply not only to the specific case under consideration, but also to all similar cases faced by other physicians. Guidelines are stronger than rules of thumb that provide advice but are not binding. Many philosophers regard ethical guidelines as *prima facie* binding: they should be followed unless they conflict with stronger obligations or guidelines or unless there are compelling reasons to make an exception (5). The burden of argument is on those who claim that an exception to the guideline is warranted. Furthermore, when *prima facie* guidelines are overridden, they are not simply ignored. People often experience regret or even remorse that guidelines are being broken. Thus, people should minimize the extent to which *prima facie* guidelines are violated and mitigate the adverse consequences of doing so.

Conflicts Among Guidelines

In many situations, following one ethical guideline would require the physician to violate or compromise another guideline. Respecting a patient's refusal of treatment might clash with acting in the patient's best interests. Maintaining confidentiality might conflict with preventing harm to third parties. Allocating resources equitably might conflict with doing what is best for an individual patient. The practice of medicine would be much easier if there were a fixed hierarchy of ethical guidelines; for example, if patient autonomy always took priority over beneficence. Life is not so simple, however. In some clinical situations, respecting a patient's wishes should be paramount, whereas in others, a patient's best interests should prevail. Physicians need to understand why an ethical guideline should take priority in one situation but not in others.

The ability to make prudent decisions in specific situations has been described as *discernment* or *practical wisdom*. Discernment involves an understanding of how ethical guidelines are relevant in a variety of situations and to the particular case at hand.

PRINCIPLES, RULES, AND DUTIES

This book uses the term *guidelines* to refer to ethical generalizations that guide action because other terms, such as *principles*, *rules*, and *duties*, have undesirable connotations. According to the dictionary, *principle* connotes a "basis for reasoning or a guide for conduct or procedure." However, many philosophers use the term in a more restricted sense, to refer only to a comprehensive ethical theory that explains how to resolve conflicts among different precepts (5). A unified theory would also presumably provide clear, specific rules for action and a justification of those rules.

Philosophers have devoted considerable effort to developing comprehensive ethical theories. The two main types of ethical theory are consequentialist and deontologic. *Consequentialist* theories judge the rightness or wrongness of actions or guidelines by their consequences. Utilitarianism, the most prominent consequentialist theory, considers actions and rules appropriate when the overall benefits to all parties outweigh the overall harms. For instance, a utilitarian would consider it justified to tell a lie, breach confidentiality, or break a promise if, on the whole, the benefits of doing so outweigh the harms. In contrast, *deontologic* theories claim that the rightness or wrongness of an action depends on more factors than the consequences of an action. To a deontologist, actions such as telling a lie, breaching confidentiality, and breaking promises are inherently wrong. They would be morally suspect if they produced no harmful consequences or if they led to beneficial ones.

Comprehensive theories of clinical ethics, however, are problematic (5). Utilitarian theories are flawed because they condone seemingly harmful actions that are not detected. For example, utilitarians might condone breaking a promise when no one else knows it is broken. Furthermore, acts that maximize the benefits for society as a whole may be considered acceptable even though they impose grave harms on individual persons or groups. In a utilitarian analysis, harms to individuals might be outweighed by a sufficiently large benefit to society. Such an inequitable distribution of benefits and harms, however, might be unfair.

Deontologic theories can be criticized because they cannot provide a satisfactory account of which principles or rules take priority over others in cases of conflict. For example, deontologic theories would have difficulty determining whether beneficence or confidentiality would prevail when a patient with HIV infection refuses to notify his or her partner that he or she is at risk.

Detailed and lucid expositions of ethical theories and their critiques are available (5). Many writers, myself included, believe that a comprehensive and consistent theory of clinical ethics cannot be developed. This book avoids reference to ethical theories and to the term *principle* not only because of these conceptual problems, but also because ethical theories and principles are too abstract to guide physicians in specific cases.

The term *rule* is used in ethics to refer to generalizations that are narrower in scope than principles. The term is helpful because it focuses on individual conduct in specific situations, rather than on abstract generalizations. However, rules are generally regarded as binding, often prohibiting certain behaviors. In common language, *rule* might imply restrictions on individual conduct to maintain order in the group or for the sake of a goal. We speak of rules for a game or an institution. The implication might be that rules can be applied in a straightforward manner, as when disputes in a game are settled by referring to the rules. In this sense, rules may be arbitrarily imposed to establish clear expectations for everyone. For example, rules for visiting hours may be established in a hospital to provide clear guidance for conduct, without any claim that one choice of hours is superior to another. The term *rule* is misleading in clinical ethics because exceptions need to be made and guidelines are not arbitrary conventions, but reflect important values.

Finally, this book avoids the term *duty*, which might connote legal and ethical obligations. Ethical obligations, however, differ from legal duties imposed by legislation, regulations, or court rulings, as Chapter 22 discusses.

OTHER APPROACHES TO ETHICS

Because ethical theories and principles often do not help people resolve conflicts, other approaches to clinical ethics have been suggested.

Casuistry

Instead of constructing or relying on theories, some writers focus on how to resolve specific cases (6, 7). According to these writers, people resolve dilemmas in everyday life by "looking at the concrete details of particular cases" (6). In this view, moral rules are not absolute; they merely create presumptions that may be rebutted, depending on the particular circumstances. The strategy is to compare a given case with clear-cut, paradigmatic cases. The key issue is whether the given case so closely resembles a paradigmatic case that it should be resolved in a similar manner or whether it can be distinguished and, therefore, treated differently. In some cases, the application of ethical maxims will be clear-cut. In more difficult cases, it might be unclear whether a guideline applies or whether different guidelines might provide conflicting advice. Proponents of case-based ethics emphasize the need for what Aristotle called practical wisdom, the ability to make appropriate decisions given the particular circumstances of the case. In educational terms, casuistry teaches by case analyses, starting with paradigmatic cases in which principles clearly apply and moving to complex, ambiguous cases over which reasonable people may disagree.

A case-based approach to clinical ethics takes into account the complexity of real-life decisions and offers readers a vicarious experience in resolving ethical problems (7a). Dilemmas in clinical ethics generally present as specific decisions in clinical care, not as clashes of abstract philosophical principles. This book emphasizes how to approach difficult cases and how to weigh different considerations in reaching a decision.

However, case-based analyses face a serious challenge: to provide a convincing basis for weighing some factors more heavily than others in reaching a decision. Indeed, casuistry runs the risk of ad hoc reasoning and inconsistent decisions. To avoid such pitfalls, this book will continually refer back to the ethical guidelines described in this chapter and explain why particular factors will be decisive in some situations, whereas different considerations will weigh most heavily in other circumstances.

Ethics of Caring

Some feminist writers argue that principles and rules provide an incomplete and inadequate conception of ethics. In this perspective, more attention is needed on maintaining or restoring relationships among individuals and avoiding interpersonal conflicts. Responding to the needs and welfare of individuals with whom one has close relationships might be more important than acting in accord with abstract standards. For example, when family members make decisions for an incompetent patient, traditional ethics might undervalue the need for the family members to get along and live with the consequences of their decisions. In some situations, it might be more important to prevent serious family disputes than to follow the patient's prior directives. Such caring and responsiveness is often claimed to be a typically "feminine" orientation, as contrasted with a "masculine" orientation toward rules and principles. However, empirical studies do not support the hypothesis of gender-related orientations to ethics (8).

The emphasis on caring and on the well-being of others is welcome in medicine and other helping professions. Caring is essential in the doctor–patient relationship, and in clinical practice sympathy and compassion might be more important than following ethical guidelines mechanically. It is also important, however, to move beyond a sensitivity and commitment to caring to a specific description of how caring should impact decisions in particular clinical situations. Furthermore, attending to the welfare of others might conflict with other important ethical imperatives, such as respecting the patient's autonomy.

Virtue Ethics

Some writers point out that merely following guidelines might lead to a thin view of ethics. Physicians might perform the right actions but lack the spirit that should animate the medical profession. Virtue ethics emphasizes that the physician's characteristics are ultimately more important than the doctor's specific actions and their congruence with ethical principles (9-11). In this perspective, the essential questions are whether the doctor is a good physician and a good person, In one such view, the virtues of a good physician include fidelity, compassion, fortitude, temperance, integrity, and self-effacement (11).

Virtue ethics is helpful because it emphasizes the importance of qualities such as compassion, dedication, and altruism in physicians. Furthermore, in some complicated or unique situations, the physician's integrity might be a crucial factor in resolving dilemmas. Virtue ethics, however, also has serious limitations because it lacks specificity on what the doctor should do in particular circumstances. A virtuous person might still commit wrong actions. Also, virtues might conflict with each other. In a given case, some people may believe that the physician's integrity is paramount, whereas others believe that the actions to do so would fall short in compassion or fidelity to the patient.

SUMMARY

1. Ethical guidelines include showing respect for persons, avoiding deception, maintaining confidentiality, keeping promises, acting in the best interests of patients, and allocating resources justly.
2. These guidelines need to be applied to particular cases with discretion and judgment.

References

1. Beauchamp TL, Childress JF. *Principles of Biomedical Ethics*. 7th ed. New York: Oxford University Press; 2013:101-149.
2. Jonsen AR. Do no harm. *Ann Intern Med* 1978;88:827-832.

3. Brewin TB. Primum non nocere? *Lancet* 1994;344:1487-1488.
4. Pellegrino ED. Toward a reconstruction of medical morality. *Am J Bioeth* 2006;6:65-71.
5. Beauchamp TL, Childress JF. *Principles of Biomedical Ethics*. 7th ed. New York: Oxford University Press; 2013:19-29.
6. Sunnstein CR. *Legal Reasoning and Political Conflict*. New York: Oxford University Press; 1996.
7. Jonsen AR, Toulmin S. *The Abuse of Casuistry: A History of Moral Reasoning*. Berkeley: University of California Press; 1988.
7a. Lo B, Jonsen AR. Ethical dilemmas and the clinician. *Ann Intern Med* 1980;92:116-117.
8. Bebeau MJ, Brabeck M. Ethical sensitivity and moral reasoning among men and women in the professions. In: Brabeck MM, ed. *Who Cares? Theory, Research, and Educational Implications of the Ethic of Care*. New York, NY: Praeger; 1989:144-163.
9. Sulmasy DP. Edmund Pellegrino's philosophy and ethics of medicine: an overview. *Kennedy Inst Ethics J* 2014;24:105-112.
10. Pellegrino ED, Thomasma DG. *The Virtues in Medical Practice*. New York: Oxford University Press; 1993.
11. Pellegrino ED. Toward a virtue-based normative ethics for the health professions. *Kennedy Inst Ethics J* 1995;5:253-277.

ANNOTATED BIBLIOGRAPHY

1. Beauchamp TL, Childress JF. *Principles of Biomedical Ethics*. 6th ed. New York, NY: Oxford University Press; 2008.
   Comprehensive and lucid presentation of the philosophical foundations of biomedical ethics. Excellent references for further reading in the philosophical literature.
2. Jonsen AR, Toulmin S. *The Abuse of Casuistry: A History of Moral Reasoning*. Berkeley, CA: University of California Press; 1988.
   Offers a cogent rationale for a case-based approach to ethics and provides an overview of the accomplishments and downfall of casuistry.

3

CHAPTER

Informed Consent

Although informed consent is legally required, many physicians are skeptical because patients rarely understand medical situations as well as doctors and because doctors can often persuade patients to follow their recommendations. In some situations, however, therapeutic options differ dramatically in terms of their side effects and impact on the patient, and no option is clearly superior. In these situations, the patient's values and preferences will be decisive. This chapter discusses the definition of informed consent, its justification, its requirements, and problems with informed consent. In complex decisions, physicians should go beyond the minimum legal requirements of informed consent to promote shared decision-making with patients.

CASE 3.1	Mastectomy or lumpectomy for localized breast cancer

Ms. B was a 58-year-old woman who was found to have a small breast cancer, stage T1N0M0. Her surgeon recommends mastectomy and informs her of the benefits and risks of the operation, including side effects such as lymphedema of the arm. The surgeon says that a less extensive operation may not remove all the tumor. Ms. B's daughter searched the Internet for information about breast cancer and learned that her mother's cancer could also be effectively treated with lumpectomy plus radiation therapy, which would avoid disfiguration and lymphedema.

Case 3.1 illustrates that patients or families may obtain medical information from sources other than the physician and may consider options that the physician has not mentioned. Moreover, patients and relatives may take a more active role than is traditional, raising new options and advocating for them. Evidence-based practice guidelines recommend breast-conserving surgery for early breast cancer. Survival and disease-free survival are similar for mastectomy and lumpectomy plus radiation. The percentage of women who receive breast-conserving surgery, however, varies strikingly by geographical region, and many women may not participate in decisions regarding surgery to the extent they wish (1). Before a mastectomy, the legal duty of informed consent requires surgeons to disclose the nature of the operation, its risks, and the alternatives.

Case 3.1 illustrates, however, that a narrow vision of informed consent, although meeting legal standards, may result in suboptimal patient care decisions.

WHAT IS INFORMED CONSENT?

Discussions about informed consent are often confusing because people use this term in different senses.

Agreement with the Physician's Recommendations

Patients usually agree with physicians' recommendations, particularly in acute illness or injury, when the goals of care are clear, one option is superior, the benefits are great, and the risks are small. For example, a patient who suffers a wrist fracture needs a cast to heal. A patient with urinary tract infection needs antibiotics. In such situations, informed consent seems tantamount to obtaining the patient's agreement to the proposed intervention. Physicians often speak of "consenting the patient," implying that it is a foregone conclusion that the patient will agree, and indeed almost all patients do agree. However, even with clinical decisions that are predominantly technical, patient preferences may be important, for example choosing among effective antibiotic regiments that have different durations of treatment.

Right to Refuse Interventions

Patients have an ethical and legal right to be free of unwanted medical interventions and bodily invasions. Many early court cases on consent involved patients who had undergone surgery or invasive procedures and suffered serious adverse effects. The patients claimed that they would not have agreed to the intervention had they been told about these risks. Legally, competent patients must be informed of the risks of the proposed care and have the right to reject their physicians' recommendations. This right to refuse also extends to noninvasive care, such as diagnostic tests and medications.

Choice Among Alternatives

More broadly, patients should have the positive right to choose among medically feasible options, in addition to the negative right to refuse unwanted interventions. For instance, Case 3.1 involves a choice between two very different treatment plans.

Shared Decision-Making

A still more comprehensive view is shared decision-making by the physician and the patient (2, 3). Both parties play essential roles in clinical decisions. The physician has medical knowledge and experience. Patients can ascertain their values and preferences for, for example, what risks and side effects are acceptable. Shared decision-making is a back-and-forth process. Decision aids may facilitate patient comprehension and shared decision-making. The physician can also help educate patients, correct misunderstandings, help them deliberate, make recommendations, and to try to persuade them to accept the recommendation most consistent with their values (4).

Shared decision-making is a continuum (5). The physician may simply explain the medical options or may also make a recommendation based on the patient's goals and values. In a more fully engaged model of decision-making, the patient and physician may be equal partners and deliberate together. Patients may have different preferences for decision-making procedures for different kinds of decisions or at different times in their course of illness. For instance, the choice of mastectomy versus lumpectomy and radiation will depend on how the patient trades off breast conservation to the patient versus the return visits for radiation therapy. However, most patients want the surgeon to make decisions regarding the type of sutures used and the positioning and removal of drains.

REASONS FOR INFORMED CONSENT AND SHARED DECISION-MAKING

Several ethical and pragmatic reasons justify a broader conception of informed consent (6).

Respect Patient Self-Determination

People want to make decisions about their bodies and health care in accordance with their values and goals. One court declared, "Every human being of adult years and sound mind has a right to determine what shall be done with his own body" (7). In most clinical settings, interventions have both potential benefits and risks, and outcomes are uncertain. Patients differ in what likelihood of risk and what adverse effects they find acceptable.

In Case 3.1, most women choose lumpectomy because it is less disfiguring and has fewer side effects. For some older women, however, conservation of the breast may be unimportant, and returning for a course of radiation therapy may be burdensome. Physicians cannot accurately predict patients' preferences. For example, patients with newly diagnosed cancer are more likely than physicians, nurses, and the general public to prefer intensive chemotherapy with little chance of cure.

Enhance the Patient's Well-Being

The goal of medical care is to enhance patient well-being, which can be judged only in terms of the patient's goals and values. The patient's values are particularly important if various treatment approaches have very different characteristics or complications and involve trade-offs between short-term and long-term outcomes, if one option carries a small chance of a serious complication, if the patient has strong aversions toward risk or certain outcomes, or if there is uncertainty and disagreement among physicians (8). The choice between mastectomy and lumpectomy/radiation in Case 3.1 has many of these characteristics. In addition, participation in decisions might have other beneficial consequences for patients, such as increased sense of control, self-efficacy, and adherence to plans for care.

REQUIREMENTS FOR INFORMED CONSENT

Ethically and legally, informed consent requires discussions of pertinent information, obtaining the patient's agreement to the plan of care, and freedom from coercion (6).

Information to Discuss With Patients

Physicians need to discuss with patients information that is relevant to the decision at hand (Table 3-1). Most court decisions and legal commentaries use the term *disclose*, and, when summarizing legal doctrine, this book also uses this term. In general, however, we prefer the term *discuss* to emphasize that a dialog with the patient is preferable to a monolog by the physician.

Patients must be told the *nature* of the intervention, the expected *benefits*, the *risks*, and the likely *consequences*. Risks that are common knowledge, already known to the patient, of trivial impact, or very infrequent do not need to be discussed, for example the risks of venipuncture. For invasive interventions, courts have ruled that physicians need to discuss rare but serious risks, such as death or stroke.

Patients also need to understand the *alternatives* to the proposed test or treatment and their risks, benefits, and consequences. In particular, alternatives that are recommended in the medical literature and by evidence-based consensus guidelines need to be offered, even if the physician personally disagrees. The alternative of no intervention needs to be discussed. If a patient declines the recommended intervention, the physician needs to explain the adverse consequences of the refusal. In a case where a woman refused a Pap smear, the court ruled that the physician needed to discuss how the test could diagnose cancer at an early stage and avert death through early treatment.

The extent of disclosure will depend on the clinical context. For conditions such as appendicitis or fracture, where there is only one realistic option and it is highly effective, relatively safe, and strongly recommended, a detailed discussion of alternatives offers little benefit to patients (9). However, the physician still needs to tell the patient the nature of the treatment, the risks, and the consequences, such as the course of convalescence.

Physicians must take the initiative in discussing information rather than wait for patients to ask questions. Patients might be uncomfortable asking questions or not even know what questions to ask.

TABLE 3-1. Information to Discuss with Patients
The nature of the test or treatment
The benefits, risks, and consequences of the intervention
The alternatives and their benefits, risks, and consequences

Discussions about the proposed test or treatment and the alternatives should be conducted by the attending physician or by the physician performing the intervention.

The process of communicating information to patients has been revolutionized by the development of decision aids that present balanced evidence information to patients about the options for care, as well as the benefits, risks, and consequences of each option. Decision aids can be presented to patients on line, over the Internet, and on video. Some decision aids incorporate stories that tell patients how people like them have experienced an option. Information about medical conditions, treatments, and patient experiences is widely available on the Internet. Physicians may need to identify and respond to misunderstandings that might result from such information.

It is controversial whether physicians need to inform patients of alternatives for care that they do not believe are medically indicated. Obviously, physicians do not need to mention treatments that have no scientific rationale, would provide no medical benefit, or are known to be ineffective or harmful. However, physicians should inform patients of alternatives that other reasonable physicians would recommend, particularly if there is strong evidence of effectiveness and safety.

CASE 3.1	*Continued*

Ms. B's surgeon needs to discuss alternatives to the mastectomy he is recommending. Because lumpectomy plus radiation therapy has fewer complications and equivalent long-term outcomes, it needs to be offered. Physicians' recommendations should be supported by published evidence and evidence-based guidelines. Even if Ms. B's surgeon believed that mastectomy was the best approach, he still should inform her about the option of lumpectomy plus radiation therapy and tell her that it is recommended in evidence-based guidelines. He can then explain why he thinks mastectomy is better for her. The surgeon should not expect Ms. B or her daughter to take the lead in asking about alternatives to mastectomy. From the patient's perspective, the Internet may be an invaluable source of information about cancer treatments. The National Cancer Institute, the American Cancer Society, and medical school websites offer reliable information.

Some kinds of information that the law does not require be disclosed may still be ethically desirable to disclose, as the following case illustrates. That is, the law sets a minimum for information to disclose, but ethical standards may require additional information.

CASE 3.2	**Disclosure of prognostic information**

Mr. A was a 50-year-old man who, after resection of a carcinoma of the pancreas, was recommended to have adjuvant chemo- and radiation therapy. He had indicated to his oncologist that he wished "to be told the truth about his condition." The doctor told him that most patients with pancreatic cancer die of the disease, and that there was a serious risk of recurrence. He died a year later, and his family sued, claiming that had he been told outcomes data, he would have declined chemo- and radiation therapy and put his business affairs in order. In 1993, the California Supreme Court ruled that physicians did not need to give patients statistical data on outcomes. "Statistical morbidity values derived from the experience of population groups are inherently unreliable and offer little assurance regarding the fate of the individual patient."
Based on Arato v. Avedon, 858 P.2d 598 (Cal. 1993)

After resection for pancreatic cancer, the median survival is about 20 months for patients receiving adjuvant chemotherapy, a few months longer than in patients treated only with surgery. Quantitative information may be material to patients' decisions, notwithstanding the court's ruling. Physicians can explain why an individual patient might be expected to do better or worse than average. Even if not legally required, it is ethically desirable for physicians to provide such information to patients.

Other information may also be ethically desirable to discuss, although not legally required. The hospital's *experience* might be pertinent to a patient's decision, because increased volume is associated with significantly better outcomes for some operations and surgeons have a "learning curve" for new procedures. For example, the mortality for pancreatic resection is over 12% higher in low-volume hospitals than in high-volume hospitals (10). Similarly, patients might find it pertinent to know the *outcomes* of a surgical procedure at a given institution or by a particular surgeon, not outcomes reported in the literature. Some states make such surgeon- and hospital-specific, risk-adjusted outcome data for coronary artery bypass surgery publicly available. For cardiology procedures, it was recommended that patients receive information about clinician and institutional outcomes, with benchmark comparisons, or, at a minimum, information about experience and procedure volumes (11). Although some courts have ruled that physician-specific experience needs to be disclosed for some operations, other courts have not. The majority of surgical patients regard knowing the surgeon's experience with highly innovative procedures as essential to their decision to have surgery (12). Another issue that many patients might find pertinent is the *role of trainees* in their care, particularly with invasive or surgical procedures, as Chapter 36 discusses.

CASE 3.2   *Continued*

Although the courts do not require physicians to offer to present outcomes statistics to patients, there are good ethical reasons to do so. Although statistics cannot predict what will happen in a particular case, they do provide estimates of the likelihood of outcomes. Physicians can always discuss with patients the features of the individual case that make it likely that their prognosis is better or worse than the numbers in the literature.

Public health experts and evidence-based guidelines are now advocating that patients calculate individualized probabilities of outcomes to help them guide decisions about their care. The Framingham cardiac risk index and the World Health Organization fracture risk tool are available online for patients to use to guide their decisions regarding treatment of cardiac risk factors or treatment for osteoporosis. Case 3.2 illustrates how ethical standards for informed consent may be higher than legal requirements.

Patient Agreement with the Treatment Plan

Patients must agree with the intended plan of care. For major interventions, such as surgery, obtaining explicit written authorization is standard. Written consent signals to the patient that the decision is important. In ambulatory care, oral agreement to the plan of care is usual because the risks are lower and patients can choose to discontinue medications (13, 14).

Agreement Should Be Voluntary

Coercion and manipulation undermine free choices by patients. Coercion involves threats that are intended to control patients' behavior and that patients find irresistible (15, 16). An example is a threat to discharge a patient from the hospital if he or she does not agree with the recommended care. Manipulation of information might also thwart informed decisions. For example, physicians might misrepresent the patient's condition or the nature of the proposed intervention. Coercion and manipulation contrast with persuasion, which is an attempt to convince the patient to act in a certain way by providing rational arguments and accurate data. Persuasion respects patient autonomy and, indeed, enhances it by improving the patient's understanding of the situation.

Certain constraints on patients' choices are not coercive. The patient's prognosis might be so grim that all alternatives are undesirable and the patient has no "real choice." Warnings by the physician about the outcomes of choices or about the natural history of the illness are also not coercive because the physician makes no threat to bring about undesirable outcomes. Indeed, physicians would be ethically remiss if they did not point out to patients the consequences of unwise choices.

If patients lack the capacity to make informed decisions (*see* Chapter 10), the patient's values and preferences, expressed through appropriate surrogates, should guide decisions (*see* Chapters 12 and 13).

PROBLEMS WITH INFORMED CONSENT

Physicians need to understand common problems with informed consent so that they can take steps to minimize them.

Patients Do Not Understand Medical Information

Patients often do not recall information they have discussed with physicians, even basic information about the proposed treatment. Patients considering knee/hip replacement and lower back surgery have poor knowledge about the surgery. Fewer than 50% of patients could answer basic questions about the procedure (17). For back surgery, only 14% of patients knew how many will not improve after surgery and only 33% knew how many will experience complications of surgery. Furthermore, patients facing common medical decisions cannot accurately assess how well informed they are (18).

Physicians Do Not Provide Key Information

In audiotaped office visits, orthopedic surgeons discussed the nature of the decision to be made in 92% of cases, alternatives in 62%, and risks and benefits in 59%. They rarely discussed the patient's role in decision-making (14%) or assessed the patient's understanding (12%) (19). For outpatient decisions involving a new medication or change in dose, physicians described the decision in 75% of cases, but checked patient preferences in only 27% of cases. For complex decisions such as PSA screening or counseling regarding surgery, physicians discussed alternatives in only 30% of cases and pros and cons in only 26% (20). Furthermore, doctors often use technical jargon that is incomprehensible to laypeople, and informed consent forms are usually difficult to read and understand.

Some Patients Do Not Want to Make Decisions

Some patients might not want to make decisions, but instead defer to physicians or family members.

CASE 3.3   **Reluctance to make a decision**

Mr. T was an 88-year-old man with severe chronic obstructive pulmonary disease (COPD), coronary artery disease, and peptic ulcer disease. He developed an adenocarcinoma of the lung, which could be treated with surgery or radiation therapy. His physician was reluctant to recommend surgery because of the patient's increased operative risk. In addition, his COPD was so severe that he might be dyspneic after a pneumonectomy. When his doctor discussed alternatives for treatment, Mr. T said, "Do what you think is best. You're the doctor."

Like Mr. T, about 25% to 50% of Americans prefer to leave medical decisions to their physicians, depending on the physician (21). Women and more educated and healthier people are more likely to prefer an active role in decision-making. Furthermore, persons from cultures where informed consent is not as important as in the United States may defer to physicians.

Patients Might Want Families Make Decisions

In some cultures, patients might be expected to involve their families in medical decisions rather than make decisions as individuals. Women might traditionally be expected to defer decisions to their husbands or fathers. Clearly, physicians need to allow patients to involve others in their medical decisions if they wish to do so, recognizing that individuals within a culture vary in their preferences for decision-making.

Patients Cannot Anticipate Their Future Reactions

People cannot accurately predict how future situations will affect their preferences (22, 23). Healthy patients underestimate the quality of life that patients with illness or disability report. When people imagine what it would be like to have a severe illness or disability, they overlook the many activities they might still be able to enjoy and do not appreciate how patients adapt to their circumstances (24). The concern is that people will make important decisions based on transient feelings or inaccurate perceptions of how they will feel in future states of illness.

LEGAL ASPECTS OF INFORMED CONSENT

Court rulings have shaped the doctrine of informed consent, with particular focus on what information must be disclosed to patients (6).

Malpractice

Physicians who do not obtain informed consent might be found liable in civil suits for battery or negligence. *Battery*, the harmful or offensive touching of another person, includes surgery without the patient's consent or beyond the scope of patient consent. For instance, a physician might be liable for performing a mastectomy on a patient who had consented to only a biopsy, even if the intervention was medically appropriate, skillfully performed, and beneficial. This battery model, however, fits medicine poorly. Many cases do not involve physical touching of the patient, for example making a diagnosis or prescribing drugs. In addition, battery requires that the physician intended to provide care without the patient's consent. Most cases of malpractice, however, are unintentional.

The modern approach to malpractice, which has supplanted the battery model, is to hold physicians liable for *negligence*: the physician breached a duty to the patient, the patient suffered harm, and the breach of duty caused the harm. The patient needs to prove that the physician failed to disclose a risk that should have been disclosed, that the patient would not have consented had the risk been discussed, and that the risk occurred and caused harm. A crucial issue in malpractice law, therefore, is what risks should be discussed.

Standards for Disclosure

Full or complete disclosure of all information that physicians know about a particular condition is impossible. Thus, the issue is not *whether* physicians should limit the amount and types of information they discuss with patients, but rather *what* information to discuss or omit.

Courts have used several standards to determine what information to disclose to patients (6). About half of the states have adopted a *professional standard*: The physician must disclose what a reasonable physician of ordinary skill would disclose in the same or similar circumstances. This is equivalent to providing the information that colleagues customarily provide. The professional standard has been criticized because it is based on what physicians customarily discuss, not on what information patients need (25). In Case 3.1, a physician would not be liable for failing to inform a patient of breast-conserving surgery if surgeons in the area had not adopted it, even if there is rigorous evidence and evidence-based practice guidelines favoring it.

Other states have adopted a patient-oriented standard for disclosure. Physicians should disclose what a *reasonable patient* in the same or similar situation would find material to the medical decision; that is, what would influence the decision. Generally, this standard requires more disclosure than the professional standard and is more consistent with the goal of promoting patient decision-making and choices. However, this standard has been criticized because it does not take into account how patients vary in their preferences regarding what information is relevant (25).

Some patients might desire more information than the standard "reasonable" patient. For example, a carpenter might be particularly concerned that a new medication might impair his or her dexterity or alertness. In clinical practice, as a practical matter, physicians need to answer direct questions from patients to maintain the doctor–patient relationship. A few states have adopted a subjective standard for disclosure: The physician must provide information that the *individual patient* would find pertinent to the decision. This subjective standard for disclosure is problematic in malpractice litigation. If a rare, undisclosed complication occurs, the patient might claim that he or she would not have consented to the intervention if the physician had mentioned that particular risk. In hindsight, it might be difficult to decide whether this assertion is plausible.

In some states, laws specify that certain risks need to be disclosed—for example, "brain damage" or "loss of function of any organ or limb" (6).

From the perspective of shared decision-making, physicians and health care institutions can provide information about options to care through printed, video, or Internet-based decision aids, to supplement face-to-face discussions with the patient.

Consent Forms

The consent form documents that the patient agreed to treatment. In some states, a signed consent form provides a legal presumption of valid consent. A signed consent form, however, is not equivalent to informed consent because the discussion of the risks, benefits, alternatives, and consequences might be inadequate. Physicians should document in the progress notes that the indications, risks, benefits, and alternatives were discussed and that the patient agreed to the care.

Laws Restricting Physician Discussions with Patients

Several states have passed laws that forbid or mandate what physicians may say to patients. A Florida law prohibiting physicians from asking about firearms in the home was mostly stuck down by the courts as unconstitutional in 2017, thus upholding the free speech of physicians to patients (26). Several states mandate specific language that physicians must use in talking with women who seek an abortion. For example, the physician may be required to say that depression and suicide are risks of abortion, although there is no credible scientific evidence that this is the case (27). Backers of these laws say that they assure that women have information needed to make an informed decision. Critics object that the law violates a physician's First Amendment right to be free of government-mandated speech to patients that is ideological, misleading, or false (27).

EXCEPTIONS TO INFORMED CONSENT

Several exceptions to informed consent illustrate how acting in the patient's best interests might supersede patient self-determination. These exceptions need to be carefully limited so that they do not undermine informed consent.

Lack of Decision-Making Capacity

When patients lack decision-making capacity, an appropriate surrogate should give permission or refusal, following the patient's previously stated preferences or his or her best interests (*see* Chapter 4).

Emergencies

In an emergency, delaying treatment to obtain informed consent might jeopardize the patient's life or health. Courts have recognized a doctrine of *implied consent*: because reasonable persons would consent to treatment in such emergency circumstances, physicians may presume that the patient in question also would consent. Few people would object to treatment for life-threatening emergencies, such as impending airway obstruction due to anaphylaxis, without the patient's explicit consent. It is often possible to abbreviate the process of disclosure and concurrence while the treatment is being started in an urgent situation, rather than dispense with it altogether. In addition, the process of informed consent can often be initiated while the treatment is being started.

The emergency exception should not be used when informed consent is feasible or if it is known that a particular patient does not want the treatment. For example, terminally ill patients might have indicated that they do not want cardiopulmonary resuscitation.

Some physicians claim that consent is implied when a patient seeks care from a hospital or signs a general consent form upon admission. The implication is that informed consent for specific tests or treatments is unnecessary. However, this use of "implied consent" is unacceptable because it allows physicians to administer any type of care they choose. When patients come to a hospital, they do not give physicians *carte blanche*. Most patients would probably agree to certain interventions, such as diagnostic testing, but base further decisions on new information.

Therapeutic Privilege

Physicians may withhold information when disclosure would very likely severely harm the patient or undermine informed decision-making by the patient. For example, a depressed patient might have a history of previous suicide attempts in response to serious medical diagnoses. Telling such a patient that he or she has cancer might provoke another suicide attempt. The concept of therapeutic privilege, however, needs to be circumscribed (28). The possibility that the patient might feel sad or refuse treatment does not justify withholding a serious diagnosis.

Waiver

Patients such as Mr. T in Case 3.3 might not want to participate in making decisions about their care. Alternatively, patients might request that certain information not be disclosed. Ethically and legally, patients' requests to waive the right of informed consent should be respected. Self-determination would be undermined if patients were forced to participate in decision-making against their wishes. Shared decision-making entitles patients to participate actively in health care decisions, but does not require them to do so. To be ethically valid, a waiver of informed consent must itself be informed. Patients must appreciate that they have the right to receive information and to make decisions about their care. Patients might later decide to participate more actively in decisions.

PROMOTING SHARED DECISION-MAKING

The process of shared decision-making generally requires multiple discussions between the physician and patient (Table 3-2).

Encourage the Patient to Play an Active Role

Patients vary in their preferred role in decision-making, and this variation may depend on the nature of the problem and the stage of their condition. Doctors should try to adapt their role to the patient's preferences. Physicians can encourage patient involvement in decisions, even with patients like Mr. T in Case 3.3, who defer to their recommendations.

TABLE 3-2.   Promoting Shared Decision-Making

Encourage the patient to play an active role in decisions.
    Elicit the patient's perspective about the illness.
    Build a partnership with the patient.

Ensure that patients are informed.
    Provide comprehensible information.
    Try to frame issues without bias.
    Interpret the alternatives in light of the patient's goals.
    Check that the patients have understood information.

Protect the patient's best interests.
    Help the patient deliberate.
    Make a recommendation.
    Try to persuade patients.

Elicit the Patient's Perspective About the Illness

Physicians can elicit the patient's concerns, expectations, and values regarding medical care through open-ended questions, such as:

- "As you think about the next few years, what is most important to you?"
- "What concerns you the most about your health?"

Build a Partnership with the Patient

Physicians can acknowledge that the decision is complex and difficult (29). Moreover, doctors can affirm their dedication to working for the patient's well-being: "We'll work together to make the best decisions for you."

Ensure That Patients Are Informed

Provide Comprehensible Information

To enhance patient understanding, physicians should use simple language and avoid medical jargon. Decision aids, such as interactive CDs or computer programs, increase patients' knowledge about their condition and options and reduce their sense of conflict over decisions. For patients like Ms. B in Case 3.1, decision aids increase the use of breast-conserving surgery by about 25% (30). Decision aids do not require additional face-to-face time between physicians and patients. Talking to other patients who have experienced an intervention such as mastectomy or colectomy can help patients appreciate how they can adapt.

Try to Frame Issues Without Bias

The framing of options can introduce bias. People are more likely to accept a treatment if the outcomes are phrased in terms of survival, rather than in terms of death (31). Lung cancer patients are more likely to prefer surgery to radiation therapy if outcomes are framed as the probability of living rather than of dying (31). Moreover, surgery is more attractive when survival data are presented as the average number of years lived rather than as the probability of surviving a given time period. To minimize bias, physicians can use visual displays of the frequency of desirable and undesirable outcomes (32).

Physicians also need to consider how to discuss rare but serious risks, such as anaphylactic reactions to radiographic contrast material (33). Patients might infer incorrectly that a risk is significant because the physician has mentioned it. Physicians can put the risk in context: "I believe that this is a very small risk, compared with the information we would gain from the test."

Check That Patients Have Understood Information

Disclosure by the physician is not equivalent to comprehension by the patient. It is helpful to ask patients to repeat the information in their own words and to invite them to ask questions. This repeat back technique improves patient comprehension, while maintaining patient satisfaction, reducing anxiety slightly, and adding only 4 minutes to an ambulatory visit (34, 35).

Promote the Patient's Best Interests

The guideline of beneficence requires physicians to help patients make decisions that are in their best interests (*see* Chapter 4). In addition to providing information, physicians should help patients deliberate about their choices in complex situations.

Help Patients Deliberate

Some situations are close calls or toss-ups: various options may have similar net health outcomes, but strikingly different consequences for the patient, as in Cases 3.1 and 3.2 (32). The patient's goals and values should be decisive. The physician can help the patient clarify whether to try to prevent a complication or to accept the natural course of illness rather than severe adverse effects of interventions.

Make a Recommendation

Physicians should not merely list the alternatives and leave it to the patient to decide (36). Patients commonly ask physicians what they would do and physicians need to clarify what exactly the patient is asking (37). If the patient is asking if he or she is making the right choice, the physician needs to be supportive and compassionate. If the patient wants to know what the physician would do personally, it is helpful for physicians to describe the process of decision-making they would use, including talking with relatives, friends, and religious leaders. If the patient still wants to know what the physician would do, it is appropriate to offer a recommendation and guidance (38), based on the patient's values and goals, acknowledging that they may differ from the physician's.

Try to Persuade Patients

Physicians should also try to dissuade patients from choices that are clearly contrary to their best interests, as judged by their own values. Chapter 4 discusses this issue in depth.

CASE 3.3 **Continued**

Mr. T's doctor said, "I'd be glad to tell you what I think is best for you. But first I need to understand what is important to you." When the physician asked Mr. T what was most important to him over the next few years, he replied that he wanted to care for his sister, who had stomach cancer. The physician explained that he would be unable to care for his sister while recuperating from surgery and also that he might die from the operation. Given Mr. T's priorities, his doctor recommended radiation therapy. Mr. T tolerated radiation well and cared for his sister during her terminal illness. He had several more years of good health before he developed hemoptysis from spread of his lung cancer. He ultimately died an inpatient hospice.

SUMMARY

1. Shared decision-making respects patient self-determination.
2. For patients to make informed choices, physicians must discuss with them the alternatives for care and the benefits, risks, and consequences of each alternative.
3. Physicians need to encourage patients to play an active role in decision-making and to ensure that patients are informed.

References

1. Kuppermann M, Sawaya GF. Shared decision-making: easy to evoke, challenging to implement. *JAMA* 2015;175:167-168.
2. Barry MJ, Edgman-Levitan S. Shared decision making—pinnacle of patient-centered care. *N Engl J Med* 2012;366:780-781.
3. Elwyn G, Durand MA, Song J, et al. A three-talk model for shared decision making: multistage consultation process. *BMJ* 2017;359:J4891.
4. Emanuel EJ, Emanuel LL. Four models of the physician–patient relationship. *JAMA* 1992;267:2221-2226.
5. Kon AA. The shared decision-making continuum. *JAMA* 2010;304:903-904.
6. Berg JW, Lidz CW, Appelbaum PS. *Informed Consent: Legal Theory and Clinical Practice.* 2nd ed. New York: Oxford University Press; 2001.
7. *Schloendorff v Society of New York Hospitals*, 211 N.Y.125,105 N.E.92 (1914).
8. Kassirer JP. Incorporating patient preferences into medical decisions. *N Engl J Med* 1994;330:1895-1896.
9. Rosenbaum L. The paternalism preference—choosing unshared decision making. *N Engl J Med* 2015;373:589-592.
10. Scally CP, Yin H, Birkmeyer JD, et al. Comparing perioperative processes of care in high and low mortality centers performing pancreatic surgery. *J Surg Oncol* 2015;112:866-871.

11. Krumholz HM. Informed consent to promote patient-centered care. *JAMA* 2010;303:1190-1191.
12. Lee Char SJ, Hills NK, Lo B, et al. Informed consent for innovative surgery: a survey of patients and surgeons. *Surgery* 2013;153:473-480.
13. Braddock CH, Fihn SD, Levinson W, et al. How doctors and patients discuss routine clinical decisions: informed decision making in the outpatient setting. *J Gen Intern Med* 1997;12:339-345.
14. Diem SJ. How and when should physicians discuss clinical decisions with patients? *J Gen Intern Med* 1997;12:397-398.
15. Faden RR, Beauchamp TL. *A History and Theory of Informed Consent.* New York: Oxford University Press; 1986:337-381.
16. Beauchamp TL. Autonomy and consent. In: Miller FG, Wertheimer A, ed. *The Ethics of Consent.* New York: Oxford University Press; 2010:79-106.
17. Fagerlin A, Sepucha KR, Couper MP, et al. Patients' knowledge about 9 common health conditions: the DECISIONS survey. *Med Decis Making* 2010;30:35S-52S.
18. Sepucha KR, Fagerlin A, Couper MP, et al. How does feeling informed relate to being informed? The DECISIONS survey. *Med Decis Making* 2010;30:77S-84S.
19. Braddock C, 3rd, Hudak PL, Feldman JJ, et al. "Surgery is certainly one good option": quality and time-efficiency of informed decision-making in surgery. *J Bone Joint Surg Am* 2008;90:1830-1838.
20. Braddock CH, 3rd, Edwards KA, Hasenberg NM, et al. Informed decision making in outpatient practice: time to get back to basics. *JAMA* 1999;282:2313-2320.
21. Levinson W, Kao A, Kuby A, et al. Not all patients want to participate in decision making. A national study of public preferences. *J Gen Intern Med* 2005;20:531-535.
22. Halpern J, Arnold RM. Affective forecasting: an unrecognized challenge in making serious health decisions. *J Gen Intern Med* 2008;23:1708-1712.
23. Shaffer VA, Focella ES, Scherer LD, et al. Debiasing affective forecasting errors with targeted, but not representative, experience narratives. *Patient Educ Couns* 2016;99:1611-1619.
24. Ubel PA, Loewenstein G, Schwarz N, et al. Misimagining the unimaginable: the disability paradox and health care decision making. *Health Psychol* 2005;24:S57-S62.
25. King JS, Moulton BW. Rethinking informed consent: the case for shared medical decision-making. *Am J Law Med* 2006;32:429-501.
26. Lee TT, Curfman GD. Physician speech and firearm safety: *Wollschlaeger v Governor, Florida. JAMA* 2017;177:1189-1192.
27. Curfman GD, Morrissey S, Greene MF, et al. Physicians and the first amendment. *N Engl J Med* 2008;359:2484-2485.
28. Sirotin N, Lo B. The end of therapeutic privilege? *J Clin Ethics* 2006;17:312-316.
29. Epstein RM, Alper BS, Quill TE. Communicating evidence for participatory decision making. *JAMA* 2004;291:2359-2366.
30. Waljee JF, Rogers MA, Alderman AK. Decision aids and breast cancer: do they influence choice for surgery and knowledge of treatment options? *J Clin Oncol* 2007;25:1067-1073.
31. McNeil BJ, Weichselbaum R, Pauker SG. Speech and survival: tradeoffs between quality and quantity of life in laryngeal cancer. *N Engl J Med* 1981;305:982-987.
32. Samson P, Waters EA, Meyers B, et al. Shared decision making and effective risk communication in the high-risk patient with operable stage I non-small cell lung cancer. *Ann Thorac Surg* 2016;101: 2049-2052.
33. Brody H. *The Healer's Power.* New Haven: Yale University Press; 1992.
34. Fink AS, Prochazka AV, Henderson WG, et al. Enhancement of surgical informed consent by addition of repeat back: a multicenter, randomized controlled clinical trial. *Ann Surg* 2010;252:27-36.
35. Schenker Y, Fernandez A, Sudore R, et al. Interventions to improve patient comprehension in informed consent for medical and surgical procedures: a systematic review. *Med Decis Making* 2011;31:151-173.
36. Ubel PA. "What should I do, doc?": Some psychologic benefits of physician recommendations. *Arch Intern Med* 2002;162:977-980.
37. Kon AA. Answering the question: "Doctor, if this were your child, what would you do?" *Pediatrics* 2006;118:393-397.
38. Korones DN. What would you do if it were your kid? *N Engl J Med* 2013;369:1291-1293.

ANNOTATED BIBLIOGRAPHY

1. Beauchamp TL. Autonomy and consent. In: Miller FG, Wertheimer A, ed. *The Ethics of Consent.* New York: Oxford University Press; 2010:79-106.
   Lucid chapter on philsophical underpinings of informed consent.
2. Elwyn G, Durand MA, Song J, et al. A three-talk model for shared decision making: multistage consultation process. *BMJ* 2017;359:j4891.
   Presents guiding principles of shared decision-making and practical advice on implementing it.
3. Berg JW, Lidz CW, Appelbaum PS. *Informed Consent: Legal Theory and Clinical Practice.* 2nd ed. New York, NY: Oxford University Press; 2001.
   Comprehensive and lucid book, covering ethical, legal, and practical aspects of informed consent. Stresses the need for dialogue between doctors and patients.

Promoting the Patient's Best Interests

INTRODUCTION

Patients may reject the recommendations of their physicians, refusing beneficial interventions or insisting on interventions that are not indicated. In such cases, physicians are torn between respecting patient autonomy and acting in the patients' best interests. If physicians simply accept unwise patient decisions in the name of respecting patient autonomy, their role seems morally constricted. This chapter discusses how physicians can protect the well-being of patients while avoiding the pitfalls of paternalism. Chapter 12 addresses how to assess the best interests of a person who lacks decision-making capacity.

PATIENT REFUSAL OF BENEFICIAL INTERVENTIONS

The following case illustrates how patients may refuse beneficial interventions.

CASE 4.1	Refusal of surgery for critical aortic stenosis

Mrs. N is a 76-year-old widow with aortic stenosis. For several years she has been refusing further evaluation, saying that she would not want surgery or a heart procedure. After an episode of near-syncope, she agrees to echocardiography, mostly to humor her primary care physician. Critical aortic outflow obstruction is found. Her physician strongly recommends valve replacement. The risks of surgical or percutaneous valve replacement are unacceptable to her, particularly the risk of prolonged hospitalization, loss of independence, or neurologic or cognitive impairment after valve replacement. She deems the risks of percutaneous valve replacement unacceptable, even though they are lower than the risks of surgical replacement. Having lived a full life, she says she welcomes a sudden death. In the past, she has been reluctant to visit physicians, undergo tests, or take medications. She leads an active life, writing a resource book for senior citizens, leading several volunteer organizations, and enjoying concerts.

Mrs. N's physicians believe that her refusal conflicts with her best interests. With valve replacement, she is likely to live longer and avoid debilitating symptoms, such as chest pain and dyspnea. Refusal of valve replacement might result in what she fears most: progressive decline and loss of independence.

How can physicians respond to Mrs. N's refusal? On the one hand, it would be disrespectful, impractical, and illegal to override her refusal and operate without her consent. On the other hand, accepting her refusal without further discussion might result in severe disability that she would not want. What attempts by physicians to persuade Mrs. N to agree to surgery are warranted? To address these issues, physicians need to understand the ethical guidelines of doing no harm and acting in their patients' best interests.

DOING NO HARM TO PATIENTS

The ethical guideline of nonmaleficence requires people to refrain from inflicting harm on others. Prohibiting harmful actions is the core of morality. For instance, the Ten Commandments prohibit killing, lying, and stealing. Avoiding harm is generally considered a more stringent ethical obligation than providing benefit.

The widely quoted maxim "Do no harm" has several distinct meanings (1). First, physicians should not provide interventions that are known to be ineffective. Second, physicians should not act maliciously, as by providing substandard care because they dislike the patient's ethnic background or political views. Third, doctors should also act with due care and diligence. Fourth, the maxim sometimes is cited as "Above all, do no harm," or, more impressively in Latin, *Primum non nocere*. If physicians cannot benefit patients, they should at least not harm them or make the situation worse.

The precept "do no harm" provides only limited guidance. Many medical interventions, such as the aortic valve replacement in Case 4.1, offer both great benefits and significant risks. Literally doing *no* harm would preclude such interventions, yet many patients with serious illness may accept substantial risks to gain medical benefits. Furthermore, as we next discuss, merely doing no harm seems a limited view of the physician's role.

PROMOTING THE PATIENT'S BEST INTERESTS

The ethical guideline of beneficence requires physicians to promote patients' "important and legitimate interests" (2). This guideline arises from the nature of the doctor–patient relationship and of medical professionalism.

The Fiduciary Nature of the Doctor–Patient Relationship

Physicians have special responsibilities to act for the well-being of patients.

Reasons for the Fiduciary Relationship

Patients are vulnerable. Because illness often undermines patients' independence and judgment, people might be less able to look after their own interests when they are sick. Furthermore, the stakes are high; poor decisions might place patients' health or lives at risk.

Physicians have expertise that patients lack. Physicians have expert clinical knowledge, as well as the experience and judgment to apply it to the patient's individual circumstances. Often, patients have no previous experience in making medical decisions.

Patients rely on their physicians. Even in the era of activated patients and availability of information on the Internet, it is often difficult for patients to obtain information and individualized advice except from physicians. With serious illnesses, patients might have little time to seek second opinions. It is hard for laypeople to determine whether a physician's advice is sound or to evaluate a physician's skills. Hence, patients commonly rely on the advice of their physicians.

Definition of a Fiduciary Relationship

Legally, relationships between professionals and clients are characterized as fiduciary. The term *fiduciary* is derived from the Latin word *fidere*, to trust. Fiduciaries must act in the best interests of their patients or client, subordinating their self-interest and the interests of third parties, such as hospitals. Fiduciaries are held to higher standards than ordinary business people, who use their knowledge and skill for their own self-interest, rather than for the benefit of their customers. Ordinary business relationships are characterized by the phrase *caveat emptor*, "let the buyer beware," not by trust and reliance. Some financial and structural incentives challenge the fiduciary nature of the doctor–patient relationship, as Chapter 34 discusses.

The Nature of Professionalism

In professional codes of ethics, physicians promise to serve the best interests of patients. Literally, physicians "profess" to use their skills to heal and comfort the sick, encouraging patients to rely on them and promising to act in a fiduciary manner (3). Similarly, current discussions of medical professionalism affirm patient-centered care as a core value (4). In return for physicians acting for the good of their patients, society allows physicians to regulate themselves by, for example, selecting applicants for medical schools and postgraduate training, establishing standards for certification, and disciplining practitioners.

Professionalism is now considered a core competency for trainees and is regularly assessed during training (4). The term may refer to several different things. First, it may be a set of core values that physicians should follow, such as primacy of patient welfare, respect for patient autonomy, and integrity (5). Second, professionalism may refer to attitudes, beliefs, and skills that foster these core values, such as the ability to solve challenges to these values and a willingness to engage in reflection, deliberation, and discussions with peers. Third, it may refer to observed behaviors, particularly in clinical settings. Faculty assessments of students' professionalism has been criticized because they may be inconsistent (6) and fail to take into account attention to context and motivation in judging people's behaviors.

The relationship between professionalism and clinical ethics merits clarification. Clinical ethics helps physicians specify values and principles, decide what to do when values are in conflict in a clinical situation, and articulate reasons for their decisions and actions. Articulating reasons when people disagree over what to do is a crucial step towards agreeing on how to resolve the dilemma. Later chapters in this book focus on specific ethical dilemmas. In contrast, training in professionalism focuses more on behaviors that are unacceptable or desirable in paradigmatic situations, such as disrespectful or abusive behavior towards colleagues (7), failure to disclose errors (8), and over-ordering of well-compensated medical procedures (9). A strength of the medical professionalism literature is explicitly discussing the challenges in operationalizing professional behavior because of power discrepancies, modeling of unprofessional behavior by faculty, the hidden curriculum, and student complaints that they are being unfairly targeted by professionalism initiatives (4).

PROBLEMS WITH BEST INTERESTS

The precept that physicians should act in the best interests of patients is indisputable. In any given case, however, determining what actions are in the patient's best interests might be controversial.

Disagreements Over What Is Best for a Patient

People may disagree over the goals of care or the assessment of the benefits and burdens of an intervention relative to those goals. In Case 4.1, Mrs. N's goal is to avoid hospitalization, dependence, and physical and mental decline. Physicians and patients may weigh the risks and benefits of treatment differently. Physicians tend to focus on the prospect of long-term survival, although Mrs. N. is more concerned about the short-term risks of surgery and her quality of life (10). In Case 4.1, the physician was concerned that refusal of valve replacement increased the likelihood of a slow physical decline, which Mrs. N wished to avoid.

Quality of Life

The term *quality of life* is used in many ways. Factors that might be considered include the following:
1. The symptoms of the illness and the side effects of treatment
2. The patient's functional ability to perform activities of daily life, such as walking, shopping, and preparing meals

3. The patient's subjective experiences of happiness, pleasure, pain, and suffering
4. The patient's independence, privacy, and dignity

Competent patients usually consider their quality of life, as well as the duration of life, when making health care decisions. In some situations, a patient with a serious illness may decide that his or her quality of life is so poor that interventions are unacceptably burdensome. The principle of respect for persons requires respecting judgments about quality of life made by patients who are competent and informed. More controversy exists if other persons are making the judgments for the patient.

Quality-of-Life Judgments by Others Might Be Problematic

Quality-of-life judgments by others often differ sharply from the patient's own assessment. Persons with chronic illness, such as coronary artery disease and chronic obstructive lung disease, rate their quality of life higher than do their physicians or other healthy persons (11). Similarly, elderly patients who have survived a hospitalization in the intensive care unit view their quality of life higher than their family members do. Such discrepancies are not surprising. Many patients learn to cope with chronic illness over time, develop support systems, and continue to find substantial pleasure in life. Furthermore, quality of life might improve substantially if in-home assistance or adaptive devices are provided. In addition, assessments of quality of life made by others might be discriminatory if they are based on the patient's economic value to society or social worth.

Some people reject all quality-of-life considerations because they will lead to discrimination against people with disabilities. Proponents of the "right to life" may believe that biologic life should be prolonged, regardless of prognosis or quality of life, a position often based on religious beliefs about the sacredness of life. However, it is disrespectful for people to impose their view of quality of life on a patient who does not agree. Moreover, interventions that may prolong life also have burdens that should be taken into account (12). These disagreements illustrate how determinations of quality of life by others are problematic unless they are based on the patient's own values and priorities.

Medical Paternalism

Historically, beneficence rather than respect for persons was the dominant ethical principle for physicians. Doctors made decisions for the patient on the basis of what they believed was the patient's best interest. This approach to decision-making has been termed *medical paternalism*, analogous to how parents make decisions for their children. Deferring to the physician's recommendations is reasonable in many acute illnesses or emergencies: when cure is possible, when the benefits of therapy far outweigh the risks, and when treatment must be started promptly.

Definition of Paternalism

Paternalism is intentionally overriding a person's known preferences or actions to benefit that person. Philosophers distinguish two types of paternalism. Although *paternalism* is the term used in the medical and philosophical literature, *parentalism* would be a gender-neutral term. In weak or soft paternalism, the patient's decisions are not informed or voluntary. If a patient's autonomy is impaired or in doubt, it is appropriate for physicians to intervene, at least temporarily. The justification is that patients should be protected from harming themselves through nonautonomous decisions and actions. Intervening to determine whether a patient is competent and informed is a minimal imposition on patient autonomy, compared with the possible harms of allowing an incompetent patient to suffer adverse consequences from acting unwisely.

In strong or hard paternalism, a patient's autonomous choices are overridden. An example is withholding a diagnosis or a test result requested by a patient because the physician believes the information will greatly upset the patient. When writing about paternalism, philosophers generally mean strong or hard paternalism, which has been sharply criticized, as we discuss in the next section.

Problems with Medical Paternalism

Critics of (strong) paternalism raise several objections (2). First, value judgments are unavoidable in clinical medicine, and patients, not physicians, should make them. Physicians can define the burdens and benefits of an intervention, but in Case 4.1 only Mrs. N can decide whether the risks and adverse effects of valve replacement are worth the chance for long-term survival and relief or prevention of her symptoms.

Second, the belief that patients cannot make wise medical decisions is a self-fulfilling prophecy. If patients are not informed, they will not be able to make meaningful choices. When empowered and encouraged to make decisions, most patients ask questions, seek information, and take responsibility for difficult choices.

Third, physicians might seek to override a patient's wishes because of their own psychological and emotional reactions to the case. Some physicians are affronted and angry if patients reject their recommendations.

CASE 4.1 *Continued*

Mrs. N's physician wanted to be sure that her refusal of aortic valve replacement was informed. He explained the situation as a dilemma: without valve replacement she might have a sudden death, but she might also have progressive disability from congestive heart failure or angina. Valve replacement offered the prospect of avoiding such disability, but with a trade-off of major risks and possible recuperation. He asked how she would feel if she suffered a decline in health because she refused the procedure, as opposed to suffering a decline as a complication of medical care. He reassured her that the decision was hers to make. She agreed to speak with a cardiologist, cardiac surgeon, and several elderly patients who had undergone the procedure. Her physician also encouraged her to bring a friend (she had no close living relatives) to these meetings. Afterward, she still declined valve replacement because of the risks of the procedure. She lived several more years of active life, before developing memory loss and severe osteoarthritis.

PATIENT REQUESTS FOR INTERVENTIONS

When patients insist on medical interventions that physicians consider far more harmful than beneficial, doctors often get frustrated and angry. Such disagreements are often framed as conflicting rights: Patients claim the right to decide about their medical care, whereas the physician asserts a countervailing right to follow his or her professional judgment. However, framing the issues in this way generally leads to stalemate. A more fruitful approach is to examine the benefits and burdens for the patient.

Interventions Outside Appropriate Medical Practice

CASE 4.2 **Request to monitor side effects of a performance-enhancing drug**

A 21-year-old college swimmer is taking oral anabolic steroids, which she obtains through friends at the gym where she lifts weights. She is aware of the long-term side effects but plans to use the drugs only for the next year while she is competing. Because some competitors are using steroids, she cannot remain competitive unless she takes them also. She asks her physician to monitor her for side effects, but not to prescribe the drugs.

In this case, the patient is using drugs for enhancement, not for the treatment or prevention of illness. Many physicians believe that enhancement of normal function is not an appropriate goal of medicine. In this case, the long-term medical risks might be serious. Furthermore, using performance-enhancing drugs is unfair to other competitors and violates rules governing athletic competitions (13). Monitoring for adverse effects could condone the use of steroids or make the physician complicit.

Another perspective frames monitoring for adverse effects as preventing harm to the patient. Patients commonly use other substances that might harm their health, such as cigarettes, alcohol, and illicit injection drugs, which they obtain without prescription, and physicians continue to follow patients who use such substances, monitor them for adverse effects, and treat complications while still urging them to stop. Indeed, by maintaining a supportive doctor–patient relationship, physicians might be better positioned to persuade patients to stop taking harmful substances.

Interventions Whose Benefit Can Be Assessed Only by the Patient

CASE 4.3	Request for controlled drug for pain

Mr. R, a 56-year-old man, has been disabled by chronic back pain for 10 years despite surgery. A magnetic resonance (MR) scan shows facet arthropathy at additional sites. Surgeons have recommended no further operations. Exercises, physical therapy, and epidural injections have provided only minor improvement. After changing health insurance plans, the patient visits a new physician and requests a refill of a prescription for three 40-mg tablets of slow-release oxycodone (Oxycontin) daily. He says that he has not changed the dosage in several years. His new physician does not prescribe opioids at this strength and dosage for chronic pain. She wants to wean the patient off opioids and to help him live an active life despite the pain. The patient refuses a referral to a pain clinic. "I know that Oxycontin works. Nothing else helps me."

The fact that pain can be assessed only through the patient's self-report creates challenges for physicians. Some physicians are uncomfortable prescribing opioids, particularly when the dosage seems high, on the basis of only subjective patient symptoms. Some patients exaggerate or amplify pain symptoms, and others seek opioids. However, pain causes substantial suffering and can be undertreated by physicians. The epidemic of opioid addiction is due in part to physician overprescribing.

The ethical guideline of respecting patient autonomy and the legal doctrine of informed consent gives patients the *negative* right to refuse unwanted treatments (*see* Chapter 3). This patient, however, claims the *positive* right to receive a specific drug. Some countries allow patients to buy many drugs, including antibiotics, without a physician's prescription. In the United States, however, only physicians are licensed to order tests or prescribe medications. Prescriptions for opioids, such as oxycodone, require special physician registration numbers from the Drug Enforcement Agency and special prescription forms. In response to the epidemic of opioid abuse, federal and state governments put in place additional regulations. These new policies include required education for physicians prescribing opioids, requirements and incentives for physicians to check state Prescription Drug Monitoring Programs databases for prescriptions from multiple providers, and restrictions on electronic prescribing of controlled substances.

CASE 4.3	*Continued*

Mr. R's physician listened to his pain symptoms and empathized with his distress. She acknowledged that only he could assess the severity of pain. She offered to prescribe opioids only as part of a comprehensive plan of pain management that included referral to physical therapy, a pain specialist, and behavioral medicine for other approaches to managing the pain, regularly scheduled visits for re-evaluation and refills, no refills by other physicians (including emergency room or urgent care physicians), periodic drug testing to detect additional substances, and a signed contract in the medical record.

Intervention with Small Benefit

CASE 4.4	**Request for an expensive, low-yield test**

Ms. D, a 41-year-old bus driver, has episodes of crampy abdominal pain, episodes of diarrhea, and some constipation. One year ago, after an evaluation that included colonoscopy, she was diagnosed with irritable bowel syndrome (IBS). Dietary manipulations and increased dietary fiber have been ineffective. On the advice of a friend, she asks her doctor to order an abdominal MR scan because when the cramps are severe she fears something serious has been missed. She also says, "If doctors could only find out what is causing this, they would be able to do something about it." She refuses to discuss psychosocial issues about her illness or to try antidepressants that inhibit serotonin reuptake, saying, "My problems aren't in my head."

The physician's goal in Case 4.4 is to help Ms. D cope with a chronic medical condition and live an active life despite her symptoms. However, Ms. D's goals are relief of her symptoms and reassurance that her condition is not dangerous. Having different goals for care, Ms. D and her physician disagree on the benefits and burdens of an MR scan.

To Ms. D, a scan has little medical risk and potentially great benefit. She believes that a negative scan would provide reassurance. In the unlikely event that the scan is abnormal, her course of care would be dramatically changed. In contrast, from the physician's perspective, a negative scan result is unlikely to lead to reassurance. Patients who seek "just another test" for reassurance often request further tests in a fruitless quest for a definitive diagnosis. Articles on IBS advise against additional diagnostic tests if a thorough initial work-up is negative and the clinical course is typical (14). Unlike MR scans, for other interventions the medical risks might be substantial. If the patient in Case 4.4 had requested exploratory surgery for reassurance or to establish a definitive diagnosis, the physicians should certainly demur.

Allocating Resources Fairly

Given the soaring cost of health care, physicians have a duty to allocate resources fairly and cannot ignore the costs of patient requests (*see also* Chapter 32). Expensive, low-yield high-technology procedures, such as the MR imaging scans noted in Case 4.4, drive up the cost of medical care. In addition, MR imaging scans commonly reveal incidental findings that require further costly and sometimes risky evaluation, but ultimately prove to be clinically insignificant.

However, cost should not be the main reason for refusing patient requests. Under the current health care system, physicians have no explicit societal mandate to limit care to control costs. It is problematic for an individual physician to limit beneficial care solely on the basis of cost (*see* Chapter 32).

The primary consideration should be the benefits and risks to the patients. If the intervention's medical risks outweigh any benefits for the patient, the patient's request can be refused without reference to costs. Patients who have financial incentives to control costs—through substantial copayments—are less likely to request such interventions. Thus, when patients and physicians both have financial incentives for cost-effective medicine, situations like Case 4.4 are easier to resolve.

CASE 4.4	*Continued*

Ms. D's physician acknowledged her concerns and frustrations about a serious illness regarding a chronic illness. Rather than ordering an MR scan, the physician recommended referral to a gastroenterologist to help develop a comprehensive approach, possibly including new medications. The doctor explained how the digestive system responds physiologically to stress and anxiety. The physician also explained the problem of incidental findings on MR scans and reviewed recommendations for screening for cervical, breast, and colon cancer. She recommended that regular visits regardless of symptoms could provide reassurance that there was "nothing serious."

TABLE 4-1. Promoting the Patient's Best Interests
Understand the patient's perspective.
Address misunderstandings and concerns.
Try to persuade the patient.
Negotiate a mutually acceptable plan of care.
Ultimately let the patient decide.

Cost might determine how much time and effort physicians should spend on trying to dissuade the patient. The physician should spend more time trying to discourage an expensive MR imaging scan than in discouraging inexpensive tests. If Ms. D with IBS in Case 4.4 wanted a simple blood count that offered little benefit, few physicians would strongly object.

REACHING AGREEMENT ON BEST INTERESTS

The cases in this chapter illustrate how the patient's choices may conflict with the physician's view of the patient's best interests. Through continued discussions with patients, physicians can promote the best interests of patients while respecting patients' ultimate power to decide (Table 4-1). Chapter 14 gives detailed recommendations for such discussions. Physicians should recommend what they believe is best for the patient from the perspective of the patient's values and preferences. In shared decision-making, physicians should not merely present patients with a list of alternatives and leave them to decide.

Physicians also should try to dissuade patients from unwise decisions. Persuasion respects patients and fosters their autonomy. Persuasion might include talking to the patient about the decision on several occasions and asking the patient to talk to family members, friends, other physicians, or other patients who have had the intervention. The goal is to negotiate a mutually acceptable plan for care, while respecting the patient's right to refuse unwanted interventions. Persuasion needs to be distinguished from deception and threats, which are wrong because they undermine the patient's autonomy. Persuasion must also be distinguished from badgering the patient. Continual attempts to convince patients to change their minds are disrespectful and might also be counterproductive.

SUMMARY

1. Physicians need to respect patient autonomy and act in the patient's best interests simultaneously.
2. Doctors have a fiduciary obligation to act for the well-being of patients, as patients would define it.
3. Physicians can satisfy the ethical guidelines of beneficence and autonomy by understanding the patient's perspective, trying to persuade patients, respecting the power to refuse unwanted interventions, and negotiating a mutually acceptable plan.

References

1. Brewin TB. Primum non nocere? *Lancet* 1994;344:1487-1488.
2. Beauchamp TL, Childress JF. *Principles of Biomedical Ethics.* 7th ed. New York: Oxford University Press; 2013:202-248.
3. Pellegrino ED, Thomasma DG. *For the Patient's Good: The Restoration of Beneficence in Health Care.* New York: Oxford University Press; 1988.
4. Levinson W, Ginsburg S, Hafferty FW, et al. *A Brief History of Medicine's Modern-Day Professionalism Movement. Understanding Medical Professionalism.* Columbus, OH: McGraw-Hill Education; 2014.
5. ABIM Foundation, American Board of Internal Medicine, ACP-ASIM Foundation, et al. Medical professionalism in the new millennium: a physician charter. *Ann Intern Med* 2002;136:243-246.
6. Ginsburg S, Regehr G, Lingard L. Basing the evaluation of professionalism on observable behaviors: a cautionary tale. *Acad Med* 2004;79:S1-S4.

7. Lucey C, Levinson W, Ginsburg S. Medical student mistreatment. *JAMA* 2016;316:2263-2264.
8. Levinson W, Yeung J, Ginsburg S. Disclosure of medical error. *JAMA* 2016;316:764-765.
9. Ginsburg S, Levinson W. Is there a conflict of interest? *JAMA* 2017;317:1796-1797.
10. McNeil BJ, Weichselbaum R, Pauker SG. Fallacy of the five-year survival in lung cancer. *N Engl J Med* 1978;299:307-401.
11. Ubel PA, Loewenstein G, Schwarz N, et al. Misimagining the unimaginable: the disability paradox and health care decision making. *Health Psychol* 2005;24:S57-S62.
12. The President's Council on Bioethics. *Taking Care: Ethical Caregiving in Our Aging Society.* Washington, D.C.2005 [updated September 11, 2012. Available from: http://bioethics.georgetown.edu/pcbe/reports/taking_care/index.html.
13. Murray TH. A moral foundation for anti-doping: how far have we progressed? Where are the limits? *Med Sport Sci* 2017;62:186-193.
14. Fass R, Longstreth GF, Pimentel M, et al. Evidence- and consensus-based practice guidelines for the diagnosis of irritable bowel syndrome. *Arch Intern Med* 2001;161:2081-2088.

ANNOTATED BIBLIOGRAPHY

1. Beauchamp TL, Childress JF. *Principles of Biomedical Ethics.* 7th ed. New York: Oxford University Press; 2013. p. 202-48.
   In-depth discussion of the ethical principle of beneficence.
2. Pellegrino ED, Thomasma DG. *For the Patient's Good: The Restoration of Beneficence in Health Care.* New York, NY: Oxford University Press; 1988.
   Comprehensive exposition of the importance of beneficence in the doctor–patient relationship.
3. Levinson W, Ginsburg S, Hafferty FW, et al. *A Brief History of Medicine's Modern-Day Professionalism Movement. Understanding Medical Professionalism.* Columbus, OH: McGraw-Hill Education; 2014.
   Thoughtful and comprehensive book of medical professionalism and its implementation in academic health centers. Fair and ethical stewardship of resources is considered a core component of medical professionalism.

Confidentiality

INTRODUCTION

Patients reveal to physicians sensitive personal information, including about their medical and emotional problems, alcohol and drug use, and sexual activities. Physicians should keep patient information confidential unless the patient gives permission to disclose it. In some situations, however, exceptions to confidentiality might be warranted to prevent serious harm to third parties or to the patient (Table 5-1). The HIV epidemic, the development of computerized medical records, the explosion of genetic information, and recent mass shootings by patients with psychiatric illnesses have sharpened controversies over patient confidentiality. The federal health privacy regulations are commonly known as HIPAA regulations because they are mandated by the Health Insurance Portability and Accountability Act.

The terms *privacy*, *confidentiality*, and *security* should be distinguished (1). *Privacy* refers to patients' interest in controlling information about themselves, access to their bodies, and freedom from unwanted medical interventions. Patients may choose what information about themselves they wish to disclose to their physicians. They may regard some information as too intimate or sensitive to disclose or simply not relevant to the issue at hand. There is no single concept of privacy that is universally accepted; instead, privacy may be viewed as a bundle of overlapping and related interests, which are also related to other interests such as liberty and autonomy.

Confidentiality refers to the further disclosure of information that the patient has provided to the physician. For example, may information that a patient has disclosed to a treating physician be further disclosed to the patient's family or insurance company, public health officials, researchers,

TABLE 5-1. Exceptions to Confidentiality
Exceptions to protect third parties

Reporting to public officials
    Infectious diseases
    Impaired drivers
    Injuries caused by weapons or crimes

Warnings to persons at risk
    Violence by psychiatric patients
    Infectious diseases

Exceptions to protect patients
Child abuse
Elder abuse
Intimate partner violence

or hospital quality improvement teams? The focus of confidentiality is on what the physician may reveal to third parties, rather than what the patient chooses to disclose to the physician. In everyday conversation, the distinction between privacy and confidentiality is blurred.

Security refers to procedural and technical measures to prevent inappropriate access, use, and disclosure of personal information in health records. With electronic health records, increased security is an important means to prevent breaches of confidentiality that may affect thousands of patients. Current security standards include training of physicians and staff regarding privacy and confidentiality, restricting access to a patient's health record to those with a need to know, time-outs, audit trails, two-factor authentication, and encryption of personal health information transmitted to remote computers and mobile devices.

THE IMPORTANCE OF CONFIDENTIALITY IN MEDICINE

Reasons for Confidentiality

Respect for patients requires keeping medical information confidential (2). Maintaining confidentiality also has beneficial consequences for patients and for the doctor–patient relationship. It encourages people to seek medical care and discuss sensitive issues candidly. In turn, treatment for these conditions benefits both the individual patient and public health. Furthermore, confidentiality prevents harmful consequences to patients, such as stigmatization and discrimination, for example, by employers. Maintaining confidentiality is a strong professional tradition in medicine, and patients expect it. The legal system also holds physicians liable for unwarranted disclosure of medical information.

Difficulties Maintaining Confidentiality

Maintaining confidentiality is increasingly difficult. Many people have access to medical records, including the attending physician, house staff, students, consultants, nurses, social workers, pharmacists, billing staff, medical records personnel, insurance company employees, and quality-of-care reviewers. Breaches of computerized medical records involve extensive data on many patients. Fax and e-mail also present opportunities for confidentiality to be broken. Posting patient stories on social media may violate confidentiality, as well as disrespect the patient (3).

Many breaches of confidentiality, however, result from health care workers' indiscretions, for example when health care workers discuss patients by name in hospital elevators or cafeterias. Although many physicians take such discussions for granted, patients object to such breaches of confidentiality.

Exceptions to Confidentiality

Although confidentiality is important, it is not an absolute value. In some situations, overriding confidentiality might be justified to provide important benefits to patients or to prevent serious harm to third parties. For example, access to information might be needed to protect the public health or improve the quality of care. These exceptions require careful justification. Not every instance of benefit to patients or prevention of harm to others warrants the disclosure of identifiable medical information without the patient's permission.

The balance between preventing harm to third parties and protecting confidentiality is ultimately set by society through statutes, public health regulations, and court decisions. Setting this balance as public policy allows all points of view to be represented and is preferable to decisions by the individual physicians in their offices or at the bedside. Laws on confidentiality vary from state to state. In general, exceptions to confidentiality are warranted when all the following conditions are met (2):

- The potential harm to identifiable third parties is serious.
- The likelihood of harm is high.
- There is no less invasive alternative means for warning or protecting those at risk.
- Breaching confidentiality allows the person at risk to take steps to prevent harm.
- Harm to the patient resulting from the breach of confidentiality is minimized and acceptable.

Disclosure should be limited to information essential for the intended purpose, and only those persons with a need to know should have the information.

FEDERAL HEALTH PRIVACY REGULATIONS

Under the HIPAA privacy regulations, health care providers—both individual health care workers and institutions—must obtain patient authorization to use or disclose individually identifiable health information, with certain broad exceptions (4). Providers must make reasonable efforts to use and disclose only the minimum identifiable information that is needed to accomplish the intended purpose. In addition, health care providers must take reasonable safeguards against prohibited or incidental use or disclosure of personal health information and maintain "reasonable and appropriate" safeguards to prevent violations of the privacy regulations.

Patients may inspect and copy their medical records and request that corrections be made. They may request to receive information by alternative means and locations (such as not leaving messages on an answering machine) and to obtain a list of disclosures of their information. Health care providers must develop privacy policies and procedures and train all staff about the privacy regulations. The regulations also address how individually identifiable health information may be used or disclosed for research and marketing and by business associates of the health care provider. Because HIPAA regulations set criminal penalties for intentional violations, many risk managers interpret them conservatively. These federal regulations establish a minimum level of protection; state laws and organizational policies may be stricter.

HIPAA regulations are not intended to impede access to individual patient information needed for high-quality and efficient patient care. No patient authorization is needed to use or disclose identifiable information for treatment, payment, and operations, including quality improvement, quality assurance, and education. Furthermore, HIPAA permits required disclosures of identifiable information to public health officials, health oversight agencies, and as required by law or a court.

Good patient care requires communication among various health care providers. In the course of care, incidental disclosure of information and breaches of confidentiality might occur. Physicians should take reasonable precautions to prevent inappropriate disclosures, but should not forego communications needed in patient care (5). For example, physicians may communicate with other providers by e-mail or fax without explicit patient authorization, but should use secure e-mail systems and keep fax machines in areas where other patients cannot access them. Furthermore, physicians may discuss patients at the nursing station, provided that they keep their voices down and pause when someone such as a patient or visitor approaches.

PATIENT AGREEMENT TO WAIVE CONFIDENTIALITY

Disclosing patient information to family members, friends, or the press might raise ethical issues.

Waivers of Confidentiality

Patients commonly authorize disclosure of information about their condition, for example, to other physicians, insurers, employers, or benefits programs such as disability or workers' compensation (6). Patients might not appreciate that signing a general release allows the insurance company to further disseminate the information without restriction. Insurance companies generally place patients' diagnoses in a computerized database that is accessible to other insurance companies or to employers without further permission from the patient.

Disclosure to Relatives and Friends

Relatives and friends often ask about the patient's condition. Generally patients want the physician to talk to their family, and family members usually have the patient's best interests at heart. Moreover, relatives might provide valuable information and help with decision-making, discharge planning, or follow-up care. Often physicians do not even ask the patient's permission to talk with family members. In some cases, however, the patient might not want the information disclosed. The HIPAA privacy regulations support a presumption of informing relatives of the patient's condition. Health care providers must notify patients that relatives will be informed unless the patient requests that they not be. In ethical terms, the physician can presume that patients would want their relatives notified.

CASE 5.1   Estrangement from spouse

Ms. D, a 32-year-old woman, is admitted to the hospital after a serious automobile accident. She is disoriented and confused. Her sister requests that Ms. D's husband not be given any information. Ms. D has previously told the physician about her hostile divorce proceedings, and this is documented in the electronic health record at the hospital. The husband learns that she is hospitalized and inquires about her condition.

If the inpatient physician knows about the contentious divorce proceedings between Ms. D and her husband, he should regard them as estranged and refer the husband to Ms. D's sister. It is reasonable to expect the admitting physician to review information in the electronic record, including the social history.

How much should physicians who do not know the patient question the presumption that they may tell family members about the patient's condition? Screening family members to ask if they are estranged would be disrespectful for the vast majority of family members who care about the patient and might lead to mistrust between them and the medical team.

Information About Public Figures

The press might seek information about patients who are public figures or celebrities. The public and news media might have legitimate reasons to know medical information about a public figure. For instance, a political candidate's health is an important and valid concern for voters (7). However, famous people have a right to confidentiality, like all patients. The physician and hospital should ask the patient or appropriate surrogate what information, if any, should be released.

EXCEPTIONS TO CONFIDENTIALITY TO PROTECT THIRD PARTIES

State laws might require overriding patient confidentiality in certain situations to prevent serious harm to third parties (Table 5-1). HIPAA expressly permits these exceptions to confidentiality. The ethical guideline of nonmaleficence requires both patients and physicians to avoid harming other people and to prevent harm to others. Institutional protocols and teams are dedicated to the specific problem to help physicians fulfill their legal and ethical obligations to report.

Reporting to Public Officials

Infectious Diseases

Physicians, clinical laboratories, and hospitals are required by law to report to public health officials the names of patients with specified infectious diseases, such as tuberculosis, gonorrhea, and enteric pathogens. Such reporting allows surveillance, investigations of outbreaks, contact tracing, partner notification, and public health planning.

Certain conditions carry a greater risk of stigma and discrimination. Early in the HIV epidemic, stigma and discrimination were so severe that HIV testing received special protections, including pretest counseling, written informed consent, and alternative test sites where people could be tested for HIV antibodies anonymously. Furthermore, although AIDS cases had to be reported, HIV infection was not reportable in many states. After highly active antiretroviral therapy became available and overt discrimination decreased, HIV infection has been treated like other sexually transmitted infections, with reporting of infected persons by name to public health officials (8). Moreover, HIV viral load and CD4 counts must now be reported in some states, to better link testing with treatment. Anonymous testing, however, is still permitted.

Public health officials contact persons who may have been infected by patients with contagious conditions like tuberculosis, notify them of exposure, and recommend appropriate testing and treatment. This process is called *contact tracing*. The identity of the index case is not revealed, but contacts can often infer it. In diseases with airborne transmission, in addition to household contacts, the infected patient may have infected unknown others through casual contact, for example, on public transportation. For sexually transmitted infections, including HIV, the term *partner notification* has replaced the traditional term *contact tracing*. More partners are notified when public health officials carry out the notification than when patients do it themselves.

The cooperation of the infected patient may not be needed for diseases that can be transmitted through aerosolized particles to casual contacts. For instance, contacts of tuberculosis patients might be located by going to the index case's home and workplace. In contrast, for blood-borne and sexually transmitted diseases, sexual or needle-sharing partners can be identified only with the infected person's cooperation, and for all practical purposes partner notification must be voluntary (9). If patients do not wish to cooperate, they can deny that they have partners or give inaccurate names and addresses. Any perception that partner notification programs are punitive or disrespectful to index cases might reduce cooperation.

Impaired Drivers

Some states require physicians to report to the department of motor vehicles persons with specified medical conditions that impair their ability to drive safely. Such conditions may include epilepsy, syncope, dementia, sleep apnea, and other conditions that impair consciousness (10). Even if the underlying condition is treated, the patient might not be able to drive safely. For example, after placement of an implantable cardiac defibrillator, about 10% of patients experience syncope or near-syncope associated with defibrillation in the first year (11). The physician's role is not to stop the patient from driving or to decide whether the patient should be permitted to drive. Such determinations are properly made by the department of motor vehicles. The physician only informs officials of persons who warrant evaluation. Reporting is particularly indicated for patients who drive commercially and present greater risks because they spend more hours on the road, drive heavy vehicles, or are responsible for passengers.

Reporting of patients with conditions that might impair driving is complicated: although reporting may reduce subsequent crashes, it might also be the unintended adverse consequences of decreasing return visits to physicians, worsening care of the underlying condition, and increasing patient depression (12). Both physicians and patients might believe that doctor−patient trust has been ruptured (13).

Injuries Caused by Weapons or Crimes

Almost all states require physicians to report injuries involving a deadly weapon or criminal act (14). The rationale is to protect the public from further violence.

Warnings to Patients

The common law and laws in some states may also impose on infected persons a legal duty to notify persons whom they place at risk. In these circumstances, the overall harm to the third parties at risk is judged to be greater than the harm to the index case resulting from overriding confidentiality.

As a first step, physicians need to explain to patients how their condition might put others at risk and to advise how the patient should protect those at risk. For instance, doctors need to explain how to avoid transmitting a contagious disease. Similarly, they should warn patients about driving if they

TABLE 5-2. Situations in Which Overriding Confidentiality Is Warranted
The potential harm to third parties is serious.
The likelihood of harm is high.
No alternative for warning or protecting those at risk exists.
Breaching confidentiality will prevent harm.
Harm to the patient is minimized and acceptable.

are taking medications that might impair their alertness. Physicians should also explain if public health officials will reserve results from a clinical laboratory, for example, when titers of HIV RNA are measured to monitor therapy, and if contact tracing will be carried out.

Warnings to Persons at Risk

Physicians might also have a legal duty or option to directly warn identifiable persons whom a patient places at risk (Table 5-1).

Violence by Psychiatric Patients

In most states, mental health professionals have a legal responsibility to override confidentiality to protect persons who are potential targets of violence by psychiatric patients (*see* Chapter 42). Laws vary among states. Some require mental health professionals to notify the police or the potential victim, whereas other states give professionals permission to do so. Clinically, it may be appropriate to institute more intensive therapy or voluntary or involuntary hospitalization or to convince the patient to give up weapons.

Infectious Diseases

Courts might require physicians to warn patients with infectious diseases to take precautions to prevent their infectious disease from afflicting others. In addition, some courts require physicians to notify identified persons whom their infected patients place at risk. Generally, physicians can fulfill this duty by notifying public health officials and having them notify persons at risk.

EXCEPTIONS TO CONFIDENTIALITY TO PROTECT PATIENTS

In some situations, physicians must override confidentiality to protect the patient rather than third parties (Table 5-1). The ethical justification for intervening is that patients might not be able to protect themselves. Some physicians might have reservations about reporting because follow-up counseling, support services, and protective interventions may be poor (15). Many protective service agencies for children and elders are underfunded and understaffed, and abuse has been documented in foster care and nursing homes.

Child Abuse

All states require health care workers to report suspected child abuse or neglect to child protective services agencies (16). Parental privacy is overridden to protect vulnerable children from an imminent risk of serious harm. More than 1000 children die of neglect and abuse each year; most are under the age of 5. Health care workers might be the only people outside the family to have close contact with preschool children. State laws vary regarding the types of situations that must be reported and the kinds of persons who must report. In some states, only helping professionals, such as health care workers, school personnel, child care providers, law enforcement workers, and mental health professionals, must report; in other states, any person who suspects abuse or neglect has a mandatory duty to report.

A report should be triggered if there is reasonable belief or suspicion of abuse and neglect that justifies fuller investigation. Definitive proof is not needed (17). To encourage reporting, most states grant legal immunity when reporting is done in good faith. Intervention might enable parents to obtain enough assistance and support to prevent further abuse. In extreme cases, the child might be removed from parental custody. In evaluating possible child abuse, pediatricians should treat parents with respect, keeping in mind that most parents are trying their best to deal with the challenges of childrearing.

Elder Abuse

Elder abuse may be physical, verbal, psychological, sexual, or financial; in addition, elders may be neglected. All states except New York require health care workers to report cases of elder abuse to adult protective services (18). The goal is to identify persons who are incapable of seeking assistance on their own and to offer them help. Elderly persons who are dependent on their caretakers might be unwilling or unable to complain about physical or psychological abuse or neglect. Patients might not be aware of available in-home supportive services or might feel intimidated by caretakers. They might fear that if they complain, they will be worse off, perhaps placed in a nursing home. Most abusers of elderly persons are family members who are overwhelmed by caring for a frail elderly person. Thus, reporting and intervention might provide resources that allow the elderly person to continue to live safely at home. Elderly persons who are truly capable of making informed decisions and are free from coercion are at liberty to decline offered assistance.

Specific laws for reporting elder abuse vary from state to state. Generally, reasonable suspicion of abuse is sufficient to trigger reporting. Health care workers typically must report abuse only when they obtain information about a patient in their professional roles. Thus, although physicians as private citizens *may* report an elderly neighbor whom they suspect is abused, they are not *required* to do so. Health care workers receive legal immunity when they report suspected abuse in good faith.

Some elders who retain decision-making capacity do not attend to their own needs and well-being and refuse help with meals, cleaning the home, or bathing. Such situations are distressing for family members and physicians, but the competent patient's prioritization of independence over safety should be respected (19). Doctors can avoid setting unrealistic safety expectations and instead follow principles of reducing harm incrementally, enlisting friends or neighbors to persuade the patient to accept assistance.

Intimate Partner Violence

Intimate partner violence can be physical, sexual, or psychological assault. The vast majority of people who are assaulted are women. Intimate partner violence may occur with same-sex partners. Some states require health care workers to report suspected domestic violence or abuse, and most states require reporting of injuries caused by a deadly weapon or illegal act (20). Persons who are assaulted often are unable to take steps on their own to escape further violence. Although reporting is intended to protect the person assaulted and to hold perpetrators of violence accountable, it might be ineffective or even counterproductive in some circumstances (21). Mandatory reporting might put victims at risk of retaliation from their assailants unless police and courts respond with sensitivity and vigor to reports of abuse. Physicians might face conflicting obligations: a legal mandate to report and the patient's desire not to report the abuse because reporting might worsen the situation. Physicians and the dedicated team at the health care institution should provide emotional support, address immediate safety concerns, and refer patients to a shelter, legal and social services, and counseling. Particular concerns about an increased risk of violence should be communicated to the police when making a report (21). Whenever possible, physicians should promote the abused person's autonomy—for example, respecting a request to delay reporting until the person can find shelter.

OMITTING SENSITIVE INFORMATION FROM MEDICAL RECORDS

Patients who are concerned about breaches of confidentiality sometimes ask physicians to omit sensitive information from their medical records.

CASE 5.2	Omission of information from the medical record

Mr. N, a 41-year-old nurse in excellent health, has a routine checkup at the hospital where he works. He asks his physician not to write in the medical record that was severely depressed several years ago. Mr. N knows that many people in the hospital might see his record, and he does not want colleagues to know his psychiatric history. He also fears that he will have difficulty changing jobs if his history is known.

Physicians might fear that omitting medical information from patient records might compromise the quality of care. Important clinical information might not be available in an emergency. In addition, documentation of the patient's current condition and treatment might be required for insurance payment or authorization for services. Furthermore, it might not be feasible to exclude information from an electronic medical record. Even if a diagnosis is omitted from the record, it might be inferred from the patient's laboratory tests or medications.

The purpose of the medical record is to enhance patient well-being and quality of care. Generally, patients are the best judges of their best interests. Some patients might regard breaches of confidentiality as more threatening than the risk of suboptimal care resulting from incomplete medical records. Thus, a patient's informed preferences to exclude sensitive information from the medical record should be respected if feasible.

CASE 5.2	*Continued*

Mr. N's concerns are understandable because depression can be considered stigmatizing. Many electronic health records allow patients to limit access to some sensitive information to persons providing direct care, such as therapy notes by mental health professionals. The Americans with Disabilities Act restricts access by potential employers to a worker's health records and bans basing hiring and promotion decisions on medical conditions that do not affect job performance. Mr. N's physician should explain how the prior history helps other doctors provide good care. If Mr. N persists in his request, the physician should try to accommodate it, preferably with a note in the medical record alerting other treating physicians to contact her for additional history not in the record. However, electronic ordering of medications should not be omitted from an electronic medical record, to allow for warnings of serious drug interactions.

SUMMARY

1. Physicians should maintain confidentiality unless there are compelling reasons to override it.
2. In some situations, the law requires physicians to override confidentiality to protect third parties or patients who cannot protect themselves.
3. Even if public health reporting is required by law, it is respectful to tell patients that reporting will occur, obtain their agreement if possible, and take steps to address their concerns and minimize harm to them.

References

1. Allen A. Privacy and Medicine. In *Stanford Encyclopedia of Philosophy* [updated February 28, 2011. Available from: http://plato.stanford.edu/entries/privacy-medicine/.
2. Beauchamp TL, Childress JF. *Principles of Biomedical Ethics.* 7th ed. New York: Oxford University Press; 2013:316-323.
3. Ofri D. The passion and the peril: storytelling in medicine. *Acad Med.* 2015;90:1005-1006.
4. Department of Health and Human Services. *Health Information Privacy: HIPAA for Professionals.* Available from: https://www.hhs.gov/hipaa/for-professionals/index.html.
5. Lo B, Dornbrand L, Dubler NN. HIPAA and patient care: the role for professional judgment. *JAMA* 2005;293:1766-1771.
6. Rothstein MA, Talbott MK. Compelled disclosure of health information: protecting against the greatest potential threat to privacy. *JAMA* 2006;295:2882-2885.
7. Markel H, Stern AM. Presidential health and the public's need to know. *JAMA* 2008;299:2558-2560.
8. Fairchild AL, Bayer R. HIV surveillance, public health, and clinical medicine—will the walls come tumbling down? *N Engl J Med* 2011;365:685-687.
9. Bayer R, Toomey KE. HIV prevention and the two faces of partner notification. *Am J Public Health* 1992;82:1158-1164.
10. Gupta M. Mandatory reporting laws and the emergency physician. *Ann Emer Med* 2007;49:369-376.
11. Epstein AE, Baessler CA, Curtis AB, et al. Addendum to "Personal and public safety issues related to arrhythmias that may affect consciousness: implications for regulation and physician recommendations: a medical/scientific statement from the American Heart Association and the North American Society of Pacing and Electrophysiology": public safety issues in patients with implantable defibrillators: a scientific statement from the American Heart Association and the Heart Rhythm Society. *Circulation* 2007;115:1170-1176.
12. Redelmeier DA, Yarnell CJ, Thiruchelvam D, et al. Physicians' warnings for unfit drivers and the risk of trauma from road crashes. *N Engl J Med* 2012;367:1228-1236.
13. Rush R. Officer of the Law. *N Engl J Med* 2017;377:1610-1611.
14. Baker EF, Moskop JC, Geiderman JM, et al. Law enforcement and emergency medicine: an ethical analysis. *Ann Emer Med* 2016;68:599-607.
15. English A. Mandatory reporting of human trafficking: potential benefits and risks of harm. *AMA J Ethics* 2017;19:54-62.
16. Dubowitz H, Bennett S. Physical abuse and neglect of children. *Lancet* 2007;369:1891-1899.
17. Levi BH, Portwood SG. Reasonable suspicion of child abuse: finding a common language. *J Law Med Ethics* 2011;39:62-69.
18. Lachs MS, Pillemer KA. Elder abuse. *N Engl J Med* 2015;373:1947-1956.
19. Smith AK, Lo B, Aronson L. Elder self-neglect—how can a physician help? *N Engl J Med* 2013;369:2476-2479.
20. Choo EK, Houry DE. Managing intimate partner violence in the emergency department. *Ann Emer Med* 2015;65:447-451.e1.
21. Hyman A, Schillinger D, Lo B. Laws mandating reporting of domestic violence: do they promote patient well-being? *JAMA* 1995;273:1781-1787.

ANNOTATED BIBLIOGRAPHY

1. Allen A. *Privacy and Medicine. In Stanford Encyclopedia of Philosophy.* http://plato.stanford.edu/entries/privacy-medicine/.
   Comprehensive, thoughtful review.
2. Lo B, Dornbrand L, Dubler NN. From Hippocrates to HIPAA: confidentiality, government regulations, and professional judgment. *JAMA* 2005;293:1766-1771.
   Analyzes the federal confidentiality regulations (also known as HIPAA regulations) and how physician judgment is still required to determine what risk of a breach of confidentiality is acceptable when disclosing information to other health care workers caring for a patient.
3. Gostin LO, Wiley LF. *Public Health Law: Power, Duty, Restraint.* 3rd ed. Berkeley: University of California Press; 2016:39-68.
   Lucid discussion of overriding confidentiality to protect the public health.
4. Mosqueda L, Dong X. Elder abuse and self-neglect: "I don't care anything about going to the doctor, to be honest..." *JAMA* 2011;306:532-540.
   Comprehensive review of elder abuse.

Avoiding Deception and Nondisclosure

INTRODUCTION

Children are taught to tell the truth and avoid lies. In clinical medicine, however, the distinction between telling the truth and lying can seem simplistic. Even doctors who condemn outright lying might consider withholding a grave diagnosis from a patient, covertly administering needed medications to a severely psychotic patient, or exaggerating a patient's condition to secure insurance coverage. This chapter analyzes the ethical considerations regarding lying, deception, misrepresentation, and nondisclosure. Such actions might mislead either the patient or a third party, such as an insurance company or a disability agency.

DEFINITIONS

Case 6.1 illustrates some ways physicians might provide misleading information.

CASE 6.1	**Family request not to tell the patient she has cancer**

Ms. Z, a 70-year-old Cantonese-speaking woman with a change in bowel habits and weight loss, is found to have a carcinoma of the colon. The daughter and son ask the physician not to tell her that she has cancer. They say that people in her generation are not told this diagnosis and that Ms. Z will lose hope if she learns she has cancer. A colleague suggests that the physician tell the patient that she has a "growth" that needs to be removed.

Physicians might provide misleading information in different ways. *Lying* refers to statements that the speaker knows are false or believes to be false and that are intended to mislead the listener. For example, the physician might tell the patient that the tests were normal.

Deception is broader than lying, and it includes all statements and actions that are intended to mislead the listener, whether or not they are literally true. An example would be telling the patient that she has a "growth," hoping that she will believe her condition is not serious. Other techniques used to mislead people include employing technical jargon, ambiguous statements, or misleading statistics; not answering a question; and omitting important qualifying information.

Misrepresentation is a still broader category, including unintentional, as well as intentional statements and actions. The statements might or might not be literally true. Unintentional misrepresentation might result from inexperience, poor interpersonal skills, or lack of diligence or knowledge. For instance, a physician might not tell Ms. Z she has cancer because the physician misread the biopsy report.

Nondisclosure means that the physician does not provide information about the diagnosis, prognosis, or plan of care. For example, a physician might not tell Ms. Z she has cancer unless she specifically asks.

Many writers on medical ethics use terms such as *truth-telling* or *veracity*. This book, however, avoids these ambiguous terms because ethically difficult cases usually do not involve outright lies.

There are strong ethical objections to lying and deception. Traditional religious and moral codes forbid lying. The Old Testament, for example, exhorts people not to bear false witness. Lying and deception also show disrespect for others. Those who are lied to or deceived generally feel betrayed or manipulated, even if the liar has benevolent motives. Lying also undermines social trust because listeners cannot be confident that other statements by the doctor, or other doctors, will be truthful. This loss of trust is particularly grave in medicine because trust is essential in a doctor–patient relationship. In addition to undermining the speaker's integrity, lying is further condemned because a single lie often requires continued deception.

Lying and deception are considered *prima facie* wrong; they are presumed to be inappropriate, and they require a justification (1, 2). Many people regard lying as more blameworthy than other types of deception (1). Some "white" lies, however, may be accepted as social customs that do not deceive anyone and might prevent people from feeling rejected.

Although lying and deception by physicians are rejected today, traditional codes of medical ethics did not require physicians to be truthful or forthcoming to patients. The writings of Hippocrates urge physicians to conceal "most things from the patient while you are attending him." Until the last quarter of the 20th century, many physicians in the United States either did not tell patients about serious diagnoses, such as cancer, or deceived them (3).

GENERAL REASONS FOR AND AGAINST DECEPTION OR NONDISCLOSURE

The ethical issue is whether general prohibitions on lying also apply to deception and nondisclosure.

Reasons for Deception or Nondisclosure to the Patient

Deception and Nondisclosure Prevent Serious Harm

In cultures where patients are not told the diagnosis of cancer, it is believed that patients will lose hope, refuse medically beneficial treatment, or become depressed after learning a serious diagnosis. Another example of nondisclosure to prevent harm occurs in organ transplantation when a potential living donor does not want to donate but fears criticism from relatives. Donor evaluation teams commonly say that he or she is not a suitable donor without disclosing the specific reason to the patient or other potential donors. Case 6.2 gives another example in which deception and nondisclosure may avert serious harm.

CASE 6.2	**Covert administration of medications**

Mr. E, a 32-year-old man with bipolar disorder, discontinued his medications and developed mania. He stole money from his parents, bought a car, and planned to drive cross-country without stopping. Mr. E's sister persuaded him to come to the emergency department, but he would not let anyone touch or examine him and refused medications and admission. Staff suggested to Mr. E's sister that she inject haloperidol and lorazepam into a sealed juice container and give him the juice, without telling him.

Similar covert administration of medications may be considered for patients with moderate or severe cognitive dysfunction who are refusing medications, becoming more agitated, or having symptoms of hyperglycemia. In such cases, covert administration of medication may prevent medical and psychiatric harms to the patient.

Deception and Nondisclosure Promote Patient Autonomy

In Case 6.2, not disclosing to the patient the administration of medicines for bipolar disorder, by treating a manic episode, can restore the patient's autonomy and ability to make informed decisions.

The Alternatives Are More Problematic

In some cases, nondisclosure or deception is judged the least bad alternative in a set of bad options.

CASE 6.2 | *Continued*

Mr. E's sister said that violent confrontations with staff during previous periods of mania had caused Mr. E physical and psychological injury. She agreed to inject haloperidol and lorazepam into a sealed juice container and gave him the juice. These events were documented in the medical record. Mr. E accepted the drink, and 45 minutes later he was calmer and cooperative and agreed to psychiatric hospitalization.

Covert administration of medications may be the least bad alternative. In Case 6.2, other options, such as physical restraints or parenteral administration of medications over the patient's objections, are also ethically problematic because they violate the patient's autonomy and bodily integrity, seem inhumane, and might injure the patient and staff. The strongest case for deception in this case is as a last resort, after attempts to persuade the patient to accept beneficial care have failed.

Reasons Against Deception or Nondisclosure to the Patient

Overall Deception and Nondisclosure Cause More Harm Than Benefit

Claims about the benefits of deception and nondisclosure must be evaluated empirically. In Case 6.1, patients with cancer rarely lose hope, refuse medically beneficial treatment, or become seriously depressed, provided that they receive emotional and social support. Although sadness and anxiety might occur, major depression or suicide attempts are rare. To be sure, some patients have active major depression or have previously attempted suicide. In such cases, it would be justified to withhold the diagnosis while obtaining psychiatric consultation and assessing the likelihood of harm. In exceptional cases, the risk of harm might be so serious as to justify withholding the diagnosis until the patient's mental health improves.

In assessing the harms and benefits of deception and nondisclosure, physicians must take into account the long-term and indirect adverse consequences. Disclosure of the diagnosis and prognosis can benefit patients. In Case 6.1, patients are more likely to cooperate with plans for care if they understand the reasons for the tests and treatments. This requires being informed of their diagnosis.

Many patients with a serious diagnosis such as cancer already suspect it. Nondisclosure of the diagnosis and not discussing their prognosis and plan of care might lead them to imagine that their situation is worse than it actually is. Patients often feel relieved when their illnesses are diagnosed and they can then focus on treatment.

More Deception Will Be Required, Undermining Trust

Deception and nondisclosure usually require additional, more complex deceptions. If a patient is not told the diagnosis of cancer, deception is needed to explain the reasons for additional testing, surgery, or other treatments. As the deception becomes more complex, inconsistencies may emerge. The patient may question why he or she is being told inconsistent things or why people appear uncomfortable interacting with him or her. Ultimately, Ms. Z may begin to mistrust her health care team or even her family. In turn, such loss of trust may cause anxiety and fear.

Trust is likely also an issue in Case 7.2. Trust is an important component of high-quality psychiatric care and has implications for long-term medication use. Psychiatric patients often discontinue medications because of adverse effects; a patient who believes that his or her caregivers and relatives cannot be trusted may be even more likely to discontinue medications and precipitate another relapse.

Deception and Nondisclosure Might Be Impossible

In the long run, it is unrealistic to keep patients like Ms. Z from knowing their diagnoses. A nurse, house officer, x-ray technician, or patient transport worker might disclose that the patient has cancer. In modern medicine, a very large number of health care workers provide care to a patient. Most of them will not have been involved in a discussion at which the primary team decided to withhold Ms. Z's diagnosis. A well-meaning health care worker might try to reassure the patient by telling her about a relative with the same diagnosis who has done well or about how good the cancer doctors are at the institution. In addition, when a patient is visited by a physician whose name tag says medical oncology or when he or she has an outpatient appointment at the cancer center, the diagnosis is clear. When patients belatedly find out their diagnoses, they generally feel angry and betrayed. Thus, the practical issue is not whether to tell the patient a serious diagnosis, but rather how to tell. Physicians should not promise family members that the patient will not learn a serious diagnosis. Surgeons may decline to operate unless a competent patient gives informed consent (see Chapter 7). It is usually counterproductive to devise elaborate schemes to try to keep patients from knowing the diagnosis instead of helping them cope with the bad news.

Similarly, in Case 7.2, when Mr. E is no longer in a manic episode, he may ask how treatment was instituted or even comment on how there was no physical confrontation with health care workers to restrain him or forcibly administer medications, as in previous manic episodes. Once again, the issue is not whether to tell him about the covert administration of medications, but how to tell. In such cases, it is generally better to explain what was done when the patient's impairment has improved, why deception was judged to be the best plan for his care, and to seek his permission to do so again in a future manic episode, again with the goal of treating the mental illness without physical force.

Slippery slopes

If allowed in one case, deception may become more widely used in other cases where the level of impairment is not as serious, when persuasion has not been vigorously attempted, or when adequate staffing and facilities are not available.

DECEPTION OR NONDISCLOSURE TO THE PATIENT

Withholding Bad News from a Patient

Withholding the diagnosis of cancer from patients presents particular ethical issues beyond the general considerations discussed above.

Deception May Be Culturally Appropriate

The vast majority of patients in the United States want to know if they have a serious diagnosis. In one early survey, 94% of those asked said that they "would want to know everything" about their medical condition, "even if it is unfavorable" (4). Ninety-six percent wanted to know a diagnosis of cancer. The desire to be told a serious diagnosis is so strong in the United States that most patients want radiologists to tell them of abnormal results at the time of the imaging study rather than waiting for their primary physician to do so (5).

In many cultures, patients traditionally are not told they have cancer or other serious illness. In a 1995 study, although 87% of European American patients and 89% of African American patients wanted to be told if they have cancer, only 65% of Mexican Americans and 47% of Korean Americans wanted to be told (6). Some cultures believe disclosure of a grave diagnosis causes patients to suffer, whereas withholding information gives serenity, security, and hope (7). Being direct and explicit might be considered insensitive and cruel. Families and physicians might try to protect the patient by taking on decision-making responsibility (8, 9). However, the crucial ethical issue is whether the individual patient wants to know the diagnosis, not what most people in their culture would want. Moreover, cultural beliefs may change over time. In China and India, despite traditional beliefs, most cancer patients now say they should be told their diagnosis (10, 11). Similar trends toward patients wanting the disclosure of a cancer diagnosis have been reported in Middle Eastern countries (12).

Patients Need to Know Their Diagnosis to Give Informed Consent

For patients to make informed decisions, physicians need to disclose pertinent information (*see* Chapter 3). Under the doctrine of informed consent, doctors are expected to disclose such information without patients having to ask for it.

Resolving Dilemmas About Withholding Bad News

Table 6-1 summarizes how physicians can respond to dilemmas without resorting to misrepresentation or nondisclosure.

Anticipate dilemmas regarding deception and nondisclosure. Dilemmas regarding deception and nondisclosure can often be anticipated. When ordering a cancer test, physicians can ask whether the patient wishes to be informed of the results: "Many patients want to know their test results, while other patients want the doctor to tell a family member. I will do whatever you prefer. What do you want me to do?" After the physician has received the test results, inquiring about the patient's preferences for disclosure might reveal the diagnosis. Simply asking the question suggests that the results are abnormal because there is no reason to withhold normal results from the patient.

In bipolar disorder or schizophrenia, relapses and refusal of treatment while mentally incapacitated are common. During remission, patients can be asked whether they would accept covert administration of medications as an alternative to physical restraint if they need to be given medications to prevent grave harm.

Respect the patient's preferences. When a family requests that a patient not be told of a serious diagnosis, the physician should assess whether this is the patient's wish or the family's. Convincing evidence that the patient herself would not want to be told should be respected.

Address concerns that prompted the request for deception or nondisclosure. The physician should explore the family's concerns regarding discussing disclosing the diagnosis of cancer, respond with empathy, and work toward a joint plan for addressing those concerns directly (12, 13).

Maintain transparency and accountability. Any decision to use deception or nondisclosure and its rationale should be documented in the medical record. Such documentation fosters accountability because the physician must explain his or her reasoning and others can review it.

Minimize the amount of deception and its adverse consequences. If Ms. Z asks the physician directly what the test showed, there are strong arguments for responding forthrightly. The question indicates that the patient wants some information. Furthermore, patients realize that an evasive response is bad news because physicians do not hesitate to give normal results.

CASE 6.1	*Continued*

The physician can elicit the family's concerns by asking, "What do you fear most about telling your mother she has cancer?" Also the physician can validate the family's feelings as the natural reactions of loving relatives and explain how bad news usually can be disclosed in supportive ways that help patients cope. Physicians should soften bad news by being compassionate, responding to the patient's concerns, offering empathy, giving bad news in short chunks, and helping mobilize support. Often the physician can persuade relatives that the patient should be told of the diagnosis.

If Ms. Z chooses not to know her diagnosis, the physician should leave open the possibility that she might change her mind. Physicians should regularly ask patients if they have questions or want to discuss anything else about their condition.

Deceiving a Patient to Administer Needed Medications

Covert administration of medications in food is common in the care of patients with dementia, particularly residents of institutions (14). Patients with dementia commonly refuse medications. Many caregivers feel they have no other alternative in patients who lack decision-making capacity to

TABLE 6-1. Resolving Dilemmas About Deception and Nondisclosure to Patients
Anticipate dilemmas about disclosure.
Respect the patient's preferences.
Address concerns that prompted the request for deception or nondisclosure.
Maintain transparency and accountability.
Minimize the amount of deception and its adverse consequences.

administer drugs to treat serious medical problems, such as diabetes or infection. However, the reasons for covert administration of medications often are not documented, and explicit orders are not written. There are additional reasons for and against deception involving medications, in addition to the general ethical considerations regarding deception and nondisclosure previously discussed (15).

Additional Reasons in Favor of Deception to Give Medications

The medication would restore the patient's autonomy. In Case 6.2, untreated mania rendered Mr. E incapable of making an informed decision. Thus, although the deception violates his autonomy, its purpose was to restore it.

The patient's surrogate authorizes deception. Mr. E's sister agreed to the deception and to administer the medications that he needed. In trying to bring him to care, she acted in his best interests. As the surrogate of a patient who lacks decision-making capacity, she judges that it is better for him to receive needed care through deception than to remain in untreated mania or to have injections over his objections.

The patient previously authorized deception. While in remission, the patient may have stated that during a relapse he or she would agree to covert administration of oral medications in preference to forced injections. Such advance directives allow physicians and surrogates to follow the preferences of the patient when autonomous.

CASE 6.2   *Continued*
Mr. E's surrogate gave permission to use deception. Furthermore, if Mr. E had indicated previously that he would prefer covert medication over forced parenteral administration in this situation, ethical concerns about deception would also be assuaged.   The physician should debrief the patient after he recovers from his psychiatric crisis and address the issue of trust explicitly. Such disclosure shows respect for the patient and offers an opportunity to plan for similar situations in the future. In same states, patients can sign an advance directive naming a surrogate if he becomes unable to make informed decisions, authorizing the surrogate to agree to covert medication.

DECEPTION OR NONDISCLOSURE TO THIRD PARTIES

Physicians may consider deceiving third parties rather than patients. Patients who seek benefits, such as insurance coverage, disability, and excused absences from work, often need physicians to give information about their condition to third parties (16). Physicians might consider using deception to help them gain such benefits. Although such deception might be motivated by a desire to help the patient, it is ethically problematic. Throughout this section, it is assumed that the patient has authorized disclosure to the third party.

Reasons Supporting Deception

Physicians might claim they are acting in the best interest of patients when using deception. In doing so, physicians might regard themselves as patient advocates, helping their patients gain medical and social benefits.

CASE 6.3   Insurance coverage

Mr. M, a 42-year-old accountant, presents with a 2-month history of lower back pain that has not responded to conservative therapy with rest, nonsteroidal anti-inflammatory agents, and exercises. There are no neurologic symptoms, and the physical examination is normal. His father had prostate cancer that presented as back pain, and he is concerned that he might have a serious disease causing his symptoms. Mr. M requests a magnetic resonance imaging (MRI) scan.

Mr. M and his physician agree that an MRI scan would reassure him. His health insurance policy requires preauthorization for MRI studies, which are usually authorized only if there are neurologic findings or other findings suggesting a systemic disease. The physician considers putting on the requisition that Mr. M has numbness and weakness in his legs to obtain insurance authorization for the study.

In one survey, 39% of physicians reported that during the past year they had exaggerated the severity of a patient's condition, changed a patient's billing diagnosis, or reported signs and symptoms the patient did not have to help the patient get needed care (17). Such deception is more common if physicians believe that the care is necessary, the appeals process is burdensome, and the patient's condition is more serious (18). The physician might regard his actions as redressing a wrong rather than breaking an ethical guideline. Some doctors might state that the patient has numbness and tingling in his or her legs and rationalize it as literally true because most people have such symptoms at some time in their lives.

CASE 6.3   *Continued*

The physician should address Mr. M's fears of cancer directly and with empathy. Mr. M's physician might consider other tests if the symptoms do not resolve as expected, such as plain films of the spine or a prostate-specific antigen to rule out prostate cancer. However, these tests have their own risks, including the possibility of incidental findings of indeterminate significance and false positive and false negative results. Even if the benefits of deception for Mr. M seem to outweigh the harms, there are consequences for the doctor–patient relationship generally that need to be considered. Insurers consider such deception to be fraud and might bring legal charges.

In other situations, the harms of deception might seem very small, as in the following case.

CASE 6.4   Excuse from work

A patient asks a physician to sign a form excusing an absence from work. He says that he had a severe upper respiratory infection, from which he has now recovered. The physician did not see the patient while he was ill.

In Case 6.4, the physician might sign the form, even though the physician does not know whether the patient was actually sick. The doctor might consider the harm, inappropriate absenteeism, minor and better handled directly by the employer (16). It makes little sense for patients to visit physicians for all self-limited illnesses that keep them from work. Even if the worker was not sick, perhaps he had a good reason to stay home, to care for a sick child, for example. For these reasons, physicians commonly certify work absences even when they have not examined the patient during the illness.

Reasons Against Deceiving

Deception Undermines Trust in Physicians

Physicians dealing with a specific case might not appreciate the impact of a practice of deception in these situations. Lying and deception undermine social trust because people cannot trust that other statements are truthful. It is especially problematic for physicians to lie or intentionally deceive others because their relationship with patients and society depends on trust. If physicians are known to use deception in some situations to help patients, they might also use it in other situations for other purposes.

Third parties expect truthful information. Physicians should also avoid deceiving them, but for different reasons. The relationship between physicians and third parties is contractual rather than fiduciary. In contracts, both parties are required to avoid deception and deal fairly (19). Insurers commonly require physicians to affirm that the information provided is accurate and complete.

It is unrealistic to expect that such deception to third parties will not be discovered. Computers help insurers to identify questionable claims. Similarly, other physicians review applications for disability from Social Security and workers compensation. Once misled, third parties will mistrust other information from physicians and might require additional documentation. Physicians, who already complain of bureaucratic intrusions on the practice of medicine, might then face additional paperwork.

The Harms of Deception Outweigh the Benefits

When indirect and long-term harms are taken into account, the overall harms of deception outweigh the benefits (20). Deception about a patient's condition indirectly harms other people. Giving disability parking permits to those who do not need them makes it more difficult for persons who are truly disabled to park. Deceptive claims for disability or insurance coverage force the others patients, employers, or the public to pay higher taxes or insurance premiums.

Resolving Dilemmas About Deception to Third Parties

The following suggestions might help physicians deal with patients' requests to use deception to gain benefits (Table 6-2).

Consider Whether an Important Health Benefit Is at Stake

Physicians need to ask in what sense they are helping the patient. In some cases, health care is not the issue.

CASE 6.5	Cancellation of travel plans
A healthy patient who has bought a vacation tour wishes to change his plans. He asks his physician to write a note saying that he is ill so that he can obtain a refund.	

In Case 6.5, the patient simply wants to break a business deal with the travel agency and avoid a financial penalty. Although physicians have a duty to provide beneficial medical care, they have no obligation to help patients gain financial advantages.

In other cases, physicians might want to help patients receive disability payments to obtain food, clothing, and shelter. Such necessities are essential for good health. Physicians have an obligation to provide truthful information that will help patients get social benefits to which they are entitled, but it is not at all clear that physicians should use deception to help certain patients get social benefits for

TABLE 6-2. Resolving Dilemmas About Deception to Third Parties
Consider whether an important health benefit is at stake.
Deception might not be necessary.
Exhaust other alternatives.
Involve patients who request deception.

which they do not qualify, even though a just society would provide a larger safety net. Even if physicians believe that the current social system is unjust, deception in selective cases seems an inadequate way to address this unfairness.

Deception Might Not Be Necessary

The literal truth might resolve the dilemma. The strategy of using the literal truth is unethical if it is intended to deceive. However, employing the literal truth is appropriate if it is not deceptive and prevents harm to the patient (18). In Case 6.4, the physician was asked to certify an absence from work without having examined the patient during the illness. Some physicians simply write, "The patient reports that he was sick and unable to work" (21). This statement, which is true, shifts the dilemma back onto the patient and employer rather than having the physician take responsibility for secondhand information (16). Furthermore, this strategy obviates physician visits simply to obtain work excuses. The physician should also explain to the patient the substance of his note and the reasons for it.

Exhaust Other Alternatives

Physicians can often benefit patients without using deception. In Case 6.3, the physician has other options for reassuring the patient, as discussed above. Pursuing these alternatives requires the physician's effort, but exhausting them gives physicians a stronger ethical justification for using deception as a last resort.

Involve Patients Who Request Deception

Physicians often believe that they alone must decide how to respond to requests for deception. In fact, patients who make such requests have ethical responsibilities as well. If patients ask physicians to use deception on a disability application or an insurance bill, then physicians can frankly say that they feel caught between two ethical duties: to help the patient and to be truthful. Physicians can reflect the dilemma back to patients, saying, "If I mislead your insurer, how would my patients trust me not to mislead them in other situations?" Furthermore, the physician can point out the problems that will occur later if the insurer requests additional documentation.

DECEPTION WITH COLLEAGUES

Trainees sometimes use deception with colleagues. In one study, 19% of residents reported that they would fabricate a test result they had not checked if they were likely to be "ridiculed and reprimanded" for not checking it (22). In another scenario, 8% of residents said they would lie about checking for occult blood in a patient with anemia who had suffered a myocardial infarction. Furthermore, more than 40% of respondents reported that they had witnessed another resident lying to an attending physician or another resident during the past year (22).

Deception with other physicians is ethically troubling for several reasons. If a physician tells other physicians that a test result is normal, without actually checking the results, the patient might be harmed. If the result was actually abnormal, then needed treatment might be delayed or omitted. In addition, if physicians cannot trust information from colleagues, they may feel they need to duplicate that doctor's work, which would waste effort and cause resentment.

As discussed in more detail in Chapter 36, it is understandable that trainees want to have a good reputation. Using deception to bolster one's reputation, however, cannot be condoned.

SUMMARY

1. There are strong ethical reasons for physicians to avoid deception and nondisclosure with patients.
2. Physicians should try to avoid deception about the patient's condition to third parties, who have a right to such information.

References

1. Sokol DK. Can deceiving patients be morally acceptable? *BMJ*. 2007;334:984-986.
2. Bok S. *Secrets*. New York: Pantheon Books; 1982:116-135.
3. Novack DH, Plumer, R., Smith, R.L., et al. Changes in physicians' attitudes toward telling the cancer patient. *JAMA* 1979;241:897-900.
4. President's Commission for the Study of Ethical Problems in Medicine and Biomedical and Behavioral Research. *Making Health Care Decisions*. Washington: U.S. Government Printing Office; 1982.
5. Amber I, Fiester A. Communicating findings: a justification and framework for direct radiologic disclosure to patients. *AJR Am J Roentgenol* 2013;200:586-591.
6. Blackhall LJ, Murphy ST, Frank G, et al. Ethnicity and attitudes toward patient autonomy. *JAMA* 1995;274:820-825.
7. Gordon DR, Paci E. Disclosure practices and cultural narratives: understanding concealment and silence around cancer in Tuscany, Italy. *Soc Sci Med* 1997;46:1433-1452.
8. Surbone A. Telling the truth to patients with cancer: what is the truth? *Lancet Oncol* 2006;7:944-950.
9. Surbone A. Truth telling to the patient. *JAMA* 1992;268:1661-1662.
10. Laxmi S, Khan JA. Does the cancer patient want to know? Results from a study in an Indian tertiary cancer center. *South Asian J Cancer* 2013;2:57-61.
11. Jiang Y, Liu C, Li JY, et al. Different attitudes of Chinese patients and their families toward truth telling of different stages of cancer. *Psychooncology* 2007;16:928-936.
12. Rosenberg AR, Starks H, Unguru Y, et al. Truth telling in the setting of cultural differences and incurable pediatric illness: a review. *JAMA Pediatr* 2017;171:1113-1119.
13. Hallenbeck J, Arnold R. A request for nondisclosure: don't tell mother. *J Clin Oncol* 2007;25:5030-5034.
14. Munden LM. The covert administration of medications: legal and ethical complexities for health care professionals. *The Journal of Law, Medicine & Ethics* 2017;45:182-192.
15. Medical Welfare Commission for Scotland. *Covert Medication* 2017.
16. Toon PD. Practice Pointer. "I need a note, doctor": dealing with requests for medical reports about patients. *BMJ* 2009;338:b175.
17. Wynia MK, Cummins DS, VanGeest JB, et al. Physician manipulation of reimbursement rules for patients: between a rock and a hard place. *JAMA* 2000;283:1858-1865.
18. Everett JP, Walters CA, Stottlemyer DL, et al. To lie or not to lie: resident physician attitudes about the use of deception in clinical practice. *J Med Ethics* 2011;37:333-338.
19. Farnsworth EA. *Contracts*. 2nd ed. Boston: Little, Brown and Company; 1990:249-272.
20. Bok S. *Lying: Moral Choices in Public and Private Life*. New York: Pantheon Books; 1978.
21. Holleman WL, Holleman MC. School and work release evalutions. *JAMA* 1988;260:3629-3634.
22. Green MJ, Farber NJ, Ubel PA, et al. Lying to each other: when internal medicine residents use deception with their colleagues. *Arch Intern Med* 2000;160:2317-2323.

ANNOTATED BIBLIOGRAPHY

1. Everett JP, Walters CA, Stottlemyer DL, et al. To lie or not to lie: resident physician attitudes about the use of deception in clinical practice. *J Med Ethics* 2011;37:333-338.
   Comprehensive discussion of different types of lies that doctors make.
2. Rosenberg AR, Starks H, Unguru Y, et al. Truth telling in the setting of cultural differences and incurable pediatric illness: a review. *JAMA Pediatr* 2017;171:1113-1119.
   Discusses a family's request to not tell an adolescent patient she has cancer; the family was from a culture where telling the diagnosis has not been customary.
3. Sokol DK. Can deceiving patients be morally acceptable? *BMJ* 2007;334:984-986.
   Analysis of deception in clinical medicine.
4. Munden LM. The covert administration of medications: legal and ethical complexities for health care professionals. *The Journal of Law, Medicine & Ethics*. 2017;45:182-192.
   Discusses ethical issues of covert administration of medications, from a Canadian and British perspective, which sets more procedural safeguards than in usual in the United States.

Keeping Promises

INTRODUCTION

Keeping promises reduces uncertainty and promotes trust. All people, including patients, expect others to keep their promises and feel betrayed if promises are broken. Physicians, as human beings, make promises and are sometimes tempted to break them. Although promises are generally regarded as binding, in retrospect, some promises might seem imprudent or mistaken. The following cases demonstrate that some promises can be kept only if important ethical guidelines are violated.

CASE 7.1	Promise not to tell the patient that she has cancer

Mrs. G, a 61-year-old Mexican American widow, is found to have cancer on a needle aspiration of a breast mass. Her primary care physician agrees to a request from her daughter and son not to tell her she has cancer because they fear that she would not be able to handle the bad news. They point out that it is not customary in Mexico to tell women of her age that they have cancer. The physician refers Mrs. G to a surgeon. The surgeon believes that patients need to be involved in decisions regarding mastectomy or lumpectomy. In addition, Mrs. G asks a Spanish-speaking nurse, "Why do I need surgery? Do I have cancer?" The nurse does not want to deceive a patient who asks a direct question. However, the surgeon and nurse feel constrained by the primary physician's promise not to tell Mrs. G her diagnosis.

Case 7.1 illustrates that in some situations, keeping promises might be problematic. The surgeon and nurse believe that the primary physician's promise not to tell Mrs. G her diagnosis fails to respect her as a person. They question why they should violate their sense of moral integrity to keep someone else's promise.

CASE 7.2	Promise to schedule tests

Mr. H, a 54-year-old heavy smoker, is hospitalized for hemoptysis, weight loss, and angina pectoris. A chest x-ray shows a 2-cm proximal lung mass, with hilar adenopathy. A bronchoscopy is scheduled to obtain a biopsy. When the intern walks by his room, the patient shouts "This is outrageous. I haven't had breakfast. I haven't had lunch. Now they say they don't know when the test will be done and that I might have to go through all this again tomorrow. If this is how the hospital is run, I'm leaving." The intern, eager to appease the patient and continue with his other work, promises the patient that the test will be done that afternoon. He tells the nurse to call the bronchoscopy suite to say that the procedure needs to be done that afternoon.

In Case 7.2, the intern makes a promise so Mr. H will cooperate with getting a needed test. However, the bronchoscopy schedule is not under his control. Even though the intern's motive is beneficent—to help the patient receive needed medical care—the means of achieving his goal is ethically problematic.

THE ETHICAL SIGNIFICANCE OF PROMISES

A *promise* is a commitment to act a certain way in the future, either to do something or to refrain from doing something. Promises generate expectations in others, who, in turn, modify their plans and actions on the assumption that promises will be kept (1). In everyday social interactions, people expect others to keep the ones they make. Promises might be exchanged for other promises, as in a business contract. For example, a merchant might promise to deliver goods in exchange for the promise of payment on delivery.

Keeping promises is desirable for several reasons. It results in beneficial consequences by making the future more predictable, relieving anxiety, and promoting trust. Indeed, the dictionary definition of promise is "that which causes hope, expectation, or assurance." Keeping promises is also important even if there are no short-term beneficial consequences. Keeping promises is essential for harmonious social interactions. If promises are commonly broken, then people would be unwilling to rely on others to keep commitments.

Breaking promises may cause significant harm. The person to whom the promise was made may suffer a setback, such as inconvenience and monetary losses. It seems unfair to allow people to break promises that others have relied on (2). The very concept of promises is negated if people break them and thereby gain an advantage but expect others to honor promises (2).

Keeping promises is especially important for physicians. Because the doctor–patient relationship is based on trust, patients might feel betrayed if physicians break promises. Once betrayed, patients might be less likely to trust the individual physician or the medical profession generally. Promises by physicians might help patients cope with the uncertainty and fears inherent in being sick. In addition, promises establish mutual expectations that benefit both physicians and patients. For example, physicians promise confidentiality of medical information; in return, patients are more candid about discussing sensitive issues pertaining to their health. Thus, promises enhance the patient's well-being and facilitate the physician's work.

CHALLENGES WITH KEEPING PROMISES

None of us wants to keep all the promises we make. Some promises are made on the spur of the moment, under emotional stress, with inadequate information, or without proper deliberation (2). Foolish promises that put one at a great disadvantage are often retracted, particularly if they confer a gratuitous boon on the other person. People might excuse breaking such promises if the other person has taken no action in reliance on the promise and is no worse off than if the promise had never been made.

Clinical dilemmas occur when keeping promises would require actions that violate other ethical guidelines. In Case 7.1, the surgeon and nurse believe the initial promise not to tell the patient violates the guideline of respect for persons.

SUGGESTIONS FOR PHYSICIANS

Do Not Make Promises Lightly

A statement that the physician regards as kindly reassurance might be interpreted by the patient or family as a promise. Even if the physician does not think a promise is important, the patient might. Patients are likely to be more upset when physicians break promises than the physicians are.

Address the Concerns Underlying the Request for a Promise

If someone asks the physician to make an unrealistic promise, then the physician can elicit the underlying concerns and try to address them in other ways.

Do Not Promise Outcomes That Are Out of Your Control

Physicians should not make promises that are beyond their power to keep. Given the complex organization of modern medicine, it is misleading to make promises about the actions of other physicians and nurses, who are autonomous agents with their own moral and professional values.

Because clinical outcomes are inherently uncertain, it is unrealistic to make a promise that guarantees a good outcome or the absence of complications after a procedure.

Do Not Violate Ethical Guidelines Because of an Ill-Considered Promise

Although keeping promises is important, it is not an absolute duty. Other ethical guidelines are also important and might take priority in some situations. In some cases, breaking the promise might be the lesser of two evils. The strongest case for overriding the keeping of promises occurs when all the following conditions are met:

- Keeping the promise would violate another important ethical guideline. In Case 7.1, keeping the promise would require deception by the physician and, thereby, compromise the patient's autonomy.
- The countervailing ethical considerations were not taken into account when the promise was made.
- The clinical and ethical situation has changed significantly since the promise was made.
- Someone else made the promise. Although a person's promise can bind his or her own future actions, it need not bind others.
- The promise was stated implicitly rather than explicitly.

CASE 7.1	*Continued*

When Mrs. G's children asked that she not be told she has cancer, the primary care physician should elicit the concerns underlying their request (see also Chapter 6). The doctor should anticipate future problems if she is not told, including the possibility that other health care workers may decide to disclose the diagnosis or the patient may ask someone directly what her diagnosis is. Another health care worker, like the surgeon in this case, may decide that she cannot provide care without offering to discuss Mrs. G's diagnosis with her. In the surgeon's view, avoiding deception should prevail over keeping an ill-considered promise made by somebody else. Similarly, when asked by the patient if she has cancer, it would be disrespectful to deceive her rather than giving a direct and compassionate answer.

Case 7.2	*Continued*

Physicians should not make promises about situations they cannot control. In the short run, it might seem easier to promise that the test will be done rather than to have the patient complain. However, making a promise that may not be kept will cause more problems in the long run. It might be better simply to listen and acknowledge that the patient has every right to be angry. Realistically, the doctor can promise to look into the matter and to do his best to get the procedure done as soon as possible, for instance, by phoning the pulmonary consultant himself, rather than asking a nurse to do so.

In summary, promises can allay patients' fears and uncertainty. It is important to keep promises because other people rely on them. Breaking promises undermines trust in the individual physician and the medical profession, yet keeping promises is not an absolute ethical duty. Sometimes, respecting a promise might require the physician to violate other important ethical guidelines. In exceptional situations, breaking a promise might be justified as the lesser of two evils.

SUMMARY

1. Physicians should keep promises because other people rely on them.
2. In exceptional circumstances, breaking a promise might be justified.

References

1. Farnsworth EA. *Contracts*. 2nd ed. Boston: Little, Brown and Company; 1990:249-272.
2. Fuller L, Eisenberg M, Gergen M. *Basic Contract Law*. 9th ed. St. Paul: West Academic Publishing; 2013.

Shared Decision-Making

An Approach to Decisions About Clinical Interventions

Medical interventions may allow accurate diagnosis and effective treatment, but they may also be applied when their benefit is questionable or when patients would not want them. Physicians therefore must try to avoid two types of errors: withholding potentially beneficial tests and therapies that the patient would want and imposing interventions that are not beneficial or wanted.

This brief chapter presents an approach to decisions about clinical interventions. The general approach to ethical issues in Chapter 1 can be adapted to such decisions (Fig. 8-1). The key questions are as follows:

Is the intervention futile in a strict sense? Sound ethical judgments require accurate medical information. Physicians are under no obligation to provide interventions that are futile in a strict sense

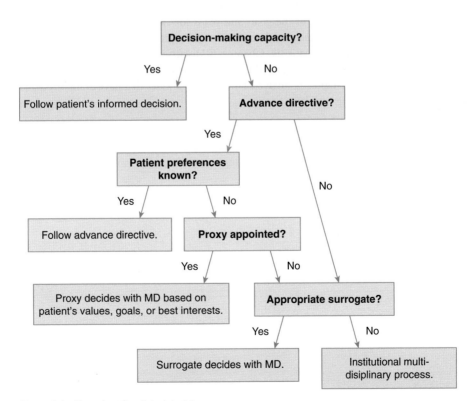

Figure 8-1. Flow chart for clinical decisions.

(*see* Chapter 14). However, in most cases in which physicians claim that an intervention is futile, it is better characterized as potentially medically inappropriate.

Does the patient have adequate decision-making capacity? This is a crucial branch point in decision-making. Chapter 9 discusses how to determine whether a patient lacks decision-making capacity.

If the patient has decision-making capacity, what is his or her informed decision? Competent, informed patients may refuse medical interventions (*see* Chapter 1). However, patients frequently lack decision-making capacity when decisions about medical interventions must be made. Chapter 10 discusses refusal of interventions by competent, informed patients.

If the patient lacks decision-making capacity, has he or she indicated her values, goals for care, and preferences in the situation? Informed preferences for specific interventions should be respected (*see* Chapter 12). In the absence of such advance directives, decisions should be based on the patient's values, preferences, or best interests (*see* Chapter 12).

If the patient has not clearly indicated what he or she would want done in the situation, who should serve as surrogate? Generally the surrogate should be a person designated by the patient or a close family member (*see* Chapter 11). If no such surrogates exist, a close friend might be an apprioriate surrogate.

The book then considers disagreements between doctors and patients over medical interventions. Chapter 13 analyzes insistence by patients or surrogates on interventions that physicians regard as inappropriate and also physician insistence of life-sustaining interventions that the patient or surrogate does not want. Chapter 14 analyzes potentially medically inappropriate interventions, formerly described as futile interventions. Chapter 15 discusses distinctions about life-sustaining interventions that are commonly drawn, but that prove misleading on closer analysis. Chapter 16 discusses how ethics committees or consultants can help physicians resolve ethical dilemmas.

Next the book analyzes life-sustaining interventions in specific situations. Chapter 17 discusses Do Not Attempt Resuscitate (DNAR) orders. Often discussions about DNAR orders are the first step in a comprehensive evaluation of the goals and plans for care. Chapter 18 discusses tube and intravenous feedings. Chapter 19 analyzes the controversial topics of physician-assisted suicide and active euthanasia for terminally ill patients. Chapter 20 discusses unresponsive wakefulness (previously called the persistent vegetative state) and the minimially conscious state. Chapter 21 discusses the determination of death. Chapter 22 analyzes landmark legal cases that have dramatized dilemmas about regarding life-sustaining interventions.

Decision-Making Capacity

INTRODUCTION

Physicians must respect the autonomous choices of patients. However, illness or medications can impair the capacity of patients to make decisions about their health care. Such patients might be unable to make decisions, or make decisions that contradict their best interests and cause themselves serious harm. Decision-making ability falls along a continuum, with no natural threshold for adequate decision-making capacity. Nevertheless, for every patient a binary decision needs to be made: either a patient has adequate decision-making capacity and his or her choices should be respected, or he or she does not and someone else should decide. The following case illustrates how it might be difficult to decide whether decision-making power should be taken away from a patient.

CASE 9.1   **Refusal to explain a decision**

Mrs. C, a 74-year-old widow with mild dementia, is admitted for congestive heart failure and chest pain and has been found to have a non-ST-elevation myocardial infarction that has progressed despite medical therapy. In the past 3 years, she has suffered two myocardial infarctions. Her physician recommends coronary angiography and, if possible, revascularization by stenting or angioplasty.

Mrs. C recognizes her primary care physician, but seldom knows the date or the name of the clinic. She has forgotten to come to several clinic appointments. Her mental functioning gets worse when she is hospitalized. A nephew, her only relative, pays a woman to shop, cook, and clean house for her. He reports that Mrs. C enjoys watching television, attending the senior center, and sitting in the park.

When asked about her wishes for care, Mrs. C says that she wants to go home. After many discussions, the cardiology team convinces her to have the angiogram. On the morning of the procedure, however, she changes her mind, saying that she doesn't want anyone to put a tube into her heart and that she has been in the hospital long enough. Her nephew believes that angioplasty would be best for her, but is reluctant to contradict her wishes because she has always been independent and stubborn. Mrs. C is generally adverse to medical interventions. She refused mammography, even though she has a family history of breast cancer. She also refused treatment for a cholesterol level of 318 mg/dL.

The team asks a psychiatrist to see her. On a mental status examination, she does not know the date, the name of the hospital, or the city. She recalls only one of five objects and cannot perform serial subtraction. She refuses to talk further with the psychiatrist, saying that she is not crazy.

In this case, Mrs. C's mental functioning is obviously impaired. Is it so impaired that her nephew should have the authority to make medical decisions for her? Her refusal did not seem so unreasonable to some physicians and nurses. Furthermore, some nurses asked why her consent to angiography was not questioned, but only her refusal.

This chapter analyzes how physicians should assess whether patients like Mrs. C have the capacity to make decisions about their care. This book uses the term *competent* to refer to patients who have the capacity to make informed decisions about medical interventions. Strictly speaking, all adults are considered competent to make such decisions unless a court has declared them *incompetent*. In everyday practice, however, physicians make *de facto* determinations that patients lack decision-making capacity and arrange for surrogates to make decisions, without involving the courts (1). This clinical approach has been defended because routine judicial intervention imposes unacceptable delays and generally involves only superficial hearings. This book uses the phrase *lacks decision-making capacity* if a physician, rather than a court, determines that the patient is unable to make informed decisions about health care.

ETHICAL IMPLICATIONS OF DECISION-MAKING CAPACITY

Caring for patients whose decision-making capacity is questionable involves two conflicting ethical guidelines. On the one hand, physicians must respect the authority of competent patients to make decisions that others might regard as foolish, unwise, or harmful (*see* Chapter 11). On the other hand, physicians should act in their patients' best interests (*see* Chapter 4). If patients who lack decision-making capacity make decisions that are contrary to their best interests, they need to be protected from serious harm. The patient's decision-making capacity is therefore crucial. If it is intact, then the patient's decisions will be respected. If it is seriously impaired, then decision-making power is taken from the patient and given to a surrogate.

Generally, a patient's decision-making capacity is not challenged if he or she agrees with the physician. On its face, this practice suggests that patients are only incapacitated when they disagree with physicians. It makes sense to raise more questions about decision-making capacity, however, when patients refuse a beneficial intervention than when they consent to it. When Mrs. C accepts angiography, her care would be the same whether or not she has decision-making capacity. If she has adequate decision-making capacity, her consent to angioplasty would be valid. If she lacks it, her physician and surrogate agree that angiography was in her best interests. Now consider Mrs. C's refusal of angiography. If she has decision-making capacity, then her refusal should be respected. If she lacks it, then a surrogate would assume decision-making power. The physician and her nephew agree that angiography is in her best interests. Hence, if she refuses, then her management hinges on whether her decision-making capacity is considered impaired. Thus, it is appropriate that Mrs. C's refusal of recommended interventions triggers questions about her capacity to make medical decisions. Such a refusal, however, does not by itself prove that she lacks such capacity.

LEGAL STANDARDS FOR COMPETENCE

The courts have not articulated clear standards for competency to make medical decisions (2, 3). Many older legal cases viewed incompetence in general or global terms. Either the patient was competent in all aspects of life or the patient was not competent in any sphere. The courts inferred incompetence from a person's overall ability to function in life, medical diagnoses, general mental functioning, and personal appearance.

In reality, a person might be capable of performing some tasks adequately but not others. For example, a person might be capable of making informed medical decisions, but not informed financial decisions. A patient with Alzheimer disease who lacked capacity to consent to a clinical trial of a new drug may still have the capacity to appoint a surrogate to make decisions for them (4). Thus, it is more appropriate to consider a person competent or incompetent for specific tasks rather than in all aspects of life (3). The modern legal and ethical consensus is that a person should be considered competent to make medical decisions if he or she is capable of giving informed consent (2); that is, he or she appreciates the diagnosis and prognosis, the nature of the tests or treatments proposed, the alternatives, the risks and benefits of each, and the probable consequences. Chapter 3 discusses informed consent in detail.

CLINICAL STANDARDS FOR DECISION-MAKING CAPACITY

A patient's decision-making capacity should be subjected to scrutiny in several situations. As in Case 9.1, the patient might refuse a treatment that the physician strongly recommends or might vacillate in making a decision. In other cases, patients might have conditions that commonly impair decision-making capacity, such as dementia, schizophrenia, or depression. Although these conditions justify closer scrutiny of the patient's decision-making capacity, they do not necessarily impair decision-making capacity. Physicians need to test directly the individual patient's ability to give informed consent for the proposed intervention. Decision-making capacity requires a cluster of abilities (Table 9-1) (5).

The Patient Makes and Communicates as Choice

A patient must appreciate that he or she—and not the physician or family members—has ultimate decision-making power. In addition, the patient must be willing to choose among the alternative courses of care. A patient who vacillates repeatedly between consent and refusal is incapable of making a decision, let alone an informed one. Such profound indecision must be distinguished from changing one's mind as the situation changes, as the patient receives more information or advice, or after the patient deliberates.

The patient must communicate his or her choice. A patient who is unable to speak because he or she is on a ventilator does not necessarily lack decision-making capacity. He or she might be able to communicate through writing messages, using an alphabet board, or blinking or nodding in response to questions.

The Patient Understands Pertinent Information and Appreciates Its Relevance

A patient needs to understand the medical situation and prognosis, the nature of the proposed intervention, the alternatives, the risks and benefits, and the likely consequences of each alternative, including no intervention. The patient also needs to appreciate that the information that the physician discussed is relevant to his or her own situation. In Case 9.1, the health care team could not determine whether Mrs. C understood that revascularization usually relieves chest pain, but has certain risks.

Decisions Are Consistent with the Patient's Values and Goals

Choices should be consistent with the patient's character and core values. If Mrs. C wants to be more active without pain, then refusing revascularization would be inconsistent with her goals. Many patients, however, do not have well-articulated health values and long-standing goals or might have multiple, conflicting goals. Mrs. C might want not only to return home but also to be more active and pain free. A course of care might be consistent with some goals, but not with others. People do not necessarily have a preexisting hierarchy of goals and values. Mrs. C might define her goals or set priorities only by deciding about angiography. Thus, physicians should not regard a patient as lacking decision-making capacity merely because she cannot articulate a set of general values or goals.

TABLE 9-1. Clinical Standards for Decision-Making Capacity
The patient makes and communicates a choice.
The patient understands the medical situation, prognosis, the nature of the recommended care and the alternatives, and the risks and benefits of each.
Decisions are consistent with the patient's values and goals.
Decisions do not result from delusions.
The patient uses reasoning to make a choice.

Decisions Do Not Result From Delusions

Some patients have delusions that preclude informed decision-making. Delusions are false beliefs or incorrect inferences in the face of incontrovertible or obvious evidence to the contrary. For instance, Mary Northern was an elderly woman who refused amputation of her gangrenous legs, denying that gangrene had caused her feet to be "dead, black, shriveled, rotting and stinking" (3). Instead, she believed that they were merely blackened by soot or dust. The court declared her incompetent because she was "incapable of recognizing facts which would be obvious to a person of normal perception." The court said that if she had acknowledged that her legs were gangrenous but refused amputation because she preferred death to the loss of her feet, she would have been considered competent to refuse the surgery.

The Patient Uses Reasoning to Make a Choice

Processing information logically is another element of decision-making capacity. Patients should compare and weigh the various options for care (3, 6, 7). This requirement does not require the patient to choose what most people consider reasonable in the situation. Unconventional decisions do not necessarily imply lack of decision-making capacity. Expectations for reasoning must take into account that many people do not deliberate, but instead rely on emotional or intuitive factors in making important decisions.

Assessments of Decision-Making Capacity Should Take Into Account the Clinical Context

Assessments must consider the patient's functional abilities, the demands of the specific clinical situation, and the harm that might result from his or her choice. Some writers have suggested that a patient who chooses an option that has great risk and little prospect of benefit should meet higher standards for decision-making capacity than a patient who chooses an option that has great prospect of benefit and little risk (5). The benefits and risks of alternatives should also be taken into account; a patient who chooses an option that has significantly less benefit and greater risk than the alternatives should be held to a stricter standard of decision-making capacity. Also, the nature of the intervention might be important. A patient might be given more leeway to refuse disfiguring surgery, such as amputation, than treatments with less drastic side effects. Such a sliding scale offers more protection to patients when the potential harm resulting from their uninformed decisions is greater. According to this view, it seems plausible in Case 9.1 to apply a more rigorous standard of capacity when Mrs. C refuses treatment for symptomatic, life-threatening cardiac disease than when she refuses screening tests or preventive measures for cardiac risk factors. Although such a sliding scale is intuitively appealing, it might be problematic in practice because people might disagree over what risks are serious and how well the patient understands the benefits and risks. A sliding scale might allow physicians to exercise inappropriate control over patients with whom they disagree. To guard against such problems, physicians should state explicitly the criteria they are using in assessing a patient's decision-making capacity.

ASSESSING THE CAPACITY TO MAKE DECISIONS

Table 9-2 offers practical suggestions for determining decision-making capacity. The assessment requires that the patient has received adequate information about his or her condition and the interventions. Physicians should keep in mind that beliefs that others consider "unwise, foolish, or ridiculous" do not render a person incompetent (8). Indeed, informed consent would be meaningless if such individualistic refusals were not respected, even though they conflicted with medical recommendations or popular wisdom.

In addition, it is helpful to talk to family and friends, nurses, and other physicians caring for the patient, particularly when the physician does not know the patient well. These persons can clarify

TABLE 9-2. Helpful Questions in Assessing Decision-Making Capacity
Does the Patient Understand the Disclosed Information?
• "Tell me what you believe is wrong with your health now."
• "What is angiography likely to do for you?"
Does the Patient Appreciate the Consequences of His or Her Choices?
• "What do you believe will happen if you do not have angiography?"
• "I've described the possible benefits and risks of angiography. If these benefits or risks occurred, then how would your everyday activities be affected?"
Does the Patient Use Reasoning to Make a Choice?
• "Tell me how you reached your decision. . . ."
• "Help me understand how you decided to refuse the angiogram."
• "Tell me what makes angiography seem worse than the alternatives."

whether the patient's mental function or choices have suddenly changed, suggesting that the impairment might be reversible.

The Role of Mental Status Testing

Clinicians often use mental status tests when assessing a patient's capacity to make medical decisions. Such tests evaluate orientation of the subject to person, place, and time; attention span; immediate recall; short-term and long-term memory; ability to perform simple calculations; and language skills.

Mental status tests are less useful, however, than directly assessing whether the patient understands the nature of the intervention, the risks and benefits, the alternatives, and the consequences. For example, Mrs. C scored poorly on standard mental status tests, but if she appreciates that angioplasty would probably improve her chest pain and shortness of breath, she has the capacity to make an informed refusal. Mental status testing is helpful when scores are very low (below 19 on the Mini Mental Status Exam), indicating such severe cognitive impairments that patients cannot appreciate the benefits of treatment and lack the ability to reason (9).

In several court rulings, patients with abnormal mental status tests were found competent to make decisions about health care. For example, a 72-year-old Robert Quackenbush, who withdrew his consent for amputation of his gangrenous legs, was found competent even though one psychiatrist found that he was disoriented to the place and people around him and had visual hallucinations (10). The probate judge found that "his conversation did wander occasionally but to no greater extent than would be expected of a 72-year-old man in his circumstances." The patient hoped "for a miracle" but realized that "there is no great likelihood of its occurrence."

In another case, 77-year-old Grace Lane was found competent to refuse amputation of her leg for gangrene (11). Testimony indicated that she was "lucid on some matters and confused on others," that her "train of thought sometimes wanders," and that "her conception of time is distorted." One psychiatrist claimed that her refusal to discuss the amputation with him indicated "she was unable to face up to the problem." The court found that she understood that in "rejecting the amputation she is, in effect, choosing death over life."

Consultation by Psychiatrists

Psychiatrists can be helpful in evaluating patients whose decision-making capacity is questionable (7). Psychiatrists are skilled at interviewing patients with mental impairment and engaging them in discussions. In addition, psychiatrists specialize in diagnosing and treating mental illnesses that might impair a decision-making capacity.

Attending physicians can readily acquire the skills to assess patients' decision-making capacity, and routine psychiatric consultation is not necessary. Ultimately, the attending physician is responsible for judging whether the patient lacks decision-making capacity.

Enhancing the Capacity of Patients to Make Decisions

Impairments in decision-making capacity might be reversible if underlying medical or psychiatric conditions are treated. In addition, physicians can enhance a patient's understanding of pertinent information by presenting information in simple language, in small chunks, slowly and repeatedly over time. Diagrams, pictographs, and videotapes might improve comprehension. Furthermore, family members or friends can help reduce anxiety, correct misunderstandings, and focus the discussion on the salient issues.

Engaging the Patient in Discussions

Patients like Mrs. C who refuse to answer questions or explain their decisions might be angry at losing control or resent being badgered. Repeated attempts to assess decision-making capacity or to persuade them might be counterproductive and frustrate health care workers. Patients need to be told clearly and sympathetically that to get the physicians to do what they want, they need to answer some questions.

DECISION-MAKING CAPACITY IN SPECIFIC CLINICAL SITUATIONS

Mental Illness Impairing Decision-Making Capacity

Many patients with mental illness are competent to make decisions about their medical care. However, loss of decision-making capacity is more common in certain psychiatric conditions. Patients with schizophrenia or depression commonly might fail to acknowledge their symptoms and diagnosis or deny the potential benefit of treatment.

Psychiatric illness might also impair decision-making capacity more subtly (5). Patients who are depressed might overemphasize the risks of treatment, underestimate the benefits, or believe that treatment is less likely to be successful for them than for others.

If psychiatric patients are gravely disabled, unable to care for themselves, suicidal, or a serious threat to others, they may be involuntarily committed (*see* Chapter 40); however, involuntary commitment does not empower physicians to give whatever medical treatment they consider advisable. If such a patient refuses treatment for medical problems, then an appropriate surrogate or a separate court order is needed to authorize treatment.

Unconventional Decisions Based on Religious Beliefs

Patients might refuse effective medical treatments because of their religious beliefs. In the United States, a person's religious beliefs are deeply respected. Religious beliefs often form the foundation of a person's value system and provide meaning in their lives. Physicians should not judge whether a patient's religious beliefs are true or false or try to change them. Because religion is based on faith, empirical evidence and rational arguments are unlikely to change people's beliefs. Doctors have no expertise in religious matters, and patients do not seek them for religious advice. Thus, refusals of treatment by competent adults on religious grounds are accepted. Parental refusals of highly effective treatment for children, however, may be overridden (*see* Chapter 37).

If, however, a patient refuses highly effective treatment for religiously based reasons, then the physician should not simply accept the refusal. Instead, the physician should respectfully explore whether the refusal is consistent with the patient's prior decisions and actions and is shared by other members of his or her faith tradition. Chapter 11 discusses how to carry out such conversations with Jehovah's Witnesses regarding refusal of blood transfusions. Furthermore, the physician should examine if other aspects of decision-making are problematic. Some patients have religious delusions or hallucinations. For example, a patient might believe that he or she is Christ and must die to redeem the world, that the devil is tempting him or her to take medicine, or that he or she should refuse surgery because it is God's will that he or she suffer. In such cases, physicians should arrange for the patient to talk with other members of the faith tradition and consider psychiatric evaluation and medication or counseling (12).

Emergencies

A patient with questionable decision-making capacity might present with an emergency condition that requires immediate treatment. Rather than evaluating the patient's decision-making capacity, physicians should provide emergency care unless it is known that the patient or surrogate would refuse such care or a conscious patient actively refuses. This approach is justified by implied consent to emergency care (*see* Chapter 3).

CARING FOR PATIENTS WHO LACK DECISION-MAKING CAPACITY

After physicians determine that a patient lacks decision-making capacity, advance directives or surrogate decision-making should guide further care (*see* Chapters 12 and 13).

Even if a patient lacks the capacity to make decisions, his or her stated preferences should be given substantial consideration. For instance, mentally incapacitated patients might balk at phlebotomy or x-rays, sometimes screaming their refusal. Even if the courts declared such a patient incompetent, it would be morally and emotionally repugnant to force interventions on an unwilling patient who cannot understand how the interventions are helping him or her. Health care workers might consider it inhumane to force a patient to undergo a highly invasive intervention when he or she cannot understand its purpose and benefits. Furthermore, future cooperation might be undermined. Physicians should try to obtain the patient's assent to interventions authorized by a surrogate or court, even if that patient cannot give informed consent. Persuasion, cajoling, and asking family members and friends to talk to the patient are acceptable ways to try to gain the patient's cooperation. Often, a patient will agree to treatment after caregivers have listened to his or her objections, modified the treatment plans, or changed the hospital routine.

SUMMARY

1. Physicians commonly determine that patients lack the capacity to make informed decisions about their care without resorting to the courts.
2. Physicians need to understand the clinical standards for decision-making capacity and be able to apply them in specific cases.

References

1. Lo B. Assessing decision-making capacity. *Law, Medicine, and Health Care* 1990;18:193-201.
2. Berg JW, Lidz CW, Appelbaum PS. *Informed Consent: Legal Theory and Clinical Practice*. 2nd ed. New York: Oxford University Press; 2001.
3. Meisel A, Cerminara KL, Pope TM. *The Right to Die*. 3rd ed. New York: Wolters Kluwer; 2014.
4. Moye J, Sabatino CP, Weintraub Brendel R. Evaluation of the capacity to appoint a healthcare proxy. *Am J Ger Psych* 2013;21:326-336.
5. Charland LC. *Decision-Making Capacity. The Stanford Encyclopedia of Philosophy.* Available from: https://plato.stanford.edu/archives/fall2015/entries/decision-capacity/.
6. Buchanan AE, Brock DW. *Deciding for Others*. Cambridge: Cambridge University Press; 1989.
7. Applebaum PS, Grisso T. Assessing patient's capacities to consent to treatment. *N Engl J Med* 1988; 319:1635-1638.
8. In re Brooks. 32 Ill.2d 361, 205 N.E.2d 435 (1965).
9. Kim SY. When does decisional impairment become decisional incompetence? Ethical and methodological issues in capacity research in schizophrenia. *Schizophr Bull* 2006;32:92-97.

10. In re Quackenbush. 156 N.J. Super. 282, 383 A.2d 785 (1978).
11. Lane v. Candura. 6 Mass. App. 377,376 N.E.2d 1232 (1978).
12. Cochrane TI. Religious delusions and the limits of spirituality in decision-making. *AJOB* 2007;7:14-15.

ANNOTATED BIBLIOGRAPHY

1. Grisso T, Appelbaum P. *Assessing Competence to Consent to Treatment: A Guide for Physicians and Other Health Professionals.* New York, NY: Oxford University Press; 1998.
   Lucid, practical, and comprehensive discussion of how to assess decision-making capacity.
2. Kim, SYH. *Evaluation of Capacity to Consent to Treatment and Research.* New York, NY: Oxford University Press; 2010.
   Detailed information on how to assess decision-making capacity.
3. Meisel A, Cerminara KL, Pope TM. *The Right to Die.* 3rd ed. New York: Wolters Kluwer; 2014.
   Comprehensive reference on legal issues regarding decisions about life-sustaining interventions, with discussions of key legal cases.
4. Charland LC. *Decision-Making Capacity. The Stanford Encyclopedia of Philosophy.* Available from: https://plato.stanford.edu/archives/fall2015/entries/decision-capacity/
   Comprehensive, accessible conceptual review of decision-making capacity.

Refusal of Treatment by Competent, Informed Patients

INTRODUCTION

Competent and informed patients may refuse interventions that their physicians recommend. In some cases, physicians may hesitate to accept refusals that jeopardize the patient's life or health. Although concern for a patient's well-being is commendable, as discussed in Chapter 4, it is important for physicians to understand the compelling ethical and legal reasons for respecting refusals by informed, competent patients. This chapter discusses the reasons for respecting such refusals, specific clinical examples of refusal of treatment, and restrictions on patient refusal.

REASONS FOR RESPECTING PATIENT REFUSALS

Respect for Patient Autonomy

Honoring refusal of treatment by competent, informed patients respects their autonomy to make decisions about their care and to be free of unwanted medical interventions. The option of declining treatment is fundamental to the concept of informed consent. If patients must consent to treatment, then logically they have the right to decline treatment. The US Supreme Court has suggested that the Constitution protects a competent patient's refusal of life-sustaining treatment (1). A large body of case law supports the right of competent, informed patients to refuse treatment (2).

Imposing Medical Interventions Would Be Impractical

On a practical level, it is difficult to impose unwanted interventions on a competent patient. Sedating or restraining patients to impose treatment over their objections seems intrusive and inhumane.

SCOPE OF REFUSAL

Competent patients are permitted to refuse virtually any treatment, even highly beneficial ones with few side effects (2). The range of interventions includes surgery, mechanical ventilation, renal dialysis, cardiopulmonary resuscitation, antibiotics, and tube feedings. Competent patients may refuse treatment even if such a refusal might shorten their lives or lead to their deaths. They are not required to have a terminal illness to refuse treatment.

Competent patients may refuse treatment even if their family, friends, or physicians disagree with them. As one court ruling declared, even decisions that are unwise or foolish might need to be respected (3). Indeed, informed consent would be meaningless unless patients could refuse interventions for highly personal reasons or make decisions that conflict with medical or popular wisdom.

Jehovah's Witness Cases

Jehovah's Witnesses do not accept blood transfusions, basing their refusal on an interpretation of the Bible (4). They believe that although a blood transfusion might save their corporeal life, it will deprive them of everlasting salvation. Their refusals usually are clearly articulated, steadfast over time, and usually are supported by their family and friends. Jehovah's Witnesses generally consent to other interventions, such as surgery, if transfusions are not used.

Reactions of Health Care Providers

Refusals of blood transfusions by Jehovah's Witnesses might distress some physicians because the clinical benefits of transfusion are great and the medical risks very small (5). Many patients are young, previously healthy, and can be restored to perfect health. Physicians might feel that Jehovah's Witnesses, by refusing transfusions but agreeing to other care, unnecessarily compromise medical outcomes and require the physician to provide substandard care. Physicians might believe that they are being asked to accomplish the goal of saving the patient's life without using the best available means. Some surgeons complain that operating on a Jehovah's Witness without transfusions is like having to operate with one hand tied behind their back or being painted into a corner because they have less margin for error or complications (5). Psychologically, some physicians resent losing control over the patient's care. Some health care workers might also blame the patient for making their jobs more complicated. Many surgeons and anesthesiologists prefer not to treat Jehovah's Witnesses. Often, however, transferring such patients to another institution or physician is impractical.

Frustrated health care workers sometimes develop ingenious plans for administering blood to Jehovah's Witnesses. Some physicians suggest waiting until such patients are unconscious and then asking if they object to a transfusion (5). Because patients are then no longer able to refuse, these physicians would administer blood. Other physicians advocate simply giving transfusions after patients are under anesthesia and not telling them about it. Such deceptive actions are unacceptable and undermine trust in physicians.

Most Jehovah's Witnesses accept bloodless medical care techniques, including blood conservation techniques, hematopoietic growth factors, artificial oxygen carriers, normovolemic hemodilution, intraoperative cell salvage, and blood conservation techniques (4). Acceptance of normovolemic hemodilution, continuous blood pathway circuits, and hemostatic products containing blood fractions is more variable (4). With these techniques, the risk from foregoing transfusion in surgery, trauma, and childbirth can be largely avoided.

Legal Issues

The courts have consistently upheld refusals of blood transfusions by competent adult Jehovah's Witnesses (2). Recent controversies have involved incompetent Jehovah's Witnesses. Many patients sign wallet cards declaring they would refuse transfusions. Some physicians, however, question whether patients have been coerced by peer pressure and whether they were informed about the risks and benefits of transfusions (6).

Practical Suggestions

Physicians caring for adult Jehovah's Witnesses should take several steps to ensure that the patient's refusal of transfusions is informed, voluntary, and steadfast. First, to minimize the possibility of undue influence, the physician should ask the patient about transfusions when no family members, friends, or religious advisors are present. When alone, some Jehovah's Witnesses will agree to transfusions (7). Second, the physician should ask patients whether they would accept transfusions if they are ordered by a court. Some Jehovah's Witnesses will accept a transfusion as long as they do not personally consent to it. Under these circumstances, many judges are willing to order that transfusions be given. Third, Jehovah's Witnesses vary in what types of transfusion they will refuse. Some refuse all blood products, but others accept various blood components. Fourth, physicians should ask whether the patient has any other concerns about receiving blood, such as a risk of HIV infection or hepatitis. If the underlying reason for refusal is really a fear of infection, this concern should be addressed directly.

Having ensured that the refusal is free and informed, health care workers should respect the patient's decision. From the point of view of a Jehovah's Witness, the decision to refuse transfusions is simple. They would be pleased to survive the hospitalization, but as one patient put it, "What good is a few years of life compared to everlasting damnation?" (8). Even if health care workers do not agree with this belief, they should respect it. Continuing to try to convince a Jehovah's Witness shows disrespect.

When an adult Jehovah's Witness who requires a transfusion lacks decision-making capacity, advance care planning that reflects informed decisions should be respected, as Chapter 12 discusses.

If the patient is a minor and parents are refusing medically indicated transfusions, physicians should ask a court to order the transfusions (*see* Chapter 37). As one court declared, parents are "not free to make martyrs of their children" (9).

Renal Dialysis

About 15% of deaths in patients on renal dialysis occur after a decision to withhold dialysis (10). The patient might have a very limited prognosis, unacceptable quality of life, or technical difficulties, such as serious shunt complications. When the possibility of withholding dialysis is considered, physicians need to ensure that the decision is informed and voluntary. Furthermore, physicians need to palliate for the symptoms of uremia (10).

Pacemakers and Implanted Defibrillators

Some patients and health care worker are reluctant to deactivate these cardiac devices because they feel that turning off the device would be suicide or euthanasia (11). Although such beliefs are understandable, respecting informed and voluntary refusal by a patient is ethically and legally distinguishable from killing the patient (*see* Chapter 15). Physicians need to ensure that the patient's decision is informed and consistent with the patient's goals for care. For example, deactivating a pacemaker, particularly a sequential dual-chamber pacemaker, may lead to symptoms of shortness of breath, dizziness, and fatigue, rather than a peaceful death from arrhythmia.

RESTRICTIONS ON REFUSAL

The right of competent, informed patients to refuse medical treatment may be limited in certain situations.

Communicable Diseases

In certain circumstances, competent patients may be required to undergo treatment against their wishes to prevent harm to third parties. For example, tuberculosis can be transmitted by casual contact. To reduce the risk of transmitting this infection to other persons, infected individuals may be required to be treated or quarantined.

Treating Competent Patients for Their Own Benefit

Providing interventions over the objections of a competent patient to prevent harm to third parties needs to be clearly distinguished from providing treatment to prevent harm to the patient. The physician's duty to prevent harm to competent patients is weaker than the duty to prevent harm to unsuspecting third parties. Physicians should try to persuade patients and to negotiate a mutually acceptable plan of care (*see* Chapter 4). They may not, however, override the informed decisions of a competent patient because they believe it would be better for that patient.

If the clinical stakes of a patient's refusal of treatment are high, physicians should spend time trying to identify underlying reasons for refusal and address them. For example, a patient may refuse treatment because of the fear of repeating a bad experience, concerns about cost, or the need to care take care of matters at home, such as caring for a family member or pet. The physician should try to negotiate an acceptable plan of care, even if it is not medically optimal (12).

In some situations, physicians might want to administer treatment to save the life of a patient who refuses treatment, for example to give antibiotics to a patient with bacterial meningitis who shows no indication of impaired decision-making capacity other than his or her refusal of treatment. Although it is troubling to allow a patient to die from an easily treatable infection, it is also ethically troubling to override a patient's refusal if the only evidence of impaired decision-making capacity is the refusal itself. It is appropriate to examine closely whether a patient refusing such life-saving treatment is competent and informed and to try to enlist family members or friends to persuade the patient to accept treatment. However, it is ethically problematic to allow physicians to override patients who cannot provide satisfactory reasons for refusing treatment.

SUMMARY

1. There are cogent ethical and legal reasons to accept refusals of treatment by competent and informed patients.
2. Physicians can try to persuade patients to accept beneficial interventions while respecting their right to refuse.

References

1. Lo B, Steinbrook R. Beyond the Cruzan case: the U.S. Supreme Court and medical practice. *Ann Intern Med* 1991;114:895-901.
2. Meisel A, Cerminara KL, Pope TM. *The Right to Die.* 3rd ed. New York: Wolters Kluwer; 2014.
3. In re Brooks. 32 Ill.2d 361, 205 N.E.2d 435 (1965).
4. Scharman CD, Burger D, Shatzel JJ, et al. Treatment of individuals who cannot receive blood products for religious or other reasons. *American J Hemat* 2017;92:1370-1381.
5. Jones JW, McCullough LB, Richman BW. Painted into a corner: unexpected complications in treating a Jehovah's Witness. *J Vasc Surg* 2006;44:425-428.
6. Migden DR, Braen GR. The Jehovah's Witness blood refusal card: ethical and medicolegal considerations for emergency physicians. *Acad Emerg Med* 1998;5:815-824.
7. Rogers DM, Crookston KP. The approach to the patient who refuses blood transfusion. *Transfusion.* 2006;46:1471-1477.
8. In re Osborne. 294 A. 2d 372 (D.C. 1972).
9. Prince v. Massachusetts. 321 U.S. 158 (1944).
10. Cohen LM, Germain MJ, Poppel DM. Practical considerations in dialysis withdrawal: "to have that option is a blessing." *JAMA* 2003;289:2113-2119.
11. Lampert R, Hayes DL, Annas GJ, et al. HRS expert consensus statement on the management of cardiovascular implantable electronic devices (CIEDs) in patients nearing end of life or requesting withdrawal of therapy. *Heart Rhythm* 2010;7:1008-1026.
12. Goldfrank LR, Wittman I. Capacity? Informed consent; informed discharge? Uncertainty! *Ann Emerg Med* 2017;70:704-706.

ANNOTATED BIBLIOGRAPHY

1. Goldfrank LR, Wittman I. Capacity? Informed consent; informed discharge? Uncertainty! *Ann Emerg Med* 2017;70:704-706.
   Describes steps physicians should take when a patient's refusal treatment may lead to great harm, including determining and addressing the underlying reasons for refusal.
2. Meisel A, Cerminara KL, Pope TM. *The Right to Die.* 3rd ed. New York: Wolters Kluwer; 2014.
   Comprehensive legal treatise that describes court rulings permitting competent patients to refuse treatment.
3. Jones JW, McCullough LB, Richman BW. Painted into a corner: unexpected complications in treating a Jehovah's Witness. *J Vasc Surg* 2006;44:425-428.
   Clear discussion of refusal of transfusions by Jehovah's Witnesses, from the perspective of a surgeon.
4. Lampert R, Hayes DL, Annas GJ, et al. HRS expert consensus statement on the management of cardiovascular implantable electronic devices (CIEDs) in patients nearing end of life or requesting withdrawal of therapy. *Heart Rhythm* 2010;7:1008-1026.
   Consensus guidelines on the deactivation of implanted cardioverter defibrillators.

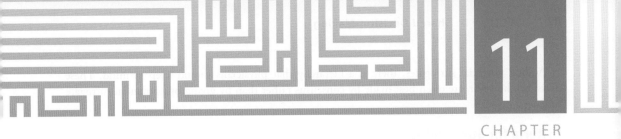

Who Serves as Surrogate When a Patient Lacks Decision-Making Capacity?

INTRODUCTION

When patients lack decision-making capacity, physicians must address two questions:

- Who should act as surrogate? This chapter addresses this question.
- What standards should be used when patients cannot give informed consent or refusal? Chapter 12 addresses this question.

When patients lack decision-making capacity, physicians need to work with their surrogates to make decisions on their behalf. Traditionally, family members serve as surrogate decision makers for such patients. This book uses the term *surrogate* for anyone who makes decisions for a patient who lacks decision-making capacity and reserves the term *proxy* for a surrogate appointed by the patient.

CASE 11.1	Disagreement between family members

Mrs. R is a 72-year-old widow with severe Alzheimer disease. She does not recognize her family, but often smiles when someone holds her hand or gives her a hug. She lives with her sister, who provides help with all activities of daily living together with an attendant. Mrs. R develops pneumonia. She had never signed an advance directive indicating what she would want in such a situation or whom she would want to make decisions for her. Her sister believes that Mrs. R would not want her life prolonged in this condition because she prized her independence, and so she asks the physician to withhold antibiotics. Mrs. R's only child is a son who visits once or twice a year. He is outraged at this request. He asserts, "Life is sacred; it's God's gift. We can't just snuff it out."

Mrs. R's sister and son both want to make decisions for her. The sister asserts priority because she has cared for Mrs. R and been close to her sister most of her life, yet the son has closer ties of kinship. What considerations justify selecting one surrogate over the other?

WHO SHOULD SERVE AS SURROGATE?

In most cases, there is no disagreement over who should serve as a surrogate for a patient who lacks decision-making capacity. Generally the family members agree on who should make decisions.

Among potential surrogates, there is a hierarchy that physicians should keep in mind. These decisions, however, are often best made by consensus rather than by giving one potential surrogate unilateral power.

Criteria for Surrogates

Ideally, surrogates should have several characteristics. First, they know the patient well and know the patient's deeply held values and goals for care at that stage of life. Second, they would know the patient's specific preferences for the medical intervention under consideration (1). Ideally, they would have discussed with the patient his or her goals, values, and the preferences he or she would want in various scenarios. Third, kinship and affection generally lead relatives to care about the patient, deliberate carefully, and do what is best. Social, cultural, and religious norms encourage family members to subordinate their own interests for the sake of relatives in need. These criteria justify the common practice of having family members serve as surrogates.

Surrogates Selected by Patients

As Chapter 12 discusses, all states allow competent patients to appoint a health care proxy with legal authority to make decisions if they lose decision-making capacity (2). Generally, the patient must complete a form and have it witnessed or notarized. In several states, a patient may appoint a proxy through an oral statement to a physician. Many patients find it easier to select who should act as proxy rather than anticipate their preference in future scenarios. Appointing a proxy can prevent disputes like that in Case 11.1.

State Laws Regarding Surrogates

Most states have laws that specify which persons have priority to act as legal surrogates for incapacitated patients who have not appointed a proxy themselves (2). Generally, the patient's spouse takes priority over adult children, followed by adult siblings. Some states give domestic partners the same authority as spouses or allow a friend as surrogate if there are no relatives. Because laws vary, physicians need to understand the law in their state. Such laws, however, might lead to ethically troubling results, such as favoring the distant son in Case 11.1 over the sister who has a closer day-to-day relationship with the patient. These laws might also be problematic when a spouse is estranged but not legally divorced or when the patient has a domestic partner who is not recognized by the surrogate statute.

Family Decision-Making

Even in the absence of explicit state laws authorizing family members to make decisions, the standard practice of family decision-making is ethically justified, as discussed in the section *Criteria for Surrogates* above. Most people want family members to make decisions for them if they cannot do so. Patients trust family members to do their best under circumstances that could not be foreseen (3).

Group Decision-Making

Many families reach decisions by consensus and do not single out one person as decision maker. Because surviving relatives will have continuing relationships after the patient's death, physicians should try to maintain family harmony. In practical terms, many proxies who are appointed by the patient are reluctant to contradict the views of close relatives. They might feel torn between what they think is best for the patient and what other family members want to do (4, 5).

Court-Appointed Guardians

Courts can declare a patient incompetent and appoint a guardian to make medical decisions for the patient (6). For patients who have lost decision-making capacity and have no family or friends, the court may have appointed a professional guardian who does not know the patient. Such guardians may have uncertain legal authority to make decisions about life-sustaining interventions and generally have no prior relationship with the patient and no knowledge of his or her goals and values (6).

Although the legal system offers procedural safeguards, involving the courts routinely in decisions has serious drawbacks (7, 8). First, the adversarial judicial system might polarize families and physicians rather than foster a mutually acceptable decision. Second, guardianship hearings are usually superficial, and courts do not monitor guardians' decisions. Finally, intolerable delays would occur if the courts were frequently involved in decisions on life-sustaining treatment. As one court decision declared, "Courts are not the proper place to resolve the agonizing personal problems that underlie these cases. Our legal system cannot replace the more intimate struggle that must be borne by the patient, those caring for the patient, and those who care about the patient" (9). Physicians and hospitals should seek court intervention only as a last resort, when disputes cannot be resolved in a clinical setting.

No Family Members Available

Decisions are most difficult when patients with impaired decision-making capacity have no advance directives and no family members—often called *unbefriended* patients (10). In some cases, a live-in partner, friend, or neighbor who has an emotional bond with the patient and a sense of the patient's values and goals would be an appropriate surrogate.

Physicians should not administer burdensome interventions that offer very little prospect of benefit to the patient just because there is no surrogate to decline them. In this situation, physicians may forego interventions that they do not consider to be in the patient's best interests. When there is no surrogate, it is advisable for physicians to consult with another physician or an institutional multidisciplinary process such as the ethics consultation service (11). Simply explaining one's reasoning to another person can clarify thinking, identify unwarranted assumptions and unconvincing arguments, and suggest new options for care.

PROBLEMS WITH SURROGATE DECISION-MAKING

Emotional Barriers to Decisions

At least one third of surrogates experience adverse emotional consequences, most commonly stress, doubt, and guilt over the decision (12). Nonetheless, actively participating in decisions allows surrogates to regain a sense of control and mitigate hopelessness and suffering. One way to do so is to ask relatives for their wishes for honoring the patient. Common responses are humanizing the medical environment, tributes, reconnecting with others, and observances. Such wishes can be implemented by the health care team and hospital (13).

Decisions Inconsistent with Patient's Values

In Case 11.1, if Mrs. R believed in the importance of prolonging life, her wishes would be followed out of respect for her (*see* Chapter 4). If, however, she disagreed with her son's beliefs about the sanctity of life, it would be inappropriate for a surrogate to impose his or her own values on the patient rather than respect the patient's values. Thus, the physician should inquire about the patient's own views about prolonging life.

Conflicts of Interest

In some cases, relatives might promote their own interests, not the patient's (14). Unscrupulous family members might try to gain control of an inheritance or a pension. When it comes to the basis for their decisions, surrogates are given less leeway than competent patients. For example, patients may choose to forego interventions to spare family members emotional distress or to preserve an inheritance. Such refusals are heeded to respect patient autonomy. However, claims by surrogates that the patient would refuse beneficial interventions for these reasons might be self-serving and need to be based on statements by the patient.

Family members cannot be expected to ignore their own needs and interests. Caring for a relative with serious chronic illness can cause emotional distress, fatigue, financial burdens, or conflicts with other responsibilities. Most family members subordinate their interests to those of the patient and make considerable sacrifices. Physicians should not be overly suspicious about surrogates. Respecting close family relationships is an important social value, and physicians should support families who are trying to deal with difficult situations as best as they can. Simply making sacrifices to care for a relative or being mentioned in a will is not a conflict of interest.

Disagreements Among Potential Surrogates

Case 11.1 illustrates how family members might disagree over decisions. Some physicians withhold interventions only when all family members agree. Giving every relative a veto, however, might impose interventions that are not in the patient's best interests. Furthermore, it is problematic to give distant or estranged relatives a voice equal to that of those with the closest relationship to the patient. Realistically, physicians often make decisions with family consensus rather than unanimity (15). Relatives are often willing to accept a decision made by the rest of the family, even though they would have decided differently themselves.

IMPROVING SURROGATE DECISION-MAKING

Table 11-1 provides several suggestions for improving surrogate decision-making.

Discuss the Decision-Making Process

Family meetings can help relatives understand and accept the medical situation (16, 17). Physicians should acknowledge that decisions are difficult and that people with good intentions might disagree. Doctors can help families express their preferred role in decision-making, articulate their emotions, and cope with their grief. In an ICU, the vast majority of surrogates of intubated patients want to play an active role in decision-making (18). Physicians should remind everybody that decisions should be based on the patient's preferences and interests, not on what surrogates or doctors would choose for themselves.

Give a Recommendation

Physicians should not merely list options and leave it to surrogates to decide. Doctors can help surrogates deliberate by summarizing and reframing surrogates' statements about the patient's values and linking those values to decisions at hand (19). Going further, doctors should offer to make a recommendation on the basis of if he or she knows about the patient's preferences and values. About 40% of surrogates, however, prefer not to receive a recommendation (20). In some cases, it may be helpful for physicians to give the family permission to let the patient die if that is consistent with the patient's values. In rare cases, when surrogates are supportive of limiting life-sustaining interventions but do not want to take responsibility for the patient's death, the physician might take responsibility for writing such an order unless the surrogates object (21). That is, the surrogates need only assent to foregoing life-sustaining interventions.

TABLE 11-1.   Suggestions for Improving Surrogate Decision-Making
Discuss the decision-making process.
Give a recommendation.
Get help from other health care workers.

Get Help from Other Health Care Workers

A nurse, social worker, or chaplain can often help the family address their spiritual and emotional needs, accept the medical situation, and work through past antagonisms with the patient or among themselves.

CASE 11.1 | *Continued*

Mrs. R's physician first asked the family what they believed Mrs. R's medical situation was and what concerns they had about her condition. The doctor then framed the task as making decisions consistent with her values and best interests, which might not be what the family would want for themselves. He asked what she would regard as important to consider in this situation and asked specifically about prior statements she had made and her religious views. He also said that the situation is usually hard for family members and asked how they were feeling. He planned to have repeated discussions with them and suggested they might talk to others who might have insight about her views, for example, her religious or spiritual advisor.

SUMMARY

1. Surrogates should be willing to respect the patient's values and goals and interpret them in the context of the decision at hand.
2. In most cases, the standard clinical practice of family decision-making is ethically and legally appropriate.
3. When family members disagree, physicians should try to achieve consensus.

References

1. Brudney D. The different moral bases of patient and surrogate decision-making. *Hastings Cent Rep* 2018;48:37-41.
2. DeMartino ES, Dudzinski DM, Doyle CK, et al. Who decides when a patient can't? Statutes on alternate decision makers. *N Engl J Med* 2017;376:1478-1482.
3. Arnold RM, Kellum J. Moral justifications for surrogate decision making in the intensive care unit: implications and limitations. *Crit Care Med* 2003;31:S347-S353.
4. Alpers A, Lo B. Avoiding family feuds: responding to surrogates' demands for life-sustaining treatment. *Journal of Law, Medicine & Ethics* 1999;27:74-80.
5. Vig EK, Starks H, Taylor JS, et al. Surviving surrogate decision-making: what helps and hampers the experience of making medical decisions for others. *J Gen Intern Med* 2007;22:1274-1279.
6. Cohen AB, Wright MS, Cooney L, Jr., et al. Guardianship and end-of-life decision making. *JAMA Intern Med* 2015;175:1687-1691.
7. Lo B, Rouse F, Dornbrand L. Family decision-making on trial: who decides for incompetent patients? *N Engl J Med* 1990;322:1228-1231.
8. Bandy RJ, Helft PR, Bandy RW, et al. Medical decision-making during the guardianship process for incapacitated, hospitalized adults: a descriptive cohort study. *J Gen Intern Med* 2010;25:1003-1008.
9. In re Jobes. 529 A. 2d 434 (N.J. 1987).
10. Farrell TW, Widera E, Rosenberg L, et al. AGS position statement: making medical treatment decisions for unbefriended older adults. *J Am Geriatr Soc* 2016.
11. Bosslet GT, Pope TM, Rubenfeld GD, et al. An official ATS/AACN/ACCP/ESICM/SCCM policy statement: responding to requests for potentially inappropriate treatments in intensive care units. *Am J Respir Crit Care Med* 2015;191:1318-1330.
12. Wendler D, Rid A. Systematic review: the effect on surrogates of making treatment decisions for others. *Ann Intern Med* 2011;154:336-346.

13. Cook D, Swinton M, Toledo F, et al. Personalizing death in the intensive care unit: the 3 Wishes Project: a mixed-methods study. *Ann Intern Med* 2015;163:271-279.
14. Lo B. Caring for the incompetent patient: is there a doctor in the house? *Law, Medcine, & Health Care* 1989;17:214-220.
15. Torke AM, Alexander GC, Lantos J, et al. The physician-surrogate relationship. *Arch Intern Med* 2007; 167:1117-1121.
16. Curtis JR, White DB. Practical guidance for evidence-based ICU family conferences. *Chest* 2008; 134:835-843.
17. Lilly CM, Daly BJ. The healing power of listening in the ICU. *N Engl J Med* 2007;356:513-515.
18. Johnson SK, Bautista CA, Hong SY, et al. An empirical study of surrogates' preferred level of control over value-laden life support decisions in intensive care units. *Am J Respir Crit Care Med* 2011;183:915-921.
19. White DB, Malvar G, Karr J, et al. Expanding the paradigm of the physician's role in surrogate decision-making: an empirically derived framework. *Crit Care Med* 2010;38:743-750.
20. White DB, Evans LR, Bautista CA, et al. Are physicians' recommendations to limit life support beneficial or burdensome? Bringing empirical data to the debate. *Am J Respir Crit Care Med* 2009;180:320-325.
21. Curtis JR, Burt RA. Point: the ethics of unilateral "do not resuscitate" orders: the role of "informed assent." *Chest* 2007;132:748-751; discussion 755-756.

ANNOTATED BIBLIOGRAPHY

1. DeMartino ES, Dudzinski DM, Doyle CK, et al. Who decides when a patient can't? Statutes on alternate decision makers. *N Engl J Med* 2017;376:1478-1482.
   Recent analysis of state laws regarding surrogate decision making.
2. Cook D, Swinton M, Toledo F, et al. Personalizing death in the intensive care unit: the 3 Wishes Project: a mixed-methods study. *Ann Intern Med* 2015;163:271-279.
   Asking family members how to honor the patient helps shift the focus from medical interventions to humanizing the end of life and reaching closure.
3. Arnold RM, Kellum J. Moral justifications for surrogate decision making in the intensive care unit: implications and limitations. *Crit Care Med* 2003:31:S347-S353.
   Clear and thoughtful review of surrogate decision-making.
4. Farrell TW, Widera E, Rosenberg L, et al. AGS position statement: making medical treatment decisions for unbefriended older adults. *J Am Geriatr Soc* 2016.
   Recommendations on making decisions for patients who have no surrogate and have carried out no advance care planning.

Standards for Decisions When Patients Lack Decision-Making Capacity

INTRODUCTION

In the past 10 years, the approach to making decisions for patients who have lost decision-making capacity has shifted from advance directives to advance care planning. The focus is now on facilitating discussions between the physician and surrogate that are guided by the patient's values and goals, rather than documenting patient wishes regarding specific interventions.

ADVANCE DIRECTIVES

History of Advance Directives

Advance directives are legal documents in which competent patients indicate *what* interventions they would accept or refuse if they should lose their decision-making capacity and *who* should act as their proxy decision-maker. The rationale for advance directives was to respect patients: their choices should guide care even when they can no longer make informed decisions.

Proof of principle and feasibility of advance directives were established early in the AIDS epidemic (1). Before antiretrovirals were developed, persons with AIDS commonly died from opportunistic infections. Many persons with AIDS had watched friends die and had strong, informed preferences to forego mechanical ventilation for *Pneumocystis carinii* pneumonia or antibiotics for central nervous system opportunistic infections, preferring palliative care instead. Only by executing a durable power of attorney for health care could homosexual men with AIDS make such preferences legally binding and appoint their partner or a close friend as proxy, instead of relatives who did not know about their medical condition, were not familiar with AIDS, or from whom they were estranged. Lawyers volunteered to help patients complete these legal documents.

The ruling in the Nancy Cruzan case (*see* Chapter 22) made a big conceptual jump. Advance directives are extremely useful when a competent patient has foreseen the clinical situation that later occurs and makes an informed refusal of an intervention in that situation. However, it does not follow that the only justification for limiting life-sustaining interventions in patients who lack decision-making capacity is a written advance directive or an oral statement declining the intervention in the specific clinical situation (*see* Chapter 22). The Cruzan case spurred measures to encourage written advance directives, including new state laws authorizing them and the federal Patient Self-Determination Act to inform patients about them.

Types of Advance Directives

Oral Statements to Family Members or Friends

Conversations with relatives or friends are the most common advance directives and, in clinical practice, frequently guide decisions for patients who have lost decision-making capacity. In 16 states, such statements have legal force (2).

Oral Statements to Physicians

Discussions with physicians are more common than written advance directives. Unlike some oral statements to relatives or friends, directives to physicians are not casual comments. Moreover, physicians can check whether directives are informed, such as by asking the patient follow-up questions about specific clinical scenarios. For instance, in Case 12.2 Mrs. A's physician might point out that many patients with moderate dementia appear to enjoy activities and interactions with friends and family. In some states, oral statements to physicians appointing a proxy are legally binding for the duration of the illness or hospitalization.

Written Documents

All states have laws authorizing living wills or health care proxies (2). Patients complete a formal legal document that must be witnessed or notarized. A lawyer is not needed to complete these documents. Many states honor forms from other states. Caregivers who follow written directives are given immunity from civil and criminal liability and professional disciplinary actions. Requirements for witnesses or notarization may present barriers to patients who are homeless, lack surrogates, or are institutionalized (2). Because statutes vary from state to state, caregivers and patients need to be familiar with their state's laws.

The courts consider written advance directives more reliable evidence of patient choices than oral statements because legal formalities make patients more likely to think seriously and appreciate the consequences.

Living wills. Patients direct their physicians to withhold or withdraw life-sustaining treatment if they develop a terminal condition or, in some states, enter a persistent vegetative state (PVS). Various states define *terminal condition* differently, usually only in general terms. In most states, living wills would not cover conditions such as Alzheimer disease. Patients typically may refuse only interventions that "merely prolong the process of dying." People might disagree on whether this includes common scenarios such as antibiotics for pneumonia or sepsis. Some states do not allow patients to decline artificial nutrition and hydration through living wills. Living wills allow patients only to withhold interventions and only in some circumstances and thus are less flexible and comprehensive than the health care proxy.

Health care proxy. Competent patients may appoint a health care proxy or agent, typically a relative or close friend, to make medical decisions if they lose decision-making capacity. In some states, this process is called executing a durable power of attorney for health care. As long as patients remain competent, they continue to make their own health care decisions. Because of conflicts of interest, certain people may not serve as surrogates, such as the treating physician or employees of the treating physician or institution unless they are relatives of the patient. The health care proxy applies to all situations in which the patient is incapable of making decisions, not just terminal illness. Proxy decisions must be consistent with the patient's previously expressed choices or best interests. No additional evidence of the patient's wishes, however, is required.

Physician orders for life-sustaining treatment (POLST). This standardized one-page form gives first responders orders regarding such interventions as CPR and transport to hospital in urgent situations where there is no time to contact the responsible physician or proxy. The POLST form applies in all settings, including the patient's home and nursing homes and can accompany a patient from one setting to another. Patients can appoint a health care proxy to make decisions for them if they cannot do so themselves. Patients can articulate goals of care, as well as specific preferences for interventions. It is signed by the patient or surrogate, as well as by the physician.

POLST is more flexible than "do not attempt resuscitation" or "do not hospitalize" orders. There are three options regarding goals of care:

1. Comfort measures only; transfer to hospital only if comfort needs cannot be met in the current setting.
2. Limited additional measures, including antibiotics and other medical treatment as indicated, but no intubation and generally avoiding intensive care; an additional checkbox may be checked to transfer to hospital only if comfort needs cannot be met in the current setting. This option acknowledges that the goal of patient comfort might require hospitalization or limited noninvasive care.
3. Full treatment as indicated, including intensive care.

Most states have authorized POLST forms. Physicians should be familiar with their state laws and forms, which can vary from state to state. The website of The National POLST Paradigm at polst.org provides state-specific information.

POLST is now the preferred means of providing written advance directives. As we discuss later, POLST should be regarded as a means of encouraging and facilitating discussions among the patient, surrogate, and treating physician. It is not a substitute for such conversations and does not avoid the need for additional discussions at the time an actual decision must be made for a patient. For instance, physicians vary in how they interpret POLST forms in specific clinical situations other than no CPR or full treatment (3). Moreover, although patients may have stable preferences to decline CPR and hospitalization, their preferences for other medical interventions may emerge only when considering a specific decision (3).

Written advance directives are particularly useful if patients have strong preferences about specific medical interventions or anticipate disagreements over who should serve as surrogate.

Limitations of Advance Directives

Advance Directives Might Not Be Informed

Even after discussions with physicians, patients commonly have serious misconceptions about life-sustaining interventions (4). Only 33% of patients know that patients on a ventilator cannot talk, and about one half believe that ventilators are oxygen tanks. More than one fourth cannot identify any basic characteristics of CPR, such as chest compressions or assisted breathing. Only one third know that if CPR succeeds in restarting the heart, a breathing machine is usually needed. Thus, patients may express "strong preferences about treatments that they did not understand" (4).

Patients commonly overestimate their prognosis. In a cohort of patients with metastatic lung or colon cancer, who had a 6-month survival of 45%, most patients were decidedly overoptimistic: 59% believed that their chance of surviving 6 months was greater than 90% (5).

People generally cannot predict how they will respond to future medical conditions, underestimating the extent to which people cope and adapt to new situations (6). Their choices when healthy may differ from what they would decide later if they actually are in the situation. Furthermore, many people do not have preexisting preferences regarding life-prolonging interventions in various clinical situations, developing them only when faced with an actual decision (3).

Patients Might Change Their Minds

Patient willingness to accept potentially life-sustaining therapy that is highly burdensome or would result in a severely disabled condition is only moderately stable over time (7, 8). Although some of this change may be related to declines in health, there is considerable unexplained variation.

Advance Directives Need to Be Discussed During an Acute Situation

Except for orders for first responders, such as "No CPR" orders, advance directives need to be discussed with surrogates in light of the new medical situation that requires a decision. Nursing homes commonly contact family members when an acute situation arises in a patient with "do not hospitalize" orders to discuss the situation and the potential benefits and risks of hospitalization (9). For example, the nursing home may be unable to keep the patient comfortable and seek hospitalization for palliative care, or the new event is unrelated to the condition that led to the do not hospitalize order. Furthermore, some families change their minds when a crisis occurs and decide on hospitalization.

Problems Interpreting Advance Directives

Vague terms. Advance directives sometimes contain vague terms such as *heroic* or *extraordinary* care. Physicians might be directed to refuse interventions when "the burdens outweigh the benefits of care." These terms must be interpreted. When does "senility" commence: When Mrs. A, in Case 12.2, can no longer pursue her favorite activities, such as reading? When she sometimes, usually, or almost always does not recognize family members? Or only when she no longer responds at all? Patients' choices in specific scenarios cannot be accurately predicted from their general preferences and goals (10).

Application to other situations. When giving advance directives, patients may have had one situation in mind but later developed a different condition. Patients differ in how much leeway surrogates should have. In one study, 39% of patients wanted their directives to be followed literally, but 31% of patients wanted their surrogates to override their advance directives if their surrogates believed it was best for them (11).

Unrealistic expectations. Advance directives enable patients to have some control over health care decisions if they lose decision-making capacity. It is unrealistic, however, for patients to expect to control all future care through advance directives. No one can anticipate what specific clinical decisions will need to be made in the future, or whether his or her overall health or life situation will change significantly.

Conflict Between Advance Directives and Best Interests

Following a patient's advance directives might not be in his or her current best interests. For example, surrogates and physicians might wish to override prior refusal of care if the benefits of an intervention will outweigh the burdens in the context of the patient's values and goals, the patient's prior directives do not fit well with the situation at hand, and the surrogate represents the patients best interest well (12). Alternatively, wishes to receive an intervention may become impractical if the patient no longer takes oral medicines regularly or cannot cooperate with a postoperative regimen. In addition, when giving advance directives, patients make implicit assumptions about their prognosis or situation that later may no longer hold true.

Despite many limitations, advance directives and advance care planning are valuable to facilitate important discussions about end-of-life care among patients, family members, and physicians. They promote respect for patients as unique individuals. Furthermore, they offer a means for patients to express strongly held, informed choices that they want surrogates to follow closely.

Trustworthiness of Advance Directives

In light of the limitations of advance directives, physicians and surrogates need to assess how much weight to give them when patients no longer have decision-making capacity. Advance directives are more trustworthy and should be given more weight if

- The directive covers both general *goals* and *values* what *specific treatments* the patient would want or not want *in particular clinical situations*
- The directive is *informed*, for example, because the patient has experienced the intervention or discussed it with a physician
- The directive is *repeated* over time, in different situations, to various individuals
- The directive does not clearly contradict the patient's current best interests.

Even when discussions occur, they may not give patients enough information to make informed decisions (13). When discussing hypothetical scenarios with patients, physicians usually pose dire scenarios in which patients would not survive outside an intensive care unit or reversible scenarios in which patients are expected to recover their previous health. Physicians seldom pose more difficult—and more common—situations, such as when recovery is uncertain or serious disability might persist.

Physicians also use vague language, asking patients what they would want if they were "very, very sick" or "had something that was very serious." Doctors rarely define such terms or ascertain how patients interpret them. Physicians commonly discuss specific interventions, usually CPR or mechanical ventilation, without learning what patients know about them. In discussing outcomes, physicians seldom give numerical probabilities of success or mention outcomes other than death and complete recovery.

Physicians rarely elicit patients' values, goals for care, and reasons for choices. Most commonly, physicians simply ask whether patients want interventions in scenarios without exploring their reasoning. Even when reasons are discussed, physicians rarely ask patients to clarify what they mean by a poor quality of life or being a burden to their family, which are frequent reasons for refusing interventions.

Advance Care Planning

Because advance directives overemphasize legal formalities and specific interventions, an alternative approach called advance care planning focuses instead on (14):

- Discussions among patients, physicians, and surrogates, rather than legal documents
- The patient's values, goals, hopes, and fears. Starting with these topics generally makes it easier to reach an agreement on specific decisions and may not take much more time
- The patient's preferences and hopes for a "good death," such as how the patient would like to be remembered, what they would like to say to their family, and what they would like the family to say to them. This shifts attention from withholding of medical interventions to reaching closure at the end of life. These discussions also help address the emotional needs of the patient and family
- The need for surrogates to exercise judgment and interpret the patient's previous statements, not simply implement literally the patient's directives
- The need for further discussion when a clinical decision must be made. Surrogates should anticipate the need to make difficult decisions and use the advance care planning discussions as a starting point

Improving Advance Care Planning Discussions

Physicians can resolve many problems with advance care planning by explicitly addressing the following issues (Table 12-1):

TABLE 12-1. Topics to Discuss in Advance Care Planning
Which patients should be invited to discuss advance care planning?
Who should serve as proxy?
What are the patient's goals and values?
What are the patient's preferences in specific situations?
How should directives be interpreted?
What do patients want to tell family members?
Continue discussions over time
Recommend POLST forms

Which Patients Should Be Invited to Discuss Advance Care planning?

Physicians should routinely discuss advance care planning not only with patients who are *terminal* or in a downhill course but also with those with a serious chronic illness, such as congestive heart failure, with those whose course is not so predictable, and with patients who have multiple chronic illnesses and functional limitations (15). Patients usually want discussions to occur earlier in their illness and in the patient–physician relationship (16).

In some cultures, advance care planning discussions might be problematic. Many traditional Chinese patients believe that giving directives implies that they do not trust their family to make decisions for them (17). Moreover, patients might believe that designating one person to make decisions violates the expectation of family decision-making. Furthermore, some patients believe that talking about future illness will anger ghosts or spirits, who will then bring about the illness or cause bad luck. Such reluctance to discuss advance care planning needs to be respected.

Who Should Serve as Proxy?

Most patients find it easier to discuss the choice of proxy than to discuss preferences regarding care. Straightforward questions can broach the topic: "I ask all my elderly patients how they want decisions to be made. Who would you want to make decisions for you in case you are too sick to talk with me directly?" Patients who do not wish to discuss this topics can easily demur. Patients need to select someone whose judgment they trust. It is unrealistic to think that the proxy can simply follow the patient's previous statements.

What Are the Patient's Goals and Values?

Although many physicians focus on specific medical decisions, such as Do Not Attempt Resuscitation (DNAR) orders, discussing the patient's values and goals first improves quality of care, deceases use of life-sustaining interventions near death, leads to earlier hospice referrals, and promotes care consistent with patient preferences (18). Open-ended questions help elicit the patient's perspective (19, 20):

- "When you think of serious illness, what concerns you the most?" Alternatively, "When you think of serious illness, what is most important to you?" "What do you hope for?" "What do you fear?"
- "Sometimes your family might need to make decisions about your medical care. What things would you want them to take into account?" These questions elicit how the patient defines his or her best interests or an acceptable quality of life.
- "Are there situations in which you would not want life-prolonging interventions?"

It is unrealistic to try to discuss all future medical situations. The goal of discussions is not to be exhaustive, but to elicit informed choices about highly likely scenarios and to understand what considerations are important to the patient.

What Are the Patient's Preferences in Specific Situations?

Instead of discussing dire or completely reversible situations, physicians should discuss common scenarios in which the outcome is uncertain, serious disability might persist, and interventions are burdensome (4). What types of intervention would the patient be willing to accept, for how long, with what burdens, and for what likelihood, magnitude, and duration of improvement?

Physicians need to describe interventions and their likely outcomes. For mechanical ventilation, patients need to understand that they will have a tube in their throat, will not be able to speak, and will need sedation. Discussions should be tailored to the patient's condition. With elderly patients, physicians should discuss severe dementia and stroke. Would the patient want infections treated with antibiotics or intensive care? Would the patient want a feeding tube if unable to swallow food? How would the patient characterize severe dementia or serious stroke?

Are the Patient's Preferences Informed?

Physicians can help assure that the patient's preferences are informed and consistent with his or her general goals and values. For example, a woman with lung cancer metastatic to liver and bone might say that she wants everything done. In such cases, physicians should explore expectations, concerns, and emotions, using open-ended questions. The physician could say, "What do you think happens to patients whose cancer spreads like that?" or "I wish that were the case. Unfortunately when cancer has spread that much, even breathing machines don't help patients live much longer" (19, 21).

In some cases, physicians can point out that patients often adapt to situations that seem devastating to healthy persons. For instance, many patients with dementia or stroke find enjoyment and value in their lives, even though they would not have chosen that situation (22).

How Should Directives Be Interpreted?

Because advance care planning cannot cover all contingencies, it is important to understand how the patient would want the surrogate and physician to interpret his or her preferences. Physicians need to clarify ambiguous statements: "Can you tell me what you mean by 'no heroic treatment'?" Other common phrases that need to be specified include "being a burden to their family" and "having a poor quality of life."

Physicians should also ask patients how much leeway they would allow surrogates to interpret their statements, extrapolate directives to unforeseen situations, take into account unforeseen changes in their situation, or override their directives if it seemed in their best interests (23). The patient might want their directives simply to be preferences or suggestions to be taken into account, but not binding. Alternatively, the patient may want directives followed unless there are persuasive reasons to do the opposite. Finally, there may be some specific directives that the patient wants to be followed literally, even if the proxy believes they are contrary to what is best for the patient. Doctors should clarify, however, that it might not be possible to carry out directives, as discussed later.

What Do Patients Want to Tell Family Members?

Physician can help patients move toward closure. Patients might want their families to know that "I love them," "I wish to be forgiven for the times I might have hurt them," or "I forgive them for what they have done to me" (24). In addition, patients can indicate how they want to be remembered. These issues shift the focus from making clinical decisions to reaching closure at the end of life.

Continue Discussions Over Time

Physicians should not expect advance care planning to be completed in a single conversation. In addition, patients' choices and values might change as their illness or life situation changes. Most important, physicians will need to advise patients or surrogates that further discussion will be needed when a specific clinical decision needs to be made, to make sure they understand the new clinical situation, the options and their risks and benefits, and how those options relate to the patient's values and goals.

Recommend POLST Forms

Physicians should tell patients about the advantages of POLST forms for providing orders to emergency medical personnel and encourage patients to complete them. When completed, POLST forms should be uploaded into the electronic health record.

Document Discussions in the Medical Record

The physician's note should describe the patient's decision-making capacity as well as the issues in Table 12-1.

SUBSTITUTED JUDGMENT

Often patients who have lost decision-making capacity have given only general directives or no indication of their preferences. In the absence of clear and specific advance directives, surrogates can try to construct the decision that the patient would make under the circumstances, taking into account the patient's values and goals. The surrogate might imagine that the patient miraculously regains decision-making capacity temporarily. What care would the informed patient choose under the circumstances? Reconstructing patients' choices is ethically justified because it respects their individuality to the extent that this is possible. It respects the integrity, authenticity, and coherence of the patient's life as a unique individual (25). The metaphor of narrative has been suggested—the more coherent the narrative, the better.

CASE 12.1   Disagreements over substituted judgment

Mr. S, a 76-year-old widower, suffers a massive stroke and aphasia. One week later, he still has paralysis of his right arm and leg. He does not respond consistently to simple requests or questions, but sometimes smiles when his hand is held. He develops pneumonia.

Throughout his life, he had been reluctant to see physicians and did not regularly take prescribed medications to lower his cholesterol. He loved to take walks and work in his garden. When his wife died of a sudden heart attack, he said, "Death isn't the enemy. She wanted to be active and healthy to the end, and the good Lord granted her wish." He was a proud and independent man who was reluctant to accept help from others. He has given no oral or written advance directives. His son and daughter believe Mr. S would refuse antibiotics for his pneumonia, even though he might still improve from his stroke. "He disliked being dependent on others and would hate being in a nursing home. In this condition, he can't do any of the things he loved in life."

Problems with Substituted Judgment

Inconsistency

Reasonable people acting in good faith may disagree over what the patient would want. For example, Mr. S's sister might believe that he would want antibiotics. "He's been a fighter all his life and never gave up." She recalled that as a young man, Mr. S had overcome tremendous odds to come to America and get a college education.

Inaccuracy

Neither family members nor physicians can accurately state a competent patient's choices regarding future life-sustaining treatment (26). About one third of surrogates incorrectly state the patient's preferences (26). This level of agreement between proxies and patients would be expected by chance alone. Proxies' statements about patients' preferences are closer to what *they* would want in the situation than to what the patient actually wants (27). Even an intensive intervention to facilitate discussions between the patient and proxy about the patient's wishes for end-of-life care failed to increase the level of immediate agreement (28).

Questionable Considerations

A competent patient might not want to be a burden or might want to spare the family the expenses and stress of terminal care. A patient also might prefer to provide a college fund for a granddaughter than to spend down savings to cover nursing home costs. It seems reasonable for surrogates to consider these factors when the patient himself has already done so, but it might be self-serving for surrogates to consider them when patients have not indicated their importance (29). Family members might confound what they would want with what the patient would want.

Unavoidable Speculation

Substituted judgments are inherently less certain than advance directives (30-32). Mr. S's comments about his wife cannot be assumed to express his own desires for medical care without additional contextual information. In Case 12.1, the children's reasoning is unconvincing when applied to the converse situation. If a patient had seen physicians regularly and had taken medications faithfully, it would not be logical to infer that he wanted all life-sustaining interventions in his current situation. With regard to the idea that a substituted judgment should complete the narrative arc of a patient's life, there might be a number of endings that are consistent with the patient's life story, and the choice of one ending among alternatives requires a subjective judgment and interpretation. Furthermore, there is the possibility that people change their values and beliefs near the end of life.

Despite the limitations of substituted judgments, they are still useful because they respect the patient's individuality as a person with unique values and preferences and focus surrogates on what the patient would want, not what they might want for themselves (33).

CASE 12.1	*Continued*

First, Mr. S's physicians need to clarify the likelihood of his recovering to his goals of being independent and doing the things he enjoyed in life. Second, even if Mr. S could no longer take walks and read, he might adapt to his illness and find life worthwhile despite disabilities. The physician should say that many people learn to accept disabilities and assistance from others. Third, the doctors need to inquire whether Mr. S's comments about his wife's care express his own choices for medical care. Finally, the physician might pose the dilemma as how much burden Mr. S would accept for what probability and degree of recovery, and for how long a time.

BEST INTERESTS

A best interests standard may be appropriate in several situations. For some patients who have not given advance directives, a substituted judgment may be so speculative that it would be more honest for the surrogate and physician to acknowledge that they are basing decisions on what they believe is best for the patient (22). The ethical guideline of beneficence requires physicians to weigh the benefits and burdens of interventions for the patient and act in his or her best interests. Best interests must be determined for the particular patient in a specific situation in light of the available options under the circumstances, which are often less than ideal (34). The best interests standard does not require physicians or surrogates to extend a patient's life as long as medically possible (22).

Assessing Best Interests

Problems arise when surrogates or physicians make judgments about what is best for the patient based on their own values and preferences, rather than the patient's. For example, other people tend to underestimate how patients perceive their quality of life (*see* Chapter 4 for more details). Other concerns arise when surrogates consider the interests of third parties, as discussed in the section on substituted judgment.

May the surrogate's own interests and needs be taken into account? Family members cannot be expected to ignore their own needs and interests. Best interests must be based on what is feasible, not on some theoretical ideal. Surrogates cannot be expected to put all their effort and resources to keeping a patient with dementia out of a nursing home, to the extent that they are unable to carry out other family and work responsibilities.

Other dilemmas occur if surrogates request painful interventions that will only prolong the patient's life for a few days because they believe that suffering serves a spiritual purpose or that biologic life should be prolonged even if the interventions required are very burdensome. Decisions based on such beliefs need to be examined carefully (35). Did the patient him- or herself hold such views, as opposed to the surrogate? Did the patient say explicitly that he or she would accept painful interventions in this situation and decline palliative relief? Many patients who believe their illness serves a spiritual purpose still decline burdensome interventions. Health care workers might believe that they are acting inhumanely and causing the patient to suffer if they do not provide standard, effective palliative care when a patient is in great distress (35, 36). The ethical guideline of nonmaleficence allows health care workers to refrain from interventions that cause significant suffering and prolong the patient's life for only a few hours or days (*see* Chapter 13).

Incompetent patients who have not given advance directives and have no surrogates, sometimes called *unbefriended patients*, pose difficult cases (37). Some doctors believe all life-sustaining interventions that are technically feasible should be provided to such patients unless they are potentially inappropriate. Insisting on life-sustaining interventions, however, simply because it is not certain that the patient would decline them would impose burdensome interventions on many patients and make them "prisoners of technology" (38). In this situation, it is appropriate for physicians to make decisions on the basis of what they believe is in the patient's best interests. Consulting with another physician or the hospital ethics committee helps assure that the decision is not an idiosyncratic reflection of the physician's own personal views.

Conflicts Between Advance Directives and Best Interests

In some cases, an incapacitated patient's advance directives may conflict with his current best interests.

CASE 12.2	What is in the patient's best interests?

Mrs. A, a 78-year-old widow with Alzheimer disease, lives in a nursing home. She needs help with dressing, bathing, and eating. Over the past few years, she has walked less and less. She no longer goes on outings. She interacts less and less with her children and staff, although much of the time she still recognizes them.

About 5 years ago, when she was able to have some sustained conversations, she told her children and friends many times that she wanted "no heroics" if she became senile. She signed a POLST form, specifying that she did not want to be resuscitated or hospitalized (except if needed for comfort measures). She also wrote by hand, NO SURGERY, NO INTENSIVE CARE. She appointed her daughter, who lives in the same city, to serve as her decision maker if she could not make decisions herself.

Mrs. A falls, has left hip pain, and cannot bear weight. In all likelihood, she has a hip fracture. The on-call physician believes that it is in Mrs. A's best interests to have her hip stabilized surgically. Without surgery, she will have pain whenever she moves her leg, including when using a bedpan and having her bedding changed, and decreased mobility and worse functioning and quality of life.

Nonoperative management in hip fractures is sometimes carried out with nursing home residents with advanced dementia. Surgically treated patients had lower mortality than nonsurgical patients (31% mortality at 6 months vs. 54%) (39). Among those who survived 6 months, surgical patients had less pain and fewer pressure sores. Few patients were ambulatory at follow-up, even those who were walking before the fracture.

In Case 12.2, physicians and surrogates should ask several questions (12).

First, how likely is surgery to achieve the patient's goals and values? Is a net benefit from the intervention likely, relative to the burdens and risks? Of note, the burdens of perioperative management may be increased because Mrs. A cannot comprehend why nurses and occupational therapists want her to use an incentive spirometer, get into a chair, and have physical therapy.

Second, how well do the advance directives fit the situation at hand? When Mrs. A made her comments, was she referring to substantially different circumstances? Have her medical condition, living situation, and preferences changed markedly?

Third, did the patient indicate how much leeway she wanted the proxy to have when making decisions? In other words, how literally did Mrs. A want her daughter to follow her statements, or did she want her to use her discretion?

The surrogate would have strong justification for overriding the POLST if the patient was willing to grant her daughter leeway in making decisions, if the patient had not envisaged that an operation might improve her quality of life, and if pain causes Mrs. A visible distress and is difficult to relieve with medications.

The mere possibility that a person's values and preferences may have changed after developing a disabling illness does not justify ignoring her advance directives. An advance directive should be followed unless there are strong reasons to override it.

Fourth, does the surrogate appear to be acting in good faith and with compassion and concern?

CASE 12.2 | *Continued*

When contacted, Mrs. A's daughter reports that when the patient completed the POLST form, there was no discussion of how surgery for a hip fracture might allow better relief of pain. After discussion with the physician and her brother, the daughter agrees to have Mrs. A transferred to the emergency department. After further discussions with the orthopedic surgeon, she agrees to internal fixation of the fractured femur. The plan is to return her to familiar surroundings and staff in the nursing home as soon as possible to minimize agitation and to forego inpatient rehabilitation, as she is unlikely to walk again in any case.

SUMMARY

1. Advance care planning encourages patients to think about what values and goals are important to them to discuss with their physicians and family members. Furthermore, advance care planning allows patients to identify whom they trust to make decisions for them.
2. POLST forms are the preferred way for patients to complete advance care planning because they are physicians' orders for emergency responders and guide decisions if the patient is transferred to an acute care hospital.
3. Surrogates often must take responsibility for making difficult decisions regarding what the patient would have wanted or what is best for the patient in his or her current situation.
4. Physicians and surrogates need to guard against two types of errors: withholding treatments that would likely provide a net benefit and continuing treatments that the patient would not want or whose burdens outweigh the benefits.

References

1. Steinbrook R, Lo B, Moulton J, et al. Preferences of homosexual men with AIDS for life-sustaining treatment. *N Engl J Med* 1986;314:457-460.
2. Castillo LS, Williams BA, Hooper SM, et al. Lost in translation: the unintended consequences of advance directive law on clinical care. *Ann Intern Med* 2011;154:121-128.
3. Moore KA, Rubin EB, Halpern SD. The problems with physician orders for life-sustaining treatment. *JAMA* 2016;315:259-260.
4. Fischer GS, Tulsky JA, Rose MR, et al. Patient knowledge and physician predications of treatment preferences after discussions of advance directives. *J Gen Intern Med* 1998;13:447-454.
5. Weeks JC, Cook EF, O'Day SJ, et al. Relationship between cancer patients' predictions of prognosis and their treatment preferences. *JAMA* 1998;279:1709-1714.
6. Halpern J, Arnold RM. Affective forecasting: an unrecognized challenge in making serious health decisions. *J Gen Intern Med* 2008;23:1708-1712.
7. Fried TR, Van Ness PH, Byers AL, et al. Changes in preferences for life-sustaining treatment among older persons with advanced illness. *J Gen Intern Med* 2007;22:495-501.
8. Kim YS, Escobar GJ, Halpern SD, et al. The natural history of changes in preferences for life-sustaining treatments and implications for inpatient mortality in younger and older hospitalized adults. *J Am Geriatr Soc* 2016;64:981-989.
9. Cohen AB, Knobf MT, Fried TR. Do-not-hospitalize orders in nursing homes: "call the family instead of calling the ambulance." *J Am Geriatr Soc* 2017;65:1573-1577.
10. Fischer GS, Alpert HR, Stoeckle JD, et al. Can goals of care be used to predict intervention preferences in an advance directive? *Arch Intern Med* 1997;157:810-807.
11. Sehgal A, Galbraith A, Chesney M, et al. How strictly do dialysis patients want their advance directives followed. *JAMA* 1992;267:59-63.

12. Smith AK, Lo B, Sudore R. When previously expressed wishes conflict with best interests. *JAMA Intern Med* 2013;173:1241-1245.

13. Tulsky JA, Fischer GS, Rose MR, et al. Opening the black box: how do physicians communicate about advance directives. *Ann Intern Med* 1998;129:441-449.

14. Sudore RL, Fried TR. Redefining the "planning" in advance care planning: preparing for end-of-life decision making. *Ann Intern Med* 2010;153:256-261.

15. Institute of Medicine. *Dying in America: Improving Quality and Honoring Individual Preferences Near the End of Life.* Washington, DC: National Academies Press; 2014.

16. Johnston SC, Pfeifer MP, McNutt R. The discussion about advance directives. Patient and physician opinions regarding when and how it should be conducted. End-of-life study group. *Arch Intern Med* 1995;155:1025-1030.

17. Bowman KW, Singer PA. Chinese seniors' perspective on end-of-life decisions. *Soc Sci Med* 2001;53:455-464.

18. Bernacki RE, Block SD. Communication about serious illness care goals: a review and synthesis of best practices. *JAMA Intern Med* 2014;174:1994-2003.

19. Tulsky JA. Beyond advance directives: importance of communication skills at the end of life. *JAMA* 2005;294:359-365.

20. Lo B, Quill T, Tulsky J. Discussing palliative care with patients. ACP-ASIM End-of-Life Care Consensus Panel. American College of Physicians–American Society of Internal Medicine. *Ann Intern Med* 1999;130:744-749.

21. Back AL, Arnold RM, Quill TE. Hope for the best, and prepare for the worst. *Ann Intern Med* 2003;138:439-443.

22. The President's Council on Bioethics. *Taking Care: Ethical Caregiving in Our Aging Society.* 2005. Available at: https://bioethicsarchive.georgetown.edu/pcbe/reports/taking_care/index.html. Accessed

23. McMahan RD, Knight SJ, Fried TR, et al. Advance care planning beyond advance directives: perspectives from patients and surrogates. *J Pain Symptom Manage* 2013;46:355-365.

24. *Aging with Dignity. Five Wishes.* Available at: http://www.agingwithdignity.org/. Accessed October 12.

25. Brudney D. Choosing for another: beyond autonomy and best interests. *Hastings Cent Rep* 2009;39:31-37.

26. Shalowitz DI, Garrett-Mayer E, Wendler D. The accuracy of surrogate decision makers: a systematic review. *Arch Intern Med* 2006;166:493-497.

27. Fagerlin A, Ditto PH, Danks JH, et al. Projection in surrogate decisions about life-sustaining medical treatments. *Health Psychol* 2001;20:166-175.

28. Ditto PH, Danks JH, Smucker WD, et al. Advance directives as acts of communication: a randomized controlled trial. *Arch Intern Med* 2001;161:421-430.

29. Lo B. Caring for the incompetent patient: is there a doctor in the house? *Law, Medicine, and Health Care* 1990;17:214-220.

30. Buchanan AE, Brock DW. *Deciding for Others.* Cambridge: Cambridge University Press; 1989.

31. Annas GJ. Quality of life in the courts: Earle Spring in fantasyland. *Hastings Center Report* 1980;10:9-10.

32. Annas GJ. The case of Mary Hier: when substituted judgment becomes sleight of hand. *Hastings Center Report* 1984;14:23-25.

33. Blustein J. Choosing for others as continuing a life story: the problem of personal identity revisited. *Journal of Law, Medicine & Ethics* 1999;27:13-19.

34. Kopelman LM. The best interests standard for incompetent or incapacitated persons of all ages. *J Law Med Ethics* 2007;35:187-196.

35. Alpers A, Lo B. Avoiding family feuds: responding to surrogates' demands for life-sustaining treatment. *Journal of Law, Medicine & Ethics* 1999;27:74-80.

36. Braithwaite S, Thomasma DC. New guidelines on foregoing life-sustaining treatment in incompetent patients: an anti-cruelty policy. *Ann Intern Med* 1986;104:711-715.

37. Farrell TW, Widera E, Rosenberg L, et al. AGS Position statement: making medical treatment decisions for unbefriended older adults. *J Am Geriatr Soc* 2016.

38. Angell M. Prisoners of technology: the case of Nancy Cruzan. *N Engl J Med* 1990;322:1226-1228.

39. Berry SD, Rothbaum RR, Kiel DP, Lee Y, Mitchell SL. Association of Clinical Outcomes With Surgical Repair of Hip Fracture vs Nonsurgical Management in Nursing Home Residents With Advanced Dementia. *JAMA Intern Med* 2018;178:774-780.

ANNOTATED BIBLIOGRAPHY

1. Castillo LS, Williams BA, Hooper SM, et al. Lost in translation: the unintended consequences of advance directive law on clinical care. *Ann Intern Med* 2011;154:121-128.
   Analyzes limitations of advance directives and argues that emphasis should be on appointing a proxy whom the patient trusts to make decisions.
2. Brudney D. Choosing for another: beyond autonomy and best interests. *Hastings Cent Rep* 2009;39:31-37.
   Analyzes standards for decisions regarding incompetent patients. Argues that authenticity rather than autonomy should be the basis for decisions for patients who lack decision-making capacity.
3. Tulsky JA. Beyond advance directives: importance of communication skills at the end of life. *JAMA* 2005;294:359-365.
   Sudore RL, Fried TR. Redefining the "planning" in advance care planning: preparing for end-of-life decision making. *Ann Intern Med* 2010;153:256-261.
   Advance care planning should focus more on goals of care than on specific treatments and address the patient's and family's emotional needs.
4. Cohen AB, Knobf MT, Fried TR. Do-not-hospitalize orders in nursing homes: "call the family instead of calling the ambulance." *J Am Geriatr Soc* 2017;65:1573-1577.
   Nursing homes usually called surrogates to discuss how a do not hospitalize order should apply to a new acute event. For a number of reasons, surrogates might agree to hospitalization.
5. The President's Council on Bioethics. *Taking Care: Ethical Caregiving in Our Aging Society.* Washington, DC: The President's Council on Bioethics; 2005.
   Discusses the difficulties in determining what is best in a specific situation for a patient who lacks decision-making capacity. Argues for a case-by-case determination at the bedside by the family and physician.

Persistent Disagreements Over Care

INTRODUCTION

Disagreements over life-sustaining interventions are common, occurring in as many as one half of ICU cases (1). Although disagreements are resolved in almost all cases, in a few cases sharp disagreements persist. This chapter discusses cases in which physicians or patients (or surrogates) insist on life-sustaining interventions that the other party considers inappropriate.

Other chapters discuss related issues. Chapter 4 analyzes patient refusals that are not in their best interests. Chapter 9 discusses demands by patients or surrogates for potentially medically inappropriate interventions, analyzing the justifications for physicians unilaterally withholding such interventions and the institutional process for addressing these disputes. This chapter focuses on physician-patient discussions of such disagreements.

PATIENT OR SURROGATE INSISTENCE ON LIFE-SUSTAINING INTERVENTIONS

Clinical Considerations

Physicians are exhorted to intensify palliative care near the end of life and help patients achieve a peaceful death (2). In some cases, however, patients or surrogates insist on life-sustaining interventions that physicians believe cause suffering.

CASE 13.1	Desire for cardiopulmonary resuscitation (CPR) and mechanical ventilation in end-stage lung disease

Mr. H was a 29-year-old man with end-stage cystic fibrosis who was admitted to the hospital for antibiotics and respiratory therapy. He was emaciated, required home oxygen, and was dyspneic walking around his home. During conversations, he often paused to catch his breath or to cough up thick secretions. Lung transplantation was not an option for him because of recurrent aspiration pneumonia. He understood that his shortness of breath would get worse. He appreciated that physicians believed that CPR or mechanical ventilation had very little chance of success. He further realized that the physicians believed that if he required intubation and mechanical ventilation, he could not be weaned off the ventilator. He responded, "My entire life has been a struggle. No one thought I would live this long. I've always beaten the odds. I've always been a fighter. I'll keep fighting until the man upstairs tells me it's time to stop."

Mr. H rejected a palliative care approach and was willing to accept CPR and mechanical ventilation for the very small hope that he could be extubated. His core values included overcoming situations that others believed were hopeless.

The SUPPORT study documented shortcomings in palliative care at the end of life. This study enrolled more than 9,000 hospitalized patients with an advanced stage of one of nine illnesses (3). These patients had a hospital mortality of more than 25% and a 6-month mortality of almost 50%. For many patients who died, their last days included "undesirable states": 38% spent at least 10 days in an intensive care unit, 46% received mechanical ventilation within 3 days before death, and 45% were unconscious during their last 3 days of life. Relatives reported that 50% of conscious dying patients experienced moderate or severe pain during their last 3 days of life (4). These findings supported the idea that many patients received too much inappropriate technology and too little palliative care near the end of life.

The SUPPORT study also showed that many seriously ill patients desire interventions that have a low likelihood of success, perhaps because of overly optimistic estimates of prognosis. One study analyzed patients with metastatic cancer whose physicians predicted a 6-month survival of 10%. Thirty-six percent of such patients preferred life-extending therapy rather than relief of pain and discomfort as the primary goal of care (5). Among those patients who believed that they had a 90% chance of surviving for 6 months, 61% wanted life-extending therapy, compared with only 15% of patients who estimated their chance for surviving 6 months to be less than 90%. More recent studies confirm that patients with over optimistic estimates of prognosis are more likely to request aggressive interventions (6).

Ethical Considerations

The ethical guideline of beneficence requires physicians to refrain from interventions that would not improve outcomes, particularly if they would cause serious suffering. In this section, we analyze three difficult situations: requests that "everything" be done, requests based on religious beliefs, and requests for interventions that cause suffering with little prospect of medical benefit.

CASE 13.2   **Family insistence that everything be done**

Bishop P is a 60-year-old African American man with diabetes, quadriplegia, and persistent infections. One year ago, he developed *Staphylococcus aureus* meningitis, epidural abscess, and pneumonia. During his hospitalization, he developed quadriplegia, respiratory failure, renal failure, and persistent fevers.

Ten months later, Bishop P was rehospitalized with urosepsis from *Enterobacter cloacae*. Hypotension, respiratory failure, renal failure, stroke, and seizures complicated his course. He required mechanical ventilation and dialysis. Despite multiple courses of antibiotics, his blood cultures remained positive for *E. cloacae*, resistant to all antibiotics. A drug reaction caused a total body rash, and his skin sheared away around his bandages and electrocardiographic leads. The physicians and nurses believed that further interventions would be inhumane and disfiguring and that he would not survive the hospitalization or attempts at CPR.

Bishop P's Pentecostalist church emphasizes faith healing. Bishop P was obtunded and could not state his preferences for care. His family insisted that everything be done because he believed that all life was sacred.

Bishop P's family wanted to act in accordance with his lifelong values, appropriately making a substituted judgment (*see* Chapter 12) (7).

Requests That "Everything" Be Done

When a patient or family requests that "everything" be done, physicians should first clarify what patients or surrogates mean by "everything" (8). Many do not want literally everything done, acknowledging that some interventions might cause more suffering or harm than benefit. It is also useful to elicit the values and concerns that animate such requests and to understand what balance of benefits and burdens of interventions are acceptable. Some patients or surrogates might be concerned that if they do not insist on interventions, beneficial treatments will be withheld. Such concerns can be addressed directly.

Insistence on Interventions Based on Religion or Culture

As in Case 13.2, many patients base decisions about life-sustaining interventions on their religious, spiritual, or cultural beliefs (9, 10). Religiously-based reasons deserve special respect because they reflect a person's core values and identity. Some patients or surrogates might want any intervention that prolongs life, even for a very short time. They may believe that life is a good in itself, regardless of its quality, and that human beings must preserve and prolong life until God determines its end. Other patients or surrogates might believe that a miraculous recovery will occur if their faith is strong enough (11). Insisting on interventions might be a way of demonstrating their faith.

To many African Americans, spiritual beliefs are an important source of comfort and a means of coping with illness (12). Many believe prayer has the power to promote healing and that miracles might occur. See Chapter 44 for a more extensive discussion of how cultural factors lead many African Americans to insist on life-sustaining interventions that physicians regard as medically inappropriate. African Americans might mistrust physicians and hospitals because of a history of discrimination and limited access to medical care (13).

Physicians need sufficient information about the patient's religious beliefs to understand their impact on specific clinical decisions. Individual beliefs might differ from official doctrines. People who hold the same general belief, such as the sacredness of life, may differ in their preferences regarding specific interventions. To inquire how religion shapes a patient's decisions, a physician might say, "I understand that religion plays an important part in your father's life. Please tell me more about his beliefs." Physicians might need to understand the patient's specific beliefs regarding miracles, prayer, and divine intervention (14).

Request for Interventions That Cause the Patient Suffering

In Case 13.2, the family's request for CPR troubled caregivers, who believed that further medical interventions were causing pain and mutilation without improving the patient's prognosis. The ethical guideline of nonmaleficence, as well as professional integrity, allows health care workers not to provide interventions that cause significant suffering but prolong the patient's life only briefly (15). This rationale justifies overriding surrogate preferences and withholding interventions in exceptional cases.

Some surrogates state that the patient believes suffering serves a spiritual purpose. Caregivers should examine carefully surrogates' claims about the redemptive nature of suffering. The family's views might differ from the patient's. Many patients who believe their illness serves a spiritual purpose will still accept medications for pain and decline highly burdensome interventions (9).

Recommendations

Physicians can respond to requests by patients or families for life-sustaining interventions in several constructive ways (Table 13-1). The suggestions in Chapter 5 on informed consent might also be helpful.

TABLE 13-1. Recommendations for Responding to Requests for Life-Sustaining Interventions
Understand the patient's or surrogate's perspective.
Respond to the patient's or surrogate's needs and emotions.
Be sensitive to cultural and religious issues.
Use time constructively.
Find common ground for ongoing care.

Understand the Patient's or Surrogate's Perspective

When patients or surrogates continue to request life-sustaining interventions that the physician considers inadvisable, the doctor should first try to understand their perspective, including their understanding of the illness, concerns, goals, and expectations for care (8). This approach is generally more effective than immediately or persistently trying to persuade them about specific clinical decisions such as a Do Not Attempt Resuscitate order. Open-ended questions are helpful to elicit the patient's concerns and emotions (16):

- "What concerns you most about your illness?"
- "How is treatment going for you (your family)?"
- "As you think about your illness, what is the best and the worst that might happen?"
- "What has been most difficult about this illness for you?"
- "What are your hopes (your expectations, your fears) for the future?"
- "As you think about the future, what is most important to you (what matters the most to you)?"

Respond to the Patient's or Surrogate's Needs and Emotions

Empathic comments, which reflect the speaker's emotions, encourage patients or surrogates to explore emotions and to discuss difficult topics (16-18). In Case 13.1, when Mr. H has difficulty completing sentences, the physician might say, "It can be frightening to not get enough air." Some physicians might fear that exploring emotions might arouse in the patient and family feelings of anger, hopelessness, or sadness that doctors are powerless to alleviate. Patients and families, however, will have these emotions whether or not physicians choose to probe them. After these emotions are discussed openly, the patient and family no longer need to face them alone. Talking about emotional reactions to serious illness is frequently therapeutic, helps patients and families accept a grave prognosis, and increase their trust in the physician. Furthermore, anxiety and depression can be treated once they are identified. In turn, patients and families who feel they are understood might then be more willing to listen to the physician's perspective.

Physicians can respond to unrealistic expectations without destroying hope. One approach is to "Hope for the best, and prepare for the worst" (19). Also, physicians can use "I wish statements" to align with hopes of the patient or family, while suggesting that the desired outcome is unlikely (19, 20). In Case 13.1, the physician might say, "I wish I could make the odds be in your favor."

Be Sensitive to Cultural and Religious Issues

Bishop P and his family are African Americans, who might mistrust physicians and hospitals because of a history of discrimination and limited access to medical care. In Case 13.2, rather than leave concerns about discrimination and undertreatment unspoken, physicians might ask explicitly about the underlying issue of trust. "Many African Americans worry that they will not receive the care they need. Have you ever experienced that?" Physicians should not immediately try to reassure the family that all appropriate care will be provided (16). Reassurance is premature and generally ineffective until patients have discussed their concerns and emotions in detail (21).

Other cultural and religious traditions also have beliefs about the nature of suffering, the definition of death, the refusal of life-sustaining interventions, or the acceptance of pain (22, 23). Physicians cannot be expected to have in-depth knowledge of every culture or religion; however, doctors can ask open-ended questions to understand the cultural and religious values that impact a patient's or family's decisions (9): "How does religion or spirituality play a role in your life?" Or, "In your religion or culture, is there anything that should be done now? Is there any ceremony that should be carried out?"

Use Time Constructively

Patients or surrogates frequently have little time to adjust to a new situation before making decisions about life-sustaining interventions. Rather than trying to make a definitive decision immediately, physicians might consider how to use time to help persuade them to reconsider life-sustaining interventions that are more burdensome than beneficial. Physicians might suggest a time-limited trial of interventions, setting parameters for improvement or worsening and a time frame to reassess outcomes (24). Also, physicians can direct attention to palliative care. Doctors might say, "Your father is so seriously ill that it's possible that he might die in the hospital. Are there things that would be left undone if he were to die suddenly?" Social workers, chaplains, or the hospital ethics committee can also help the family reach closure.

Find Common Ground for Ongoing Care

The process of negotiation requires that both sides are willing to compromise (25). When patients or surrogates insist on life-sustaining interventions, a common compromise is to not add or increase interventions but also to not withdraw them. Although law and ethics do not distinguish between withholding life support and withdrawing it, the emotional difference might be significant to families.

In almost all cases, physicians eventually can reach an agreement with patients or surrogates on an acceptable plan of care. In rare instances, physicians might conclude, after repeated discussions and an ethics committee consultation, that they cannot agree with the patient's or surrogate's request. Physicians who are considering unilateral decisions to forego life-sustaining interventions should follow the procedures suggested in Chapter 9 to convene an interdisciplinary hospital committee to review the case.

CASE 13.2 | *Continued*

It is helpful to schedule regular family meetings, have one physician serve as spokesperson, and have different teams give consistent messages. Physicians should try to spend more time listening than talking. To ascertain the perspective of Bishop P's family and their needs, the physician might ask, "What are your feelings when you see your father so sick?" The doctor can also ask what they understand his skin condition is and whether they think it is painful. The physician should ask about their preferred role in making decisions. Because many surrogates find it stressful to make decisions, physicians might say, "Tell me what is most difficult about making decisions for your husband." If emotions like anxiety, fear, or guilt are identified, they should be explored further.

The physician should also ask if the family is hoping for a miracle. If so, the doctor should acknowledge that many families hope for that but also ask the family to clarify what they mean by a miracle (11). Rather than flatly disagreeing with the family's hopes, the physician might say, "I wish that we had more effective medicines for his infection."

While continuing life support, doctors might also "prepare for the possibility that the treatment doesn't work out as we all hope" (19). They might also say, "Your father is so seriously ill that no one would be surprised if he died in the hospital. What would be left undone if he were to die suddenly?"

After the health care workers have put a lot of time into listening to the family, the relatives may be more willing to listen to the perspectives of physicians and nurses. "It's very hard for us to take care of him. Every time we take his blood pressure or change his EKG leads, his skin comes off, leaving a new raw area. We feel that we're causing him more pain." Consultation with palliative care or an ethics committee generally is helpful.

PHYSICIAN INSISTENCE ON LIFE-SUSTAINING INTERVENTIONS

Physicians and hospitals might seek to administer life-sustaining interventions to an unwilling patient. This section focuses on insistence on interventions based on the physician's conscience or religious beliefs. Chapter 24 discusses conscience-based refusals to provide medical interventions.

| CASE 13.3 | **Withdrawal of mechanical ventilation** |

William Bartling was a 70-year-old man with chronic obstructive lung disease. A needle aspirate of a new pulmonary nodule revealed adenocarcinoma. After the procedure, he suffered a pneumothorax and required a chest tube and mechanical ventilation. During the next 2 months, he could not be weaned from the respirator. Mr. Bartling requested that the respirator be disconnected and he signed a living will, a durable power of attorney for health care, and a declaration of his wishes. His family also signed documents releasing the physicians and hospital from liability.

The hospital and physicians refused Mr. Bartling's request, arguing that they had an ethical duty to preserve life and that withholding life-sustaining treatment was incompatible with their own born-again Christian prolife beliefs. Attempts to transfer the patient to another hospital that would comply with his wishes were unsuccessful. The Bartling case posed the question of whether the caregivers may insist on providing life-sustaining interventions over a patient's refusal, based on their own religious views (26, 27).

Arguments for Insistence by Caregivers on Interventions

Respect the Autonomy of Caregivers

Health care professionals are moral agents with values, rights, and consciences. In this view, just as patients have the right to refuse interventions, physicians should also have the right to refuse to violate their professional ethics or personal morality. Because the United States respects freedom of religion, it would be particularly repugnant to require health care workers to carry out actions that violate their religious beliefs. Also, it would be counterproductive to require physicians to act against their moral views. A grudging or antagonistic doctor–patient relationship would not be therapeutic.

Respect the Mission of Health Care Institutions

Health care institutions might have a mission statement that expresses their goals and values. Hospices have an explicit philosophy of palliative care. Catholic hospitals have policies that forbid abortions. Many people believe that a pluralistic society should encourage such statements of mission so that patients can seek care at institutions whose moral and spiritual views match their own (28, 29).

Objections to Insistence by Caregivers on Interventions

Insistence by caregivers on providing interventions over the informed objections of patients is ethically troubling for several reasons (Table 13-2).

Undermining the Right of Refusal

If caregivers could insist on treatment, the right of patients to refuse medical interventions would in effect be nullified. In Case 13.3, the court ruled that the patient's refusal of treatment must be respected: "If the right of the patient to self-determination as to his own medical treatment is to have any meaning at all, it must be paramount to the interests of the patient's hospital and doctors" (27).

Confusion Between Negative and Positive Rights

Philosophers make a distinction between negative and positive rights. *Negative rights* are claims to be left alone, to be free from unwanted interference or intrusions. They are justified on the grounds

TABLE 13-2. Objections to Caregivers' Insistence on Life-Sustaining Interventions
Undermining the right of refusal
Confusion between negative and positive rights
Lack of timely and clear notification of patients

of respecting persons and their autonomy. An example is the constitutional right to be free of unreasonable searches and seizures. Negative rights might require other people to refrain from intervening, exerting control, or thwarting the person holding the rights. Patients have the negative right to be free of unwanted medical interventions because of the guideline of respect for patient autonomy and doctrine of informed consent (*see* Chapter 3). To be exercised, this negative right requires physicians to refrain from providing interventions that patients do not want.

Positive or *affirmative rights*, on the other hand, are claims to receive something or act in a certain way. Positive rights might require others to take action or provide means or resources, not simply to refrain from interfering (30). In Case 13.3, the physicians claimed the positive right to continue medical interventions, even though Mr. Bartling did not want it.

Negative rights are generally considered to carry more moral weight than positive rights (31). Usually, negative liberty is limited only by promises or special role-specific obligations; for example, parents cannot claim a negative right to be freed from providing their children's basic needs. The physician's role, however, does not give them the right to carry out interventions on unwilling patients. For example, surgeons have no right to insist on transfusions to save the life of a patient with severe intra-abdominal bleeding after an automobile accident if the patient is a Jehovah's Witness and refuses transfusions. In contrast, positive rights are more difficult to justify and enforce because they generally require other people to do something or interfere with the negative rights of others.

Recommendations When Physicians Insist on Interventions

Timely and Clear Notification of Patients

Physicians who work in a situation in which this conflict is likely to arise should make their position known before starting a doctor–patient relationship. Such notification would enable patients to make informed plans for their care and to seek another provider. Similarly, institutions that have policies insisting on certain interventions should describe them in their publicity and informational materials and notify patients on admission. Patients may have no option to seek another provider if they are brought by ambulance or are restricted by insurance.

Transferring Care of the Patient

Health care workers should be permitted to withdraw from a case in which they have deep moral objections to the plan of care, but they also have professional obligations not to abandon patients (*see* Chapter 24). Thus, they should facilitate transfer of the patient to a health care worker or an institution that is willing to forego withdrawal of the intervention in question in accordance with the patient's wishes.

Some physicians might not want to inform the surrogate of the option of transfer of care because they believe this would constitute cooperation with an immoral act. Physicians have an obligation under the informed consent doctrine, however, to inform patients (or surrogates) of alternatives to the proposed treatment. Generally, even if a physician personally would not carry out a medical intervention, the physician still needs to mention it if a respected minority of physicians would do so. The obligation would be even stronger if the intervention were generally considered an acceptable or standard option. If the physician did not want to provide the information personally, then he or she could ask another physician or a member of the ethics committee to do so.

Even when transfer of care can be arranged, it might be very burdensome for patients or their families. Patients might face a tragic choice if they must either accept unwanted interventions or else leave caregivers with whom they have developed a long-term relationship. Beverly Requena, a 57-year-old woman with amyotrophic lateral sclerosis wanted tube feedings withheld if she could no longer swallow. The hospital asserted that her decision conflicted with its prolife values and sought to transfer her to another local hospital that would respect her decision. When she refused to accept the transfer, the hospital went to court to force her to leave. The court ruled that because she had lived in the hospital for 17 months transfer would be upsetting and burdensome for her. The trial court judge suggested that "by rethinking their own attitudes," the hospital staff "might find it possible to be more fully accepting and supportive of Ms. Requena's decision." The court continued, "It is fairer to ask the health care workers to bend than to ask Ms. Requena to bend" (27).

SUMMARY

1. Health care workers almost always can find common ground with patients or surrogates.
2. In disagreements, physicians should start by listening to and understanding the patient's or surrogate's perspective.
3. As a last resort, physicians may withdraw from the case and transfer care to another provider.

References

1. Breen CM, Abernethy AP, Abbott KH, et al. Conflict associated with decisions to limit life-sustaining treatment in intensive care units. *J Gen Intern Med* 2001;16283-289.
2. Institute of Medicine. *Dying in America: Improving Quality and Honoring Individual Preferences Near the End of Life: National Academies Press*; 2014. Available from: http://www.iom.edu/Reports/2014/Dying-In-America-Improving-Quality-and-Honoring-Individual-Preferences-Near-the-End-of-Life.aspx
3. The SUPPORT Investigators. A controlled trial to improve care for seriously ill hospitalized patients. *JAMA* 1995;274:1591-1598.
4. Lynn J, Teno JM, Phillips RS, et al. Perceptions by family members of the dying experience of older and seriously ill patients. *Ann Intern Med* 1997;126:97-106.
5. Weeks JC, Cook EF, O'Day SJ, et al. Relationship between cancer patients' predictions of prognosis and their treatment preferences. *JAMA* 1998;279:1709-1714.
6. Feemster LC, Curtis JR. "We understand the prognosis, but we live with our heads in the clouds": understanding patient and family outcome expectations and their influence on shared decision making. *Am J Resp Crit Care Med* 2016;193:239-241.
7. Alpers A, Lo B. Avoiding family feuds: responding to surrogates' demands for life-sustaining treatment. *Journal of Law, Medicine & Ethics* 1999;27:74-80.
8. Quill TE, Arnold R, Back AL. Discussing treatment preferences with patients who want "everything." *Ann Intern Med* 2009;151:345-349.
9. Lo B, Ruston D, Kates LW, et al. Discussing religious and spiritual issues at the end of life: a practical guide for physicians. *JAMA* 2002;287:749-754.
10. Geros-Willfond KN, Ivy SS, Montz K, et al. Religion and spirituality in surrogate decision making for hospitalized older adults. *J Rel Health* 2016;55:765-777.
11. Widera EW, Rosenfeld KE, Fromme EK, et al. Approaching patients and family members who hope for a miracle. *J Pain Symptom Manage* 2011;42:119-125.
12. Johnson KS, Elbert-Avila KI, Tulsky JA. The influence of spiritual beliefs and practices on the treatment preferences of African Americans: a review of the literature. *J Am Geriatr Soc* 2005;53:711-719.
13. Crawley LM, Marshall PA, Lo B, et al. Strategies for culturally effective end-of-life care. *Ann Intern Med* 2002;136:673-679.
14. Lo B, Kates LW, Ruston D, et al. Responding to requests regarding prayer and religious ceremonies by patients near the end of life and their families. *J Pall Med* 2003;6:409-415.
15. Braithwaite S, Thomasma DC. New guidelines on foregoing life-sustaining treatment in incompetent patients: an anti-cruelty policy. *Ann Intern Med* 1986;104:711-715.
16. Lo B, Quill T, Tulsky J. Discussing palliative care with patients. *Ann Intern Med* 1999;130:744-749.
17. Suchman AL, Markakis K, Beckman HB, et al. A model of empathic communication in the medical interview. *JAMA* 1997;277:678-682.
18. Scheunemann LP, Arnold RM, White DB. The facilitated values history: helping surrogates make authentic decisions for incapacitated patients with advanced illness. *Am J Resp Crit Care Med* 2012;186:480-486.
19. Back AL, Arnold RM, Quill TE. Hope for the best, and prepare for the worst. *Ann Intern Med* 2003;138:439-443.
20. Quill TE, Arnold RM, Platt FW. "I wish things were different": Expressing wishes in response to loss, futility, and unrealistic hopes. *Ann Intern Med* 2001;135:51-55.

21. Maguire P, Faulkner A, Booth K, et al. Helping cancer patients disclose their concerns. *Eur J Can* 1996;32A:78-81.
22. Firth S. End-of-life: a Hindu view. *Lancet* 2005;366:682-686.
23. Sachedina A. End-of-life: the Islamic view. *Lancet* 2005;366:774-779.
24. Quill TE, Holloway R. Time-limited trials near the end of life. *JAMA* 2011;306:1483-1484.
25. Fisher R, Ury W. *Getting to Yes*. 2nd ed. New York: Penguin; 1991.
26. Lo B. The Bartling case: protecting patients from harm while respecting their wishes. *J Am Geriatr Soc* 1986;34:44-48.
27. Meisel A, Cerminara KL, Pope TM. *The Right to Die*. 3rd ed. New York: Wolters Kluwer; 2014.
28. Miles SH, Singer PA, Siegler M. Conflicts between patients' wishes to forgo treatment and the policies of health care facilities. *N Engl J Med* 1989;321:48-50.
29. Engelhardt HT. *The Foundations of Bioethics*. New York: Oxford University Press; 1986.
30. Collopy BJ. Autonomy in long term care: some crucial distinctions. *Gerontologist* 1988;28:10-17.
31. Beauchamp TL, Childress JF. *Principles of Biomedical Ethics*. 7th ed. New York: Oxford University Press; 2012.

ANNOTATED BIBLIOGRAPHY

1. Lo B, Quill T, Tulsky J. Discussing palliative care with patients. *Ann Intern Med* 1999;130:744-749.
   Back AL, Arnold RM, Baile WF, et al. Approaching difficult communication tasks in oncology. *CA Cancer J Clin* 2005;55:164-177.
   Quill TE, Arnold R, Back AL. Discussing treatment preferences with patients who want "everything." *Ann Intern Med* 2009;151:345-349.
   Suggestions for communicating with patients and families, emphasizing how physicians can use open-ended questions and empathic comments to understand their perceptions of illness, concerns, and emotions.
2. Lo B, Ruston D, Kates LW, et al. Discussing religious and spiritual issues at the end of life: a practical guide for physicians. *JAMA* 2002;287:749-754.
   Lo B, Kates LW, Ruston D, et al. Responding to requests regarding prayer and religious ceremonies by patients near the end of life and their families. *J Palliat Med* 2003;6:417-424.
   Suggestions for how physicians might respond in disagreements in which the patient's religious concerns or beliefs are salient.
3. Curtis JR, Vincent JL. Ethics and end-of-life care for adults in the intensive care unit. *Lancet* 2010; 376:1347-1353.
   Suggestions for improving family meetings about end-of-life decisions.
4. Sachedina A. End-of-life: the Islamic view. *Lancet* 2005;366:774-779.
   Keown D. End-of-life: the Buddhist view. *Lancet* 2005;366:952-955.
   Firth S. End-of-life: a Hindu view. *Lancet* 2005;366:682-686.
   Articles on how three non-Christian faith traditions approach end-of-life decisions.

14

Potentially Inappropriate Interventions

INTRODUCTION

Patients or surrogates sometimes request medical interventions that physicians consider pointless. The concept of futility seems an appealing way to resolve such disagreements. The term *futility* comes from a Latin word meaning "leaky" (1). In classical mythology, the gods condemned the daughters of Danaus to carry water in leaky buckets. No matter how hard they tried, they could never achieve their goal of transporting water. By analogy, futile medical interventions would serve no meaningful goal, no matter how often they are repeated. Because the term *futility* gives so much decision-making power to physicians, however, it must be used with great caution.

Some physicians claim that their judgments of futility are based on professional expertise and that they therefore do not need to share decisions about futility with patients or surrogates. These physicians contend that they should not be required to provide interventions that will not benefit patients. However, the physician's professional responsibilities need to be balanced against respecting the goals and values of patients and their surrogates.

Because the term *futility* has been used inconsistently and in confusing ways, the term *potentially inappropriate* is now preferred. The latter term conveys that these assessments involve contested value judgments and are usually not solely matters of medical expertise.

STRICT DEFINITIONS OF FUTILITY

Physicians use the term *futility* in different ways (2). In some cases, an intervention cannot accomplish the desired physiologic goals, and unilateral decisions by physicians to withhold the intervention are justified.

CASE 14.1 **Futile interventions in progressive septic shock**

A 74-year-old woman has progressive septic shock with methicillin-resistant *Staphylococcus aureus* (MRSA) infection despite treatment with appropriate antibiotics, fluids, and vasopressors. The patient's family requests an antibiotic that they learned about on the Internet, to which the patient's organism is resistant.

In this situation, there is no pathophysiologic rationale for the antibiotic, and no physiologic or clinical benefit can be achieved. Even if the family insists on the drug, there is no medical reason to administer it.

CASE 14.2 | **Progressive multiorgan failure and impending cardiopulmonary arrest**

The patient in Case 14.1 is now comatose, on renal dialysis and a ventilator. Despite fluid replacement and increasing doses of vasopressors, her mean arterial pressure is below 60 mm Hg. Her physicians want to write an order not to resuscitate her in case of a cardiopulmonary arrest.

In Case 14.2, cardiopulmonary arrest would occur because of progressive hypotension despite maximal support of the patient's circulation and oxygenation. If her refractory hypotension progresses to cardiopulmonary arrest, cardiopulmonary resuscitation (CPR) could not restore effective circulation.

CASE 14.3 | **No response to CPR**

A 54-year-old man suffers a cardiac arrest in the emergency room. CPR and advanced cardiac support are initiated promptly. The initial rhythm is asystole. After 30 minutes, there has not been any return of spontaneous cardiac rhythm or circulation. All measures recommended in the American Heart Association advanced cardiac life support guidelines have been attempted. His family insists that resuscitation be continued.

An adequate clinical attempt of CPR has failed to achieve the fundamental goal of restoring effective circulation and breathing. It is pointless to continue or repeat interventions that have already failed.

These three strict senses of *futility* are as compelling as the root metaphor of carrying water in leaky buckets. Such interventions will not achieve the goals set by the patient, and all physicians would agree that the interventions are useless. The determination that an intervention is futile in this strict pathophysiologic sense is based on data or judgments within the expertise of physicians. Physicians have no ethical duty to provide interventions that are futile in these strict senses; indeed, they generally have an ethical obligation *not* to provide them.

LOOSE DEFINITIONS OF FUTILITY

The term *futility* is more commonly used in several looser senses that are inconsistent, involve contested value judgments, and do not justify unilateral decisions by physicians to withhold interventions (3-5). The phrase "not medically indicated" commonly is used in similar ways.

CASE 14.4 | **Recurrent aspiration pneumonia and severe dementia**

A 74-year-old man with severe dementia is hospitalized for the third time in 6 months for aspiration pneumonia. At baseline, he sometimes recognizes his daughter and smiles when watching television or listening to music. The daughter, his only surviving relative, insists that he be treated with antibiotics. The resident exclaims, "Treating him is futile! His dementia is not going to improve, and it's inhumane to keep alive someone with such a poor quality of life." The resident also argues that a Do Not Attempt Resuscitation (DNAR) order should be written on the basis of futility because CPR is so unlikely to succeed.

The Likelihood of Success Is Very Small

Some physicians contend that an intervention should be considered futile if the likelihood of success in a given situation is extremely small—for example, no success in the last 100 attempts or less than a 1% chance of success (6, 7). There are problems, however, with a quantitative, probabilistic concept of futility. Why set the threshold at 1%? Some patients or families might consider a likelihood of success of 1% worth pursuing in some circumstances. However, some physicians might desire to make unilateral decisions to forego interventions whose likelihood of success is 2% or even 5%. Indeed, physicians commonly describe interventions as futile when the likelihood of success is far greater than 1% (7). In other words, a quantitative threshold depends on value judgments that are not universally accepted.

No Worthwhile Goals of Care Can Be Achieved

Futility can be defined only in terms of the goals of care (8). Some ethicists contend that the proper goal of medicine is not simply to correct physiologic derangements. For these writers, it is inappropriate to prolong life if a critically ill patient will not regain consciousness or leave the intensive care unit (ICU) alive (9).

Individual patients or the public, however, may have sharply different views. Some people regard life as precious even if the patient will not regain consciousness. Indeed, some states have public policies that favor prolonging life in patients who will not regain consciousness (10). Physicians need to discuss the goals of care with patients or their surrogates, and not attempt to define them unilaterally.

The Patient's Quality of Life Is Unacceptable

In some situations, some physicians might declare an intervention futile because they consider the patient's quality of life unacceptable, for example, if he or she is in a minimally conscious state (1). These physicians contend that sustaining biologic life is not an appropriate goal when the patient has no likelihood of regaining consciousness or interacting with other people. However, patients or surrogates may disagree sharply. Patients generally view their quality of life more favorably than family members or physicians. Quality of life needs to be assessed according to the goals and values of the patient and should not be determined solely by physicians.

Prospective Benefit Is Not Worth the Resources Required

An intervention might be termed futile because the expected outcomes are not considered worth the effort and resources required. Allocation of resources, however, should be decided by society as a whole, not an individual physician acting unilaterally at the bedside (*see* Chapter 32). Asserting that such interventions are futile closes off this difficult but essential debate (11).

Practical Problems with Loose Definitions of Futility

Physician Judgments of Futility May Be Problematic

Physicians often err when they claim that an intervention has a very low probability of success. One study analyzed cases in which residents had written DNAR orders on the basis of a probabilistic definition of futility (12). In 32% of such cases, residents estimated the probability of survival after CPR to be 5% or higher. In 20% of cases, the estimated probability of survival after CPR was 10% or greater. Thus, the term *futility* was applied when the probability of success was considered much greater than the 1% threshold for futility proposed in the literature. Problems also occur when determinations of futility are based on quality of life. When residents judged that CPR would be futile because of unacceptable quality of life, they did not discuss quality of life with a third of competent patients (12). It is ethically problematic for physicians to judge a competent patient's quality of life without talking to the patient because doctors underestimate the extent to which patients believe their lives are worth living (13).

Unilateral Physicians' Decisions Polarize Disagreements

Attempts by physicians to resolve disputes by claiming the power to act unilaterally commonly antagonize patients and surrogates. Many surrogates do not agree with physicians' judgments of prognosis. In one small study, almost two thirds of surrogates of patients in critical care units doubted the accuracy of physician's predictions of futility, and almost a third would continue life support with less than a 1% estimate of survival (14). A larger study illuminated why relatives might reject physician's estimates of prognosis. Almost one half of surrogates of patients on mechanical ventilation believed that that the patient's prognosis for survival was over 20% greater than the physician's estimate (15). There were several reasons for such optimism: some believed that maintaining optimism would improve patient outcomes or protect themselves from emotional distress, others believed that the patient has strengths unknown to the physicians, and still others grounded their optimism in their religious beliefs (15).

Furthermore, declaring one intervention futile might not settle other important issues in a case. For instance, a unilateral decision by physicians to withhold CPR in Case 14.2 might worsen disagreements about other interventions, such as mechanical ventilation, vasopressor support, and antibiotics for infection.

APPROACH IN CASES OF POTENTIALLY INAPPROPRIATE INTERVENTIONS

The term *potentially medically inappropriate* intervention is now preferred when there is some chance the intervention will achieve the effect sought by the patient but the physician believes that there are strong reasons to not provide the intervention (2). This term makes explicit that these cases involve conflicting value judgments. Such cases should be distinguished from cases of strict physiologic futility.

If discussions between the physician and surrogate do not reach agreement, physicians and hospitals should trigger a process for conflict resolution and continued discussion with the family (2). An impartial process reduces errors, arbitrary decisions, and unwarranted variation in judgments, de-escalates emotions, and establishes decisions as legitimate.

In the United States, the courts provide an impartial process for resolving disputes. However, courts are poorly suited to resolving disagreements over clinical decisions because judicial procedures are very time-consuming and adversarial. An institutional process of dispute resolution can provide a more impartial procedure than decisions by clinicians managing the case, while retaining the options of transfer to another hospital or judicial review if the disputes persist.

Obtain a Second Opinion

As a first step, the physician should obtain a second opinion from a colleague regarding the patient's prognosis and the appropriateness of the intervention, as well as the advice of experts in negotiation, mediation, and conflict resolution. The consultants might provide persuasive clinical information or suggest more effective ways to interact with the surrogate or patient. Chapter 13 offers suggestions for such discussions.

Begin the Institutional Conflict Resolution Process

The next step should be review of the case by an interdisciplinary hospital committee (2, 16). To enhance impartiality, no member of the committee should be involved in the patient's care, and the committee should include a community representative. The surrogate or patient should be given formal notice of the committee's process and invited to participate in the committee's deliberations. Hospitals should develop written policies regarding potentially inappropriate interventions. Institutional policies demonstrate that unilateral decisions to forego such interventions are based on carefully considered standards, not on *ad hoc* decisions.

Discussing potentially inappropriate interventions with patients or surrogates shows respect for them and clarifies their expectations, goals, values, concerns, and needs. It also helps physicians understand the patient-specific considerations that surrogates consider when they assess prognosis and set goals for care. After physicians better understand the values and goals of the patient, they may be more willing to continue the interventions. Alternatively, after such discussions patients or surrogates may agree with the physicians that the interventions are highly unlikely to achieve the patient's goals or that the burdens and risks are disproportionately heavy (17).

Determine Whether the Judgment of Medically Inappropriate Is Broadly Accepted

If the committee agrees with the physician that the intervention is medically inappropriate, the physician may discontinue the intervention after a waiting period during which the hospital should try to facilitate transfer to another physician or institution willing to provide the intervention. If transfer cannot be arranged, the surrogate may appeal the decision, for example, to the courts.

The Conflict Resolution Process in Practice

In Texas, a hospital medical or ethics committee must be convened in disputes over whether an intervention is not medically indicated, and the patient or family must be notified and invited to the meeting. If the committee agrees that the intervention is not medically indicated but the family disagrees, the hospital must try to work with the family to find another physician or institution willing to provide the intervention. After 10 days, if a transfer of the patient cannot be arranged, the physician and hospital are legally permitted to withhold or withdraw the intervention. The patient or family, however, may ask the courts to order that the intervention be continued beyond the 10-day period if it is likely that they will find a provider willing to accept the patient.

A study analyzed the nonjudicial review process by Texas committees. In 30% of cases, the committee rejects the physician's judgment of medically inappropriate (18). In the remaining 178 cases in which the committee agreed that the intervention was inappropriate, before the 10-day waiting period elapsed, the patient died in 43% of cases, and the family agreed to discontinue the intervention in 38% of cases. In 16% of cases, the patient was transferred to another hospital where treatment was continued. In 4% of cases, the patient improved. Overall the conflict resolution process identifies some cases in which the judgment of medical inappropriateness is not confirmed and the intervention is continued. In the majority of cases, the surrogate agrees to discontinue the intervention or the patient dies. The Texas process has been criticized because a disproportionately high percentage of cases involved ethnic minorities (19). To address this criticism, committees that review cases should contain members of communities that are disadvantaged and vulnerable in the health care system.

SUMMARY

1. The concept of futility is intuitively appealing but should only be used in rare cases carefully.
2. When futility is strictly defined, physicians may, and indeed should, make unilateral decisions to withhold interventions.
3. In persistent disagreements with patients or surrogates whether an intervention is medically inappropriate, an institutional process of conflict resolution should provide case review by an interdisciplinary committee and continued discussions with the surrogate or patient.

References

1. Schneiderman LJ, Jecker NS, Jonsen AR. Medical futility: its meaning and ethical implications. *Ann Intern Med* 1990;112:949-954.
2. Bosslet GT, Pope TM, Rubenfeld GD, et al. An official ATS/AACN/ACCP/ESICM/SCCM policy statement: responding to requests for potentially inappropriate treatments in intensive care units. *Am J Respir Crit Care Med* 2015;191:1318-1330.
3. Lantos JD, Singer PA, Walker RM, et al. The illusion of futility in clinical practice. *Am J Med* 1989;87:81-84.
4. Truog RD, Brett AS, Frader J. The problem with futility. *N Engl J Med* 1992;326:1560-1564.
5. Helft PR, Siegler M, Lantos J. The rise and fall of the futility movement. *N Engl J Med* 2000;343:293-296.

6. Schneiderman LJ, Jecker NS, Jonsen AR. Medical futility: response to critiques. *Ann Intern Med* 1996;125:669-674.

7. Gabbay E, Calvo-Broce J, Meyer KB, et al. The empirical basis for determinations of medical futility. *J Gen Intern Med* 2010;25:1083-1089.

8. Kite S, Wilkinson S. Beyond futility: to what extent is the concept of futility useful in clinical decision-making about CPR? *Lancet Oncol* 2002;3:638-642.

9. Kon AA, Shepard EK, Sederstrom NO, et al. Defining futile and potentially inappropriate interventions: a policy statement from the society of critical care medicine ethics committee. *Crit Care Med* 2016;44:1769-1774.

10. Cruzan v. Harmon. 760 S.W.2d 408.

11. Alpers A, Lo B. Futility: not just a medical issue. *Law, Medicine & Health Care* 1992;20:327-329.

12. Curtis JR, Park DR, Krone MR, et al. The use of the medical futility rationale in do not attempt resuscitation orders. *JAMA* 1995;273:124-128.

13. Ubel PA, Loewenstein G, Schwarz N, et al. Misimagining the unimaginable: the disability paradox and health care decision making. *Health Psychol* 2005;24:S57-S62.

14. Zier LS, Burack JH, Micco G, et al. Surrogate decision makers' responses to physicians' predictions of medical futility. *Chest* 2009;136:110-117.

15. White DB, Ernecoff N, Buddadhumaruk P, et al. Prevalence of and factors related to discordance about prognosis between physicians and surrogate decision makers of critically ill patients. *JAMA* 2016;315:2086-2094.

16. Council on Ethical and Judicial Affairs AMA. Medical futility in end-of-life care. *JAMA* 1999;281:937-941.

17. Smedira NG, Evans BH, Grais LS, et al. Withholding and withdrawing of life support from the critically ill. *N Engl J Med* 1990;322:309-315.

18. Smith ML, Gremillion G, Slomka J, et al. Texas hospitals' experience with the Texas Advance Directives Act. *Crit Care Med* 2007;35:1271-1276.

19. Truog RD. Tackling medical futility in Texas. *N Engl J Med* 2007;357:1-3.

ANNOTATED BIBLIOGRAPHY

1. Bosslet GT, Pope TM, Rubenfeld GD, et al. An official ATS/AACN/ACCP/ESICM/SCCM policy statement: responding to requests for potentially inappropriate treatments in intensive care units. *Am J Resp Crit Care Med* 2015;191:1318-1330.

   Consensus guidelines recommended an institutional process in refractory disputes between physicians and patients or families, focusing on reestablishing communication rather than unilateral decisions.

2. Bosslet GT, Lo B, White DB. Resolving family-clinician disputes in the context of contested definitions of futility. *Perspect Biol Med* 2018;60:314-318.

   Special issue on topic of futility and unilateral decisions by physicians.

3. Boyd EA, Lo B, Evans LR, et al. "It is not just what the doctor tells me": factors that influence surrogate decision-makers perceptions of prognosis. *Crit Care Med* 2010;38:1270-1275.

   Empirical study showing how the vast majority of surrogates take into account factors other than prognostic information from the physician.

4. Smith ML, Gremillion G, Slomka J, et al. Texas hospitals' experience with the Texas Advance Directives Act. *Crit Care Med* 2007;35:1271-1276.

   Empirical study of a statewide law on intractable disagreements over interventions that are not medically indicated. Disputes must be referred to the hospital ethics or medical committee, which involves the surrogate or patient in ongoing discussions.

Decisions About Life-Sustaining Interventions

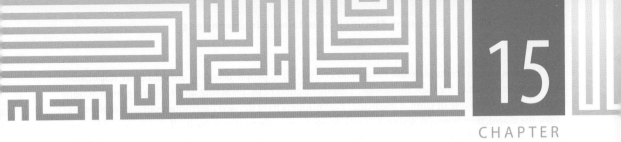

Confusing Ethical Distinctions

INTRODUCTION

In discussions about life-sustaining interventions, physicians often draw distinctions that seem intuitively plausible, but prove problematic on closer analysis. Moreover, some distinctions, although less intuitive, are nonetheless ethically valid. Failure to appreciate which distinctions are ethically meaningful and which are not leads to confusion and poor care.

CASE 15.1 | **Withdrawal of mechanical ventilation**

Mr. C, a 68-year-old man with severe chronic obstructive lung disease, developed respiratory failure. He had told his outpatient physician repeatedly that he was willing to be on a ventilator in the intensive care unit, but only for a brief period. If he did not recover, then he wanted the physicians to let him die in peace. After 2 weeks on antibiotics, bronchodilators, and mechanical ventilation, Mr. C showed little improvement and was still in respiratory failure. He asked his physicians to discontinue the ventilator and to keep him comfortable while he died. His family and primary physician believed that his decision was informed.

Some health care workers objected that although a patient may refuse life-sustaining interventions, removing them would be killing the patient. Other health care workers believed that it would be appropriate to discontinue "heroic" treatments, such as the mechanical ventilation, but that "ordinary" treatments, such as antibiotics and intravenous fluids, needed to be continued. Still others objected to the use of sedating doses of opioids for the relief of dyspnea after the ventilator was withdrawn because they would hasten death.

WITHDRAWING AND WITHHOLDING INTERVENTIONS

Many physicians and nurses are more willing to withhold interventions than to withdraw them once they have been started.

In one study, 92% of physicians agreed that physicians should comply with a competent patient's request to withdraw life-sustaining treatment (1). However, about 60% reported that it was more ethically problematic and psychologically difficult to withdraw life-sustaining interventions than to withhold them (1). Physicians who frequently attend religious services and consider religion important in their lives were more likely to find withdrawing interventions more ethically problematic than withdrawing them (although not psychologically more difficult). Physicians who had more experience caring for dying patients were less likely to report an ethical or psychological difference. Nurses are likely to have similar concerns about withdrawing life-sustaining interventions, compared to withholding them.

This distinction seems plausible because in everyday life, people generally are held more responsible for their actions than for their omissions. This distinction between acting and refraining from action, however, is not tenable in clinical medicine. Philosophers have devised ingenious examples to illustrate how the distinction between acting and refraining from acting cannot, by itself, be decisive (2). Suppose that the ventilator is accidentally disconnected from the patient. It is problematic to argue that it was permissible to refrain from reconnecting the ventilator, but not to take action to disconnect it. In either situation, the physician has an ethical obligation to respect the patient's preferences and to act in the patient's best interests as assessed from the patient's perspective. If the patient wishes the ventilator continued and the physician does not reconnect it, then it is morally wrong, even though the physician might be said to withhold the ventilator or refrain from acting. Conversely, if a patient wishes to discontinue mechanical ventilation, as in Case 15.1, then respecting the patient's wishes requires the physician to withdraw it. What is decisive is the patient's informed preferences, not the distinction between withdrawing and withholding. The considerations that justify not initiating a treatment—in Case 15.1 informed refusal by a competent patient—also justify discontinuing it.

In many cases, justifications for withdrawing treatment are actually stronger than reasons to not initiate it. Additional information might become available after treatment has started—for example, the patient did not want treatment or has end-stage disease. Furthermore, a hoped-for benefit might not materialize, as shown in Case 15.1. Typically, decisions on life-sustaining treatment must be made when the patient's prognosis is still uncertain. A time-limited trial of intensive therapy might be appropriate in this situation. If a treatment later proves ineffective, then there is no point in continuing. However, if people were unable to discontinue a treatment once it was started, then they might not even try interventions that might prove beneficial (3). The courts have consistently ruled that there is no distinction between discontinuing medical interventions and not initiating them (4). In this book, we use the term *forego* to include both withholding and withdrawing interventions.

Discontinuing implantable cardiac defibrillators (ICDs) and pacemakers raise similar ethical discomfort in health care workers (5). ICDs effectively deliver electroshocks if ventricular arrhythmias occur and can prolong survival. If deactivation of the ICD or a Do Not Attempt Resuscitation (DNAR) order is considered, the physician needs to clarify the goals for care. Discontinuing pacemakers, especially dual chamber pacemakers, may cause symptoms of light-headedness and shortness of breath. Some health care workers, patients, or family members may be reluctant to discontinue cardiac devices, particularly pacemakers because they believe it would be suicide or euthanasia; however, recent consensus guidelines carefully explain why this is not the case (6).

EXTRAORDINARY OR HEROIC CARE

People might intuitively distinguish between extraordinary and ordinary care. Interventions, mechanical ventilation, and renal dialysis, which are highly technologic, invasive, complicated, expensive, or unusual are sometimes regarded as *heroic* or *extraordinary*. In contrast, antibiotics, intravenous fluids, and tube feedings might be considered *ordinary* care. Some ordinary measures are commonly considered basic care or a standard nursing measure, such as a warm, dry bed. As in Case 15.1, some health care workers believe that extraordinary treatments may be withheld or withdrawn, but not ordinary ones.

This distinction, however, is not logical or a reliable guide to decisions (7). In some settings, such as during general anesthesia, mechanical ventilation is highly effective, desired by patients, and universally used. It is indeed appropriate to withdraw mechanical ventilation from Mr. C in Case 15.1. The reason, however, is not that the ventilator can be characterized as extraordinary or heroic, but rather that the patient does not want it and that the burdens outweigh the benefits. Instead of trying to determine whether the technology should be considered extraordinary or ordinary, physicians should examine the benefits and burdens of the intervention in the particular case, as well as the patient's preferences. The courts have rejected distinctions between ordinary and extraordinary interventions (4). Numerous rulings have declared that interventions ranging from ventilators to tube feedings may be withheld or withdrawn in appropriate circumstances (4). Chapter 20 discusses tube feedings in more detail.

RELIEVING SYMPTOMS WITH HIGH DOSES OF OPIOIDS AND SEDATIVES

Relief of pain and other symptoms in terminal illness, such as shortness of breath, is often inadequate. In the 1995 SUPPORT study of seriously ill patients, 50% of patients who died experienced moderate to severe pain in their last 3 days of life (8). In a 2018 study, almost one half of patients in a diverse urban population referred for palliative care had pain (9). Doctors might be reluctant to prescribe opioids in sufficient doses to relieve symptoms, or nurses might be reluctant to administer them (10). Some health care workers withhold high doses of opioids because they fear patients will become addicted. However, addiction should not be a primary consideration under these circumstances. Another concern is that a high dose of opioids required to relieve symptoms might hasten the patient's death by suppressing respiration or causing hypotension and, therefore, cross the line to active euthanasia or murder.

In 1996, the US Supreme Court declared, "A patient who is suffering from a terminal illness and who is experiencing great pain has no legal barriers to obtaining medication from qualified physicians, even to the point of causing unconsciousness and hastening death." Physicians, therefore, need to understand the distinctions between high-dose opioids and sedatives to relieve symptoms in patients with terminal illness and active euthanasia. One survey found that almost 90% of physicians and nurses agreed that it is appropriate to administer medication to relieve pain even if the medication hastens a patient's death (11). The doctrine of double effect, long-standing in Catholic moral philosophy, addresses this issue.

THE DOCTRINE OF DOUBLE EFFECT

Like all interventions, opioids and sedatives have both intended effects and unintended adverse effects. The doctrine of double effect distinguishes effects that are intended from those that are foreseen but unintended (12-14). In this view, intentionally causing death is wrong; however, physicians may provide high doses of opioids and sedatives to relieve suffering, provided that they do not intend the patient's death. Such high doses are permitted even if the risk of hastening death is foreseen, but not intended. The intended benefit must be proportionate to the risk of the foreseen side effect. There must be no less harmful means to accomplish the intended effect. Furthermore, the bad effect (the patient's death) may not be the means to accomplish the intended effect (relief of suffering). In addition, the unintended but foreseen bad effect must be proportional to the intended good effect. In patients who are experiencing refractory and distressing symptoms, the doctrine of double effect justifies high doses of opioids and sedatives if alternative means to relieve symptoms, such as lower doses, are ineffective and if the physician's intention is to relieve symptoms, not shorten the patient's life. If the patient is close to death because of the underlying illness, it seems unlikely that these medications significantly shorten the patient's survival.

Problems with the Double-Effect Doctrine

The doctrine of double effect, although widely accepted, presents several problems. First, people commonly have multiple intentions (15). In one study, physicians who ordered sedatives and analgesics while withholding life-sustaining interventions said they intended both to decrease pain and to hasten death in about a third of cases (16). Second, the doctrine of double effect seems to focus on what physicians say rather than on what they do. It seemingly implies that physicians may administer large doses of opioids if they can put out of mind the possibility that death might be hastened. Third, people generally are held accountable for consequences they foresee or should have foreseen, not merely for those consequences they intended.

The issue of intention is further clouded because refusal of medical interventions by a competent patient might involve the intention to hasten death in some cases. Many competent patients who forego life-sustaining interventions hope nevertheless that they can live without them. However, some patients who refuse life support want to bring about their death. There is broad agreement that physicians should respect patient refusals of interventions, even when the patient's intention is to die. Thus, although intention is central to the doctrine of double effect, it should not be the only criterion for judging an action right or wrong.

Despite problems with the doctrine of double effect, it is useful because it provides a well-accepted rationale that allows persons who strongly oppose active euthanasia to support proportionate palliative sedation. Because of controversies surrounding the doctrine of double effect, it might be helpful to give an alternative justification for high doses of opioids and sedatives to relieve refractory symptoms. When terminally ill patients experience refractory symptoms, the physician is caught between two duties: to relieve suffering and not to cause the patient's death. In balancing these conflicting duties, proportionality is crucial. The risk of hastening death is warranted if lower doses have failed to relieve severe symptoms (17). In this situation, compassion impels the physician to give higher priority to relieving refractory symptoms than to prolonging distressing symptoms for a few hours or days, or even, in our opinion, a few weeks.

Practical Aspects of Relieving Refractory Symptoms

Intention is judged by a person's actions, as well as by his or her statements. Physicians cannot simply say that they intended to relieve pain; their actions must also be consistent with their statements (18). If physicians intend to palliate symptoms, their actions must allow the possibility of relieving symptoms without hastening death. Thus, the starting dose for opioids and sedatives must not be lethal, and the criteria for increasing the dose must be reasonable.

If the physician intends only to palliate suffering, there is no warrant for increasing the dose of opioids or sedatives when the patient is comfortable (14, 19). In conscious patients, the dose can be increased if the patient reports unacceptably severe symptoms. If patients are unconscious, physicians and nurses must assess whether patients are comfortable. Reasonable criteria for increasing the dose include restlessness, grimacing, withdrawal from pain, furrowed brow, hypertension, and tachycardia (14). These are criteria that nurses and physicians commonly use to adjust the level of sedation in a patient under anesthesia in the operating room or on mechanical ventilation in a critical care unit.

RESPONSES TO REFRACTORY SUFFERING

Some terminally ill patients might experience suffering that even excellent palliative care and high-dose opioids do not relieve. Examples are uncontrollable pain, dyspnea, or bleeding and inability to swallow oral secretions in a patient with metastatic cancer. How should physicians respond in such dire situations?

Proportionate Palliative Sedation

In terminal illness, symptom relief generally is achieved with the patient remaining conscious (20). In palliative sedation, sedatives and analgesics are administered to a patient with terminal illness, with doses increased as needed to control refractory symptoms, even if unconsciousness may result. The most commonly reported refractory symptoms leading to palliative sedation are agitation or restlessness, pain, confusion, respiratory distress, and myoclonus. In addition, all life-sustaining interventions are withheld if the patient or surrogate so decides. The patient dies of the underlying illness. Death occurs a few hours to days later, depending on clinical circumstances.

The term *proportionate palliative sedation* emphasizes that increasing the dose to that of unconsciousness is a last resort used only if expert palliative care and lower doses of sedation have not relieved symptoms (21). The American Medical Association, American Academy of Hospice and Palliative Medicine, National Hospice and Palliative Care Organization, and Hospice and Palliative Care Nurses Organization all have supported proportionate palliative care sedation (21). Various other terms are used to describe what we have described as proportionate palliative sedation, in inconsistent and confusing ways, including continuous deep sedation and terminal sedation (22). Sometimes these terms signify that unconsciousness is achieved at the onset, without titration of dosage depending on symptoms. Moreover, the patient may not be required to have terminal illness. These ambiguous terms are to be discouraged. Of note, palliative sedation may be confused with active euthanasia, as has been documented in the Netherlands, where active euthanasia is permitted (23).

Broader uses of palliative sedation, however, are ethically controversial (14). Some persons object when it is combined with withdrawing other life-sustaining interventions, particularly artificial nutrition and hydration (24). Critics note that the doctrine of double effect justifies only sedation: other reasons are needed to forego artificial hydration and nutrition, such as an informed refusal by the patient or surrogate.

Palliative sedation is also very controversial when the refractory symptom is existential or spiritual suffering rather than physical symptoms (14, 24). It is difficult to establish that existential suffering is refractory, and there is a perception that death is hastened (25, 26). Physicians are often unskilled at responding to such suffering (24) and fail to consider referral to a chaplain or the patient's spiritual or religious advisor (27).

Palliative sedation sometimes is carried out without the express agreement of patients or surrogates or without explicit authorization to withhold other interventions. This violates the principle of respect for patient autonomy. Patients have different preferences regarding sedation in their last hours or days. Some will want relief from intolerable distress even if totally sedated, whereas others will prefer to have some awareness even if in some distress. Thus, the patient or the surrogate of a patient should give informed consent to palliative sedation as a means of relieving refractory symptoms, knowing that he or she is expected to die and not regain consciousness.

Palliative sedation also has limitations as a response to refractory suffering (14). First, patients who want to die in their own home might not be able to arrange palliative sedation there. Similarly, residents of board and care facilities or nursing homes who do not want to die in the hospital may not be able to have palliative sedation where they reside. Second, palliative sedation cannot relieve some symptoms, such as uncontrollable massive hemoptysis or gastrointestinal bleeding or inability to swallow secretions. Although patients are not conscious of these conditions once they are sedated, their death cannot be considered dignified or peaceful. There is a compelling ethical argument that in these exceptional situations, titration of medications is not appropriate: unconsciousness should be the immediate goal, and medication to achieve hypotension may be needed to stop massive hemorrhage.

Proportionate palliative sedation should be carefully distinguished from active euthanasia (28), which is illegal throughout the United States. Physicians commonly confuse these two actions (23), even though they are distinct ethically.

Voluntary Stopping of Eating and Drinking

In response to refractory suffering, a patient with terminal illness may voluntarily stop eating and drinking and be "allowed to die," primarily of dehydration or some intervening complication (29). Ethically and legally, the right of competent, informed patients to refuse life-prolonging interventions is firmly established. Forcibly feeding a competent patient who refuses food and fluids would violate the patient's autonomy. Stopping eating and drinking does not require the action of a physician, and hospice workers are more accepting of it than physician aid-in-dying. It is clearly voluntary. Stopping eating and drinking might seem natural because severe anorexia commonly occurs in the final stage of many illnesses.

Voluntary stopping of eating and drinking requires considerable resolve, might last for up to 2 weeks, and, therefore, might seem inhumane. Initially, the patient might experience thirst and hunger, which can be relieved by lip moisturizer and swishing and spitting artificial saliva. Sips of fluids may prolong the process. Patients should be regularly offered the opportunity to eat and drink in case they change their minds, yet such offers might be viewed as undermining the patient's resolve. Patients typically lose mental clarity toward the end of this process, which might raise questions about voluntariness or seem unacceptable to some patients or families.

EMOTIONAL REACTIONS TO THESE DISTINCTIONS

Physicians need to appreciate that the topics in this chapter raise emotional reactions, as well as philosophical disagreements. As noted, many people find stopping a treatment is much more difficult emotionally than not starting it. Health care workers, particularly nurses, might feel that they are causing the patient's death by turning down ventilator settings, discontinuing vasopressors, turning off an implanted cardiac device, administering large doses of opioids or sedatives, or increasing sedation to make the patient unconscious if patient distress persists. The shorter the time between the withdrawal of the intervention and the patient's death, the more responsible the health care worker might feel for the patient's death.

Attending physicians should anticipate questions, misunderstandings, uncertainty, disagreement, and moral distress. Physicians should routinely elicit the concerns, feelings, and objections of other health care workers about these issues, as well as those of patients or surrogates. Moreover, doctors need to acknowledge the depth and sincerity of such feelings. Team and family meetings are often helpful for this purpose.

Strong emotional reactions might be a clue that further deliberation and discussion are needed. Other team members may raise important overlooked considerations and suggest improvements in the plan of care. Health care workers should try to articulate the reasons for their reactions. However, the fact that something is emotionally difficult does not necessarily mean that it is unethical.

The concerns of nurses and house staff should be accommodated if reasonably possible. Nurses who have strong personal objections to the plan of care should not be required to carry it out. Staffing plans should allow for reasonable accommodation, and generally other nurses will volunteer to care for the patient. The attending physician should closely monitor the administration of opioids and sedatives, rather than leave it completely to the nurses and house staff. Nurses and house officers appreciate the attending physician's presence at the bedside when mechanical ventilation is withdrawn or palliative sedation initiated.

PROVIDING CARE DURING A CRISIS

A highly publicized episode during Hurricane Katrina crisis in 2005 illustrates the importance of distinguishing clearly between euthanasia and palliative sedation (30, 31).

CASE 15.2   Alleged active euthanasia during Hurricane Katrina

In August 2005, Hurricane Katrina caused widespread flooding in New Orleans. Memorial Hospital was accessible only by boat. All power was lost, so hospital equipment, computers, telephone lines, and air conditioning failed. Running water was also lost, and temperatures inside reached 100 degrees. Although some patients were evacuated, no coordinated rescue plan could be implemented.

Patients were triaged for evacuation. Highest priority was given to critically ill infants and adults and to pregnant women. A decision was made to not evacuate patients with DNAR orders. Allegations were made that physicians were injecting some patients who would not be evacuated with lethal doses of morphine. Forty-five patients died at the hospital, more than at any comparably sized hospital in the city. Eventually all patients were evacuated.

In July 2006, the Attorney General of Louisiana recommended charges of second-degree murder against Dr. Anna Pou and two nurses for administering a "lethal cocktail" of morphine and midazolam to kill four patients. Dr. Pou responded in an interview, "I did not murder those patients... I do not believe in euthanasia. I don't think it's anyone's decision to make when a patient dies. However, what I do believe in is comfort care, and that means that we ensure that they do not suffer pain." Many New Orleans residents, as well as several medical organizations, strongly defended Dr. Pou. In August 2007, the grand jury refused to indict Dr. Pou. After extensive press coverage, the coroner reviewed the cases in 2010 and called them "unclassified."

Keeping Ethical Distinctions Clear

The facts of this case may never be determined; conflicting accounts have been reported, and there has been no testimony in court under oath and cross-examination. The case illustrates that it is crucial to distinguish active euthanasia from palliative sedation. Proportionate palliative sedation to relieve intractable symptoms is always appropriate. The Katrina case illustrates that special challenges arise if it is not feasible to monitor the patient closely, to increase dosage as needed, and to document the plan for care. As Chapter 19 discusses, active euthanasia, intentionally causing or hastening a patient's death, is illegal throughout the United States. For the sake of discussion, let us assume that Dr. Pou intended to carry out palliative sedation, not active euthanasia. How might such care during an emergency have been improved?

Suggestions for Decisions During a Crisis

The Katrina case is an extreme example of how cases involving refractory suffering and palliative sedation commonly involve great stress and strong emotions. The following suggestions will help ensure that decisions are sound.

Obtain the Agreement of Other Staff

Although clear communication is important in any clinical situation, it is particularly important when palliative sedation is proposed during a crisis. The attending physician should anticipate objections and misunderstandings about palliative sedation. As in ordinary clinical care, health care workers may opt not to administer the medications for palliative sedation personally. Health care workers are more likely to work effectively toward the common goal and keep up their morale if they can voice their concerns and objections, understand the plan of care, raise important overlooked considerations, and suggest improvements in the plan. Conversely, if most members of the team remain in strong disagreement, the attending physician should reconsider the plan.

Obtain the Agreement of the Patient or Surrogate

During a crisis, staff may feel that they lack time to spend with patients. Furthermore, it may be impossible to contact surrogates of patients who lack decision-making capacity. Health care workers may wish to protect patients from grim news; however, patients who are still sentient undoubtedly already realize that their situation is dire. Competent patients should be offered a choice regarding palliative sedation, as in usual clinical care. Some patients will welcome analgesia and sedation in such a crisis, whereas others may wish to remain as lucid as possible or hope that they will survive against unfavorable odds. The Katrina case illustrates how predictions during a disaster are uncertain. Although the consequences of the hurricane were far worse than expected, the appearance of rescue teams was not anticipated when plans for the day were made.

Consider Other Actions to Relieve Distress

Palliative sedation is a means toward the goal of relieving intractable suffering, not a goal in itself. Caregivers also should consider other ways to relieve suffering. If patients will die because evacuation is not possible, then it may be critical for them to have the opportunity to reach closure, to say a prayer, or to voice their good-byes to absent family members. Even if health care workers can spend only a few minutes in a crisis, such actions may provide needed relief to the patient.

Plan for Disasters

Hurricane Katrina showed that hospitals and states need to better prepare for disasters that are inevitable in the future, for example, after an earthquake or epidemic (32, 33). Without planning and staff training, health care workers will be unprepared to make life-and-death decisions.

CASE 15.2 *Continued*

Hurricane Katrina presented unprecedented circumstances, with severe staff shortages, lack of basic resources like electricity and telephones, and great uncertainty. Although usual standards of care were impossible, fundamental ethical principles need to be observed to the extent circumstances permitted (33). The distinction between palliative sedation and active euthanasia is still important. The preferences of the patient are still crucial, as some patients who were not expected to be evacuated or to survive might prefer to be lucid rather than sedated. During a crisis, communication among caregivers regarding the goals of care and specific orders remains crucial. Although most physicians will never encounter such a crisis, clear thinking about general rules is essential before considering exceptions necessitated by an extraordinary situation.

SUMMARY

1. Several commonly held distinctions regarding life-sustaining interventions are not logically and ethically tenable.
2. Physicians should appreciate that it might be appropriate to withdraw interventions that have been started or that some persons consider ordinary care.
3. Administering increasing doses of opioids and sedatives is appropriate to relieve refractory symptoms in patients who have a terminal illness or who have refused mechanical ventilation.
4. Increasing the dose of opioids and sedatives proportionately is appropriate if lower doses have not controlled the patient's symptoms.

References

1. Chung GS, Yoon JD, Rasinski KA, et al. US physicians' opinions about distinctions between withdrawing and withholding life-sustaining treatment. *J Relig Health* 2016;55:1596-1606.
2. Brock D. Forgoing life-sustaining food and water: is it killing? In: Lynn J, ed. *By No Extraordinary Means.* Expanded edition ed. Bloomington: Indiana University Press; 1989:117-131.
3. Lo B, Rouse F, Dornbrand L. Family decision-making on trial: who decides for incompetent patients? *N Engl J Med* 1990;322:1228-1231.
4. Meisel A, Cerminara KL, Pope TM. *The Right to Die.* 3rd ed. New York: Wolters Kluwer; 2014.
5. Kramer DB, Mitchell SL, Brock DW. Deactivation of pacemakers and implantable cardioverter-defibrillators. *Prog Cardiovasc Dis* 2012;55:290-299.
6. Lampert R, Hayes DL, Annas GJ, et al. HRS expert consensus statement on the management of cardiovascular implantable electronic devices (CIEDs) in patients nearing end of life or requesting withdrawal of therapy. *Heart Rhythm* 2010;7:1008-1026.
7. President's Commission for the Study of Ethical Problems in Medicine and Biomedical and Behavioral Research. *Deciding to Forego Life-sustaining Treatment.* Washington: U.S. Government Printing Office; 1983:82-89.
8. The SUPPORT Investigators. A controlled trial to improve care for seriously ill hospitalized patients. *JAMA* 1995;274:1591-1598.
9. Dhingra L, Barrett M, Knotkova H, et al. Symptom distress among diverse patients referred for community-based palliative care: sociodemographic and medical correlates. *J Pain Symptom Manage* 2018;55:290-296.
10. Edwards MJ, Tolle SW. Disconnecting the ventilator at the request of a patient who knows he will then die: the doctor's anguish. *Ann Int Med* 1992;117:254-256.
11. Solomon MZ, O'Donnell LO, Jennings B, et al. Decisions near the end of life: professional views on life-sustaining treatments. *Am J Public Health* 1993;83:14-23.
12. Beauchamp TL, Childress JF. *Principles of Biomedical Ethics.* 7th ed. New York: Oxford University Press; 2012.
13. McIntyre A. The double life of double effect. *Theor Med Bioeth* 2004;25:61-74.
14. Lo B, Rubenfeld G. Palliative sedation in dying patients: "we turn to it when everything else hasn't worked." *JAMA* 2005;294:1810-1816.

15. Quill TE. Doctor, I want to die. Will you help me? *JAMA* 1993;270:870-873.
16. Wilson WC, Smedira NG, Fink C, et al. Ordering and administration of sedatives and analgesics during the withholding and withdrawal of life support from critically ill patients. *JAMA* 1992;267:949-953.
17. President's Commission for the Study of Ethical Problems in Medicine and Biomedical and Behavioral Research. *Deciding to Forego Life-sustaining Treatment*. Washington: U.S. Government Printing Office; 1983:73-89.
18. Alpers A, Lo B. The Supreme Court addresses physician-assisted suicide: can its decisions improve palliative care. *Arch Fam Pract* 1999;8:200-205.
19. Kamdar MM, Doyle KP, Sequist LV, et al. Case records of the Massachusetts General Hospital. Case 17-2015. A 44-year-old woman with intractable pain due to metastatic lung cancer. *N Engl J Med* 2015;372:2137-2147.
20. Sykes N, Thorns A. The use of opioids and sedatives at the end of life. *Lancet Oncol* 2003;4:312-318.
21. Quill TE, Lo B, Brock DW, et al. Last-resort options for palliative sedation. *Ann Intern Med* 2009;151:421-424.
22. Twycross R. Second thoughts about palliative sedation. *Evid Based Nurs* 2017;20:33-34.
23. Lo B. Euthanasia in the Netherlands: what lessons for elsewhere? *Lancet* 2012;380:569-570.
24. Jansen LA, Sulmasy DP. Sedation, alimentation, hydration, and equivocation: careful conversation about care at the end of life. *Ann Intern Med* 2002;136:845-849.
25. Taylor BR, McCann RM. Controlled sedation for physical and existential suffering? *J Palliat Med* 2005;8:144-147.
26. Rousseau P. Palliative sedation in the control of refractory symptoms. *J Palliat Med* 2005;8:10-12.
27. Lo B, Ruston D, Kates LW, et al. Discussing religious and spiritual issues at the end of life: a practical guide for physicians. *JAMA* 2002;287:749-754.
28. Lo B. Beyond Legalization—Dilemmas physicians confront regarding aid in dying. *N Engl J Med* 2018;378:2060-2062.
29. Quill TE, Ganzini L, Truog RD, et al. Voluntarily stopping eating and drinking among patients with serious advanced illness-clinical, ethical, and legal aspects. *JAMA Intern Med* 2018;178:123-127.
30. Fink S. *The deadly choices at Memorial*. 2009. Available at: http://www.propublica.org/article/the-deadly-choices-at-memorial-826. Accessed June 25, 2018.
31. *Katrina One Year Later: For Dear Life*. A five-part series from The Times-Picayune. 2006. Available at: https://www.nola.com/katrina/index.ssf/2006/08/for_dear_life_part_1.html. Accessed June 25, 2018.
32. Curiel TJ. Murder or mercy? Hurricane Katrina and the need for disaster training. *N Engl J Med* 2006;355:2067-2069.
33. Altvogel B, Stroud C, Hanson SL, et al. *Guidance for Establishing Crisis Standards of Care for Use in Disaster Situations*. 2009. Available at: http://www.nap.edu/catalog.php?record_id=12749&m=0003000740. Accessed June 25, 2018.

ANNOTATED BIBLIOGRAPHY

1. Quill TE, Dresser R, Brock DW. The rule of double effect—A critique of its role in end-of-life decision making. *N Engl J Med* 1997;3337:1768-1771.
   Analysis of the doctrine of double effect and its application to decisions on life-sustaining interventions.
2. Lo B, Rubenfeld G. Palliative sedation in dying patients: "we turn to it when everything else hasn't worked." *JAMA* 2005;294:1810-1816.
   Analysis of palliative sedation and the doctrine of double effect, which justifies it even for persons who believe that intentionally hastening death is unethical.
3. Quill TE, Ganzini L, Truog RD, et al. Voluntarily stopping eating and drinking among patients with serious advanced illness-clinical, ethical, and legal aspects. *JAMA Intern Med* 2018;178:123-127.
   Analysis of an option that some patients with serious advanced illness choose.
4. Lampert R, Hayes DL, Annas GJ, et al. HRS expert consensus statement on the management of cardiovascular implantable electronic devices (CIEDs) in patients nearing end of life or requesting withdrawal of therapy. *Heart Rhythm 2010;7:1008-1026.*
   Comprehensive analysis of withdrawal of life-sustaining cardiac devices.
5. Okie S. Dr. Pou and the hurricane—Implications for patient care during disasters. *N Engl J Med* 2008;358:1-5.
   Analysis of palliative sedation versus active euthanasia in the context of Hurricane Katrina.

Ethics Consultations and Ethics Committees

INTRODUCTION

Ethical dilemmas in clinical practice can lead to deep disagreements and strong emotions. The Joint Commission requires health care institutions to have a mechanism to address ethical issues in patient care, such as an ethics committee or an ethics consultation service. Ethics case consultations might be carried out by the full ethics committee, by a smaller team, or by an individual consultant; we thus use the term *ethics consultant* to refer to all of these options. Compared with court proceedings, such consultations are timelier and less adversarial. This chapter reviews the goals, problems, and effective procedures of ethics consultations. Although ethics committees usually have several tasks, such as educational activities and development of institutional policies, this chapter focuses only on their work as consultants.

GOALS OF ETHICS CONSULTATIONS

The goal of ethics consultations is to analyze and help resolve ethical problems in clinical care (1). Ethics consultations in intensive care unit (ICU) cases involving value conflicts reduce the length of hospitalization for patients who die during hospitalization and are viewed as helpful by family members (2, 3).

CASE 16.1   **Disagreement between family and health care teams**

A 76-year-old widower with severe Alzheimer disease is cared for by his two daughters and their families. He does not engage in conversations, but usually responds appropriately to simple questions. He often smiles when playing with his grandchildren and when watching television. For the third time in 6 months, he is hospitalized for pneumonia despite aspiration precautions.

The physicians believe that antibiotics are "futile" in this case and strongly recommend a palliative approach. The patient has not appointed a health care proxy, but had indicated to his primary physician that his daughters should make decisions for him. His daughters acknowledge that their father has limited life expectancy, but believe that he still has acceptable quality of life. "His family was always the most important thing to him. He always said that nothing made him happier than seeing his grandchildren grow up."

At the attending physician's request, two members of the ethics committee review the patient's medical record. They agree that antibiotics are futile in this situation. Family members are outraged. "Who are these people? They've never even spoken to us."

Clarify the Facts of the Case

The first step in ethics consultations is to gather information about the medical situation and the ethical issues in the case. Ethics consultants should not uncritically accept secondhand data, which might omit important information or views (4). Moreover, conclusions and inferences might be presented rather than primary data. For instance, physicians or nurses might describe interventions as "futile" without explaining in what sense they are using this term. In Case 16.1, the ethics consultants need to gather information about previous statements by the patient about his values and wishes for care.

Identify and Analyze Uncertainty and Conflict Over Ethical Issues

Physicians, patients, and families commonly use ethical concepts and terms without analyzing them carefully. In Case 16.1, concepts needing clarification are *futility* (*see* Chapter 9), *quality of life* (*see* Chapter 4), and *surrogate decision making* (*see* Chapter 13).

Build Consensus Among Stakeholders

Ethics case consultants should help the stakeholders arrive at decisions that are acceptable to them, within the bounds of acceptable ethical practice (5). Ethics consultants should not impose their own personal views about the course of action, but rather allow the stakeholders to reach a decision that is consistent with ethical guidelines, their own values, and the patient's values. This process usually requires discussion and negotiation (Table 16-1).

Help Stakeholders Express Their Views and Concerns

Patients and family members often feel that physicians are not listening to them. Conversely, physicians often complain that patients and family members do not hear their recommendations. Ethics consultants need to elicit the concerns and views of the various stakeholders. When patients and relatives feel their voices have been heard, they usually are more willing to listen to the physicians' assessment of the patient's prognosis and to recommendations. Moreover, physicians who hear the patient and family generally appreciate that their positions are based on deeply felt concerns and values.

Improve Communication

Many ethical dilemmas are exacerbated by breakdowns in communication. The ethics consultant can help improve communication through empathic listening and by summarizing each stakeholder's perspective. Furthermore, a frequent recommendation to health care providers is to spend more time understanding the patient's and family's concerns and needs; for example, by using open-ended questions, rather than trying to convince them to accept the physician's perspective.

Provide Emotional Support

In situations such as the one discussed in Case 16.1, emotions often are intense. In response to the patient's serious clinical situation, the children might have a variety of feelings, including grief, anxiety, and anger. The attending physician, house officers, and nurses in Case 16.1 felt frustrated

TABLE 16-1. Goals of Ethics Case Consultations
Clarify the facts of the case.
Identify and analyze uncertainty and conflict over ethical issues.
Build consensus among stakeholders.
Help stakeholders express their views and concerns.
Improve communication among clinical caregivers, patient, and family.
Provide emotional support.
Negotiate an acceptable resolution.

at the repeated hospitalizations. Unless such feelings are acknowledged and addressed, discussion of substantive issues may not be fruitful.

Negotiate an Acceptable Resolution

Ethics consultants need to know how to lead a discussion, to assure that all views are presented, and to help parties appreciate other points of view (6). Bioethics training programs sometimes fail to teach these interpersonal skills. After such a discussion, parties who had been in conflict may be willing to go along with the plan for care, even if it is not the approach they would take personally.

POTENTIAL PROBLEMS WITH ETHICS CASE CONSULTATIONS

Although ethics consultations might help resolve disputes, they might also be problematic (Table 16-2) (4, 7), as Case 16.1 illustrated.

Lack of Participation of Patients or Surrogates

Patients or relatives usually feel outraged if ethical issues are resolved "behind closed doors" without their knowledge or participation and by people whom they have never met (4). They might feel that their decision-making responsibility has been usurped.

Bias or Perceived Bias

Patients or surrogates who disagree with physicians might regard an ethics consultation as serving the interests of the physician or institution. Ethics consultants are generally employees of the hospital and might be colleagues of the health care workers in the case. Hence, families might perceive them as biased in favor of the doctors, nurses, and hospital.

Unsound Recommendations

Agreement among ethics committee members or consultants does not guarantee that their recommendations are sound. In Case 16.1, the ethics committee members adopted a view of *futility* that is highly problematic (*see* Chapter 14). Antibiotics are effective in treating the episode of aspiration pneumonia, even though they have no impact on the course of dementia or the risk of further episodes of aspiration.

Problems Beyond the Scope of an Ethics Consultation

In some cases, the problems concern legal liability, staff grievances, or discharge planning, rather than strictly ethical issues. It is unwise for ethics committees and consultants to take on the duties of risk managers, hospital administrators, psychiatrists, or social workers.

PROCEDURES FOR ETHICS CASE CONSULTATIONS

For ethics case consultations to be widely accepted, they must be regarded as accessible and fair (4, 7).

TABLE 16-2.   Potential Problems with Ethics Consultations
Lack of participation of patients or surrogates
Bias or perceived bias
Unsound recommendations
Problems beyond the scope of an ethics consultation

Who Can Request Ethics Case Consultations?

In addition to attending physicians, patients or their surrogates, nurses, and house officers should also be able to request case consultations. Disagreements over the need for a consultation generally indicate serious conflicts over patient care or ethical issues.

Who Participates in Case Consultations?

All health care workers providing direct patient care should be invited to attend an ethics case consultation, including the attending physicians, consultant, trainees, nurses, and social workers. The patient and family also should attend. Broad attendance ensures that all pertinent information is presented and all viewpoints are represented. As a practical matter, people are more likely to accept recommendations if they are allowed to express their views and to hear the reasoning behind a decision. In some cases, health care workers need to think through the ethical concerns before meeting with the patient or family.

Document Recommendations

Most consultants offer specific recommendations for resolving ethical dilemmas. For instance, in Case 16.1, the ethics consultation can recommend that more information about the patient's previous statements should be gathered. Recommendations should be written in the medical record, together with their rationale. Unwritten recommendations invite misunderstandings and reduce accountability. As with any consultation, the attending physician retains the power to follow or not follow the recommendations. Ethically and legally, the attending should act as a reasonable physician would after receiving the recommendations.

QUALITY OF ETHICS CONSULTATION

Clinical ethics consultants can speak with patients or family members, have access to confidential medical information, and make recommendations about the patient's care in the medical record. However, ethics consultants currently are the only persons with such patient care responsibilities who do not have certification or credentialing requirements. Establishment of a certification process for ethics consultants would promote quality of patient care (1, 8).

SUMMARY

1. No single approach to ethics consultations is appropriate for all hospitals and situations.
2. Persons who conduct ethics case consultations need to be aware of the potential pitfalls and the steps that can be taken to avoid them.

References

1. Dubler NN, Webber MP, Swiderski DM. Charting the future. Credentialing, privileging, quality, and evaluation in clinical ethics consultation. *The Hastings Center Report* 2009;39:23-33.
2. Schneiderman LJ, Gilmer T, Teetzel HD, et al. Effect of ethics consultations on non-beneficial life-sustaining treatments in the intensive care setting: a multi-center, prospective, randomized, controlled trial. *JAMA* 2003;290:1166-1172.
3. Lo B. Answers and questions about ethics consultations. *JAMA*. 2003;290:1208-1210.
4. Lo B. Behind closed doors: promises and pitfalls of ethics committees. *N Engl J Med* 1987;317:46-49.
5. Aulisio MP, Arnold RM, Youngner S, ed. *Ethics Consultation: From Theory to Practice*. Baltimore: Johns Hopkins University Press; 2003.
6. Arnold RM, Silver MHW. Techniques for training ethics consultants: why traditional classroom methods are not enough. In: Aulisio MP, Arnold RM, Youngner SJ, ed. *Ethics Consultation: From Theory to Practice*. Baltimore: Johns Hopkins University Press; 2003. pp. 70-87.

7. Fletcher JC, Moseley KL. The structure and process of ethics consultation services. In: Aulisio MP, Arnold RM, Youngner S, ed. *Ethics Consultation: From Theory to Practice*. Baltimore: Johns Hopkins University Press; 2003:96-120.

8. Kon AA. Clinical ethicists have an ethical obligation to create professional standards and a national certification process. *AJOB* 2016;16:30-32.

ANNOTATED BIBLIOGRAPHY

1. Lo B. Behind closed doors: promises and pitfalls of ethics committees. *N Engl J Med* 1987;317:46-49.
   Discusses potential problems with ethics committees, such as exclusion of patients and nurses, reliance on secondhand data, and groupthink.

2. Aulisio MP, Arnold RM, Youngner SJ. Health care ethics consultation: nature, goals and competencies. *Ann Intern Med* 2000;133:59-69.
   Report of an interdisciplinary task force to set standards for ethics consultations by ethics committees and individual consultants.

3. Schneiderman LJ, Gilmer T, Teetzel HD, et al. Effect of ethics consultations on non-beneficial life-sustaining treatments in the intensive care setting: a multi-center, prospective, randomized, controlled trial. *JAMA* 2003; 290:1166-1172.
   Lo B. Answers and questions about ethics consultations. *JAMA* 2003;290:298-299.
   Randomized clinical trial of ethics consultations in cases of value disagreements and accompanying editorial.

4. Dubler NN, Webber MP, Swiderski DM. Charting the future. Credentialing, privileging, quality, and evaluation in clinical ethics consultation. *Hastings Cent Rep* 2009;39:23-33.
   Argues that training, credentialing, and certification will improve the quality of clinical ethics consultations.

Do Not Attempt Resuscitation Orders

INTRODUCTION

Everyone who dies suffers a cardiopulmonary arrest. Although cardiopulmonary resuscitation (CPR) might revive some patients after unexpected cardiopulmonary arrest, in severe illness CPR is much more likely to prolong dying than to reverse death. This chapter discusses the effectiveness of CPR, appropriate reasons for Do Not Attempt Resuscitation (DNAR) orders, the interpretation of such orders, and discussions with patients or surrogates about CPR.

CPR differs from other medical interventions in several ways. When a cardiopulmonary arrest occurs, physicians or nurses who might not know the patient must decide immediately whether to initiate CPR. Otherwise, the patient will certainly die. To avoid delays, CPR is attempted in every hospitalized patient who suffers a cardiopulmonary arrest unless a prior decision has been made not to do so. Unlike other medical interventions, CPR is initiated without a physician's order. Instead, a physician's order is required to withhold CPR: the DNAR order or the No CPR order.

THE EFFECTIVENESS OF CPR

To make informed decisions about CPR, patients (or their surrogates) need to understand that CPR has limited effectiveness in many clinical situations.

Outside the hospital, when a cardiac arrest occurs, most patients were previously healthy and active. In this setting, after bystanders start CPR, 8% to 10% of persons will survive with good function.

In an acute-care hospital when CPR is attempted on an adult patient on a general hospital floor, spontaneous pulse is restored in 43% of cases (1), and about 17% survive to discharge. In other words, even when CPR is attempted, about 83% of patients die. The percentage surviving to discharge is affected by decisions after the initial resuscitation to limit life-sustaining interventions. In terms of neurologic function, 72% of survivors have a good neurologic outcome, defined as able to work with no more than a mild neurologic deficit.

In perioperative settings, CPR outcomes are better because trained personnel witness the arrest and resuscitation equipment and medications are already present. Approximately 25% of patients are alive and independent in daily activities 90 days after a perioperative arrest (2).

In certain patient groups, CPR is less beneficial. Physicians have tried to identify subgroups for which the probability of successful CPR is close to zero. However, later studies have not confirmed early reports of very low survival in patient subgroups. In recent publications, 9.3% of patients who are on vasopressors when cardiopulmonary arrest occurred and 1.9% of patients with metastatic cancer survived to discharge (3, 4). Survival to discharge is 1.3% in patients above 75 years of age and 5.5% in sepsis (4).

Complications can occur in patients who are revived by CPR. A dreaded outcome of CPR is severe neurologic impairment due to anoxic brain damage. However, 86% of those who had highest category cognitive performance before CPR remained in that category. Functional status may also be impaired (3). In patients who received CPR, 84% lived at home preadmission and 51% returned home postdischarge (3). Although only 6% of CPR recipients were admitted from a nursing home or rehabilitation, 31% were discharged to one of these sites (3). Neurologic outcomes may be better after therapeutic hypothermia. Other medical complications may also occur during CPR, including fractured ribs or sternum or flail chest.

JUSTIFICATIONS FOR DNAR ORDERS

As with other medical interventions, there are several acceptable justifications for withholding CPR.

Patient Refuses CPR

Competent, informed patients may not want CPR. Many patients wish to die peacefully rather than have physicians and nurses attempt to revive them. Such informed refusals should be respected (5).

Surrogate Refuses CPR

Appropriate surrogates may decline CPR for patients who lack decision-making capacity (5), based on the patient's values, goals of care, preferences, or best interests.

CPR Is Futile in a Strict Sense

As Chapter 14 discusses, physicians may decide unilaterally to withhold interventions that are futile in a strict sense: CPR has no pathophysiologic rationale, it has already failed in the patient, or hypotension progresses despite maximal treatment. In these strictly defined situations, physicians appropriately make the decision to stop or withhold resuscitation and CPR should not be offered to patients or surrogates (5). Instead, physicians should inform them of the DNAR order and explain the reasons.

Physicians often use futility in a looser sense to justify unilateral decisions by physicians to withhold CPR. Some physicians assert that they may withhold CPR unilaterally as "futile" when patients are highly likely to die even if CPR is attempted.

CASE 17.1   **Family wants CPR even though survival would be highly unlikely**

Mr. R is a 54-year-old bedridden man with squamous cell carcinoma of the lung metastatic to liver and bone, hospitalized for pneumonia and confusion. He has never indicated his preferences about CPR. The family insists on "full code," saying that even if he does not regain consciousness or survive the hospitalization, it is worth prolonging his life for even a few hours or days. The physicians, however, consider CPR futile because the medical literature reports that very few such patients are discharged alive after cardiopulmonary arrest. Furthermore, the doctors consider his quality of life extremely poor. In their view, prolonging the patient's life for a few hours or days is not an appropriate goal for care.

Unilateral DNAR orders based on a low likelihood of success or quality of life are problematic (*see* Chapter 14) (6). Physicians are inaccurate in predicting outcomes of CPR. One study found that physicians were no more accurate at identifying patients who would survive resuscitation than would be expected by chance alone (7). Moreover, physicians often define futility far more broadly than recommended in the literature. In a study of DNAR cases in which physicians believed CPR was futile, residents estimated the probability of the patient's survival after CPR as 5% or higher in 32% of cases (8). This threshold is far looser than what is proposed in the literature—namely, zero successes in the previous 100 cases (9, 10). In cases in which families insist on CPR that physicians believe is medically appropriate, a process of institutional conflict resolution is preferable to unilateral DNAR orders (*see* Chapters 13 and 14).

DISCUSSING DNAR ORDERS WITH PATIENTS

Patients or surrogates need to discuss CPR with physicians if they are to make informed decisions about it. Physicians cannot accurately determine patients' preferences about CPR without asking them directly. In a large multicenter study, physicians misunderstood patients' preferences about CPR in about 50% of cases (11).

Barriers to Discussions

Some physicians believe that patients do not want to discuss DNAR decisions. In fact, most ambulatory patients, between 67% and 85%, want to discuss life-sustaining treatment with physicians (12, 13). Among hospitalized patients, between 42% and 81% want to discuss end-of-life decisions with their physicians (14, 15).

Physicians sometimes hesitate to discuss DNAR orders with patients, fearing that they will lose hope, become depressed, refuse highly beneficial treatments, or even attempt suicide. Such adverse outcomes, however, rarely occur.

Targeting Discussions

Physicians typically discuss CPR only with patients whom they believe are at high risk for cardiopulmonary arrest. The prospect of cardiopulmonary arrest becomes more salient as a patient's condition worsens. If discussions are deferred, however, patients might become so sick that they are no longer capable of making medical decisions. In addition, targeting sicker patients for discussions about CPR reinforces the belief that DNAR discussions signify a bleak prognosis. For these reasons, physicians should routinely discuss CPR with all adult inpatients with serious illness. Ideally, such discussions would be initiated in the ambulatory setting as part of advance care planning. When patients lack decision-making capacity, physicians should conduct discussions about CPR with appropriate surrogates.

Patient Misunderstandings About CPR

Many patients misunderstand basic information about the nature of CPR, for example, that mechanical ventilation is usually required after CPR and that patients on a ventilator are usually conscious but cannot talk (16). Patients substantially overestimate favorable outcomes after CPR (16), perhaps because of unrealistic portrayals on television (17). Many patients who initially want CPR change their minds after they are informed about the nature and outcomes of CPR (18, 19).

Improving Discussions About DNAR Orders

Better discussions with physicians will help patients make informed decisions, as Table 17-1 summarizes.

TABLE 17-1. Improving Discussions with Patients or Surrogates About DNAR Orders
Routinely invite patients to discuss CPR.
Provide information so that patients can make informed decisions.
Make explicit recommendations about CPR.
Reassure patients about ongoing care.
Allow time for decisions.

Place Discussions in Context

It is generally better to start with a discussion of the patient's understanding of the situation and his or her concerns and goals for care rather than starting with the specific decision about CPR (20).

Routinely Invite Patients to Discuss CPR

Physicians can raise the issue of CPR in a straightforward manner. "I try to discuss with all patients what to do if they become too sick to talk with me directly. How would you feel about discussing this?" If the patient agrees, the physician can continue, "One important issue is CPR. Have you heard about CPR?"

Provide Information so that Patients Can Make Informed Decisions

Often, doctors shroud DNAR discussions in euphemisms or technical jargon (21). Physicians sometimes ask patients, "If your heart or lungs stop, would you like us to start them up again?" Such phrasing mistakenly implies that CPR is as simple and effective as jump-starting an automobile battery or changing a light bulb. The question is whether patients want doctors to *try* to revive them, even though the likelihood of death is 83% or greater. Physicians can be explicit without being blunt or offensive. To avoid bias due to framing effects, physicians should explain that if CPR is attempted, overall 17% of patients will survive the hospitalization and 83% will die. Doctors can describe CPR (including chest compressions, electroshock, and intubation) and the possible outcomes (including survival, persistent unconsciousness, and death). Some physicians try to dissuade patients from CPR by describing it in graphic detail, such as "pounding on your chest." Such biased information, however, undermines the goal of informed patient decision making. Even after discussions with physicians, patients often have serious misunderstandings about CPR. A brief video decision tool for CPR increased patient knowledge about CPR and DNAR orders before hospital discharge (22). Patients viewing the video were more likely to not want CPR and to have documented discussions with physicians about their preferences.

Make Explicit Recommendations About CPR

Physicians can offer recommendations while still allowing patients ultimate decision-making power. In rare cases, if CPR would be futile in a strict sense, then physicians should not simply offer patients or surrogates a choice but instead inform them of the DNAR order, its rationale, and the procedures families can take if they disagree.

Reassure Patients About Ongoing Care

Some patients fear that after a DNAR order, physicians will give up on them. Physicians need to emphasize plans for treating other problems, seeing the patient regularly, and providing palliative care.

Allow Time for Decisions

Patients or surrogates often need time to think about issues and deal with their emotions. Even in the emergency department, physicians usually can give them some private time to reflect and return later to resume the discussion.

Physicians can improve their skills at DNAR discussions. Doctors seldom observe more experienced physicians carry out such discussions or have colleagues watch them (23). Asking the advice of colleagues about a particular situation, role-playing, and reviewing videotapes of simulated discussions can be helpful.

| CASE 17.1 | *Continued* |

If Mr. R were to suffer a cardiopulmonary arrest, his likelihood of survival would be even lower than the 2% figure for persons with metastatic cancer. However, the physicians need to try to work with the family on a plan that is mutually acceptable. The physicians should shift the focus of discussions from CPR to the goal of care. What were Mr. R's hopes and fears? What would remain unfinished if he were to die soon? Using an approach of "hope for the best but plan for the worst" (24), physicians might ask if there are relatives who should visit and say what they have not yet said to the patient. Doctors can also ask the family for suggestions on how to make the patient more comfortable. The physicians can also ask whether religion and spirituality were important to Mr. R, to ascertain his goals for care.

Such patient-centered discussions show respect for patients and families and may make them more receptive to the physicians' recommendations about what is best for the patient.

If such discussions do not lead to a mutually acceptable plan for care, the physician may request an ethics consultation or initiate the hospital procedures for foregoing life-sustaining interventions without the concurrence of surrogates.

IMPLEMENTING DNAR ORDERS

Writing a DNAR Order

DNAR orders are common in critically and terminally ill patients. CPR is not attempted for 89% of seriously ill patients who die in acute care hospitals (25). To prevent misunderstandings, physicians should write DNAR orders in the medical record. In addition, the physician should explain in a progress note the rationale for the DNAR order, document the agreement of the patient or surrogate, and describe plans for further care. In the outpatient setting, DNAR orders may be entered on a POLST (Physicians Orders for Life Sustaining Medical Treatment) form so that the orders can be available to first responders and emergency department personnel. DNAR orders should be reviewed periodically, particularly if the patient's condition changes.

Oral DNAR orders might lead to mistakes, misunderstandings, and confusion. They create ethical quandaries and legal jeopardy for nurses and first responders to cardiopulmonary arrests. Generally considering an oral DNAR order indicates serious disagreements and a need for further discussions. A DNAR order over the telephone may be acceptable in an urgent situation, provided that the physician signs the order promptly.

Interpretation of DNAR Orders

Implications for Other Treatments

Strictly speaking, a DNAR order means only to withhold CPR. Other treatments, such as antibiotics, transfusions, and even intensive care, might still be appropriate. However, the same reasons that make CPR inappropriate might also render other interventions unsuitable. Many hospitals now require more detailed orders than simply "no CPR," for example, specifying on a checklist whether or not to provide mechanical ventilation, vasopressors, or antiarrhythmic drugs. Such detailed orders clarify whether nurses should treat abnormalities, such as hypotension or ventricular arrhythmia, or allow them to progress, perhaps to cardiopulmonary arrest.

Advances in medical technology require physicians to be even more specific about what a DNAR order means. Noninvasive ventilation, also known as noninvasive positive pressure ventilation or BiPAP, which uses a tightly fitting mask rather than intubation, may allow time for treatments directed at the cause of the episode of respiratory failure or to delay death to achieve a specific goal. Some patients find the mask unbearable, but deep sedation is not feasible. If a patient with chronic obstructive lung disease or congestive heart failure requests "no intubation," then physicians should clarify whether the patient would accept or decline noninvasive ventilation. These discussions need to be tied to goals of care and identify criteria for success or failure of the intervention (26). Patients may be willing to try noninvasive ventilation, with the understanding that it may be discontinued if it proves unsuccessful or not tolerated.

"Limited" or "Partial" DNAR Orders

Some patients or surrogates may wish to withhold aspects of advanced life support, such as defibrillation or intubation. For instance, patients with chronic obstructive lung disease may decline mechanical ventilation but agree to other resuscitative measures. Such restrictions limit chances for survival. Even if basic CPR is ineffective, advanced life support might restore circulation, breathing, and consciousness. The physician should clarify how such restrictions fit with the patient's goals of care (27). "Limited" DNAR orders are appropriate if an informed patient (or surrogate) consents to them or requests them.

Preventing Misunderstandings

Some physicians are reluctant to write DNAR orders because they fear that other health care workers—consultants, house staff, nurses, or respiratory therapists—might cease to provide needed care to the patient. Conversely, some nurses believe that after a DNAR order, physicians will stop rounding on patients or talking to them. Concerns that DNAR orders might lead to suboptimal care need to be addressed openly. Everyone needs to appreciate that DNAR orders do not mean "do not provide care."

Slow or Show Codes

"Slow codes" or "show codes" appear to provide CPR but actually do not—or do so in a way that is known to be ineffective. For example, the code team is not paged immediately, only a few chest compressions are performed, or drugs are injected into the bed rather than into the patient. Such orders are usually given orally and not written down. Slow or show codes are sometimes considered when the patient has a grim prognosis but an attending physician insists that CPR be attempted or the patient or surrogate insists that "everything" be done, as in Case 17.1. However, show codes are unacceptable because they deceive patients or families, undermine public trust, compromise the ethical integrity of health care professionals, and cause confusion and cynicism among health care workers (28) . In most cases, families recognize that the patient's prognosis is poor, but cannot bring themselves to concur with limiting CPR. Physicians should focus on compassionate communication with such families (*see* also Chapter 13). It has been recommended that they describe how CPR would not advance the patient's goals, inform them of his or her plans to withhold CPR unless they object, invite their questions and disagreements, and take responsibility for writing the DNR order without their explicit concurrence (29).

Special Settings

Anesthesia for Surgery and Invasive Procedures

Patients with DNAR orders might undergo surgery for palliation or for conditions unrelated to their primary diagnosis. Many physicians want to "suspend" DNAR orders in the operating room, when the patient's vital functions are deliberately depressed by anesthesia and maintained using techniques similar to those of advanced cardiac life support. If resuscitation were not permitted, medications might be titrated to ensure greater hemodynamic stability but at the risk of lighter anesthesia, less analgesia, and less amnesia. CPR is more successful in the operating room than in other settings. As mentioned previously, after CPR perioperative settings, approximately 25% of patients are alive and independent in daily activities 90 days after the arrest (2); this survival rate is lower than that reported in earlier studies. Another reason for suspending DNAR orders during surgery is the surgeon's sense of responsibility for intraoperative deaths (*see* Chapter 38).

If patients with DNAR orders undergo surgery or invasive procedures, physicians should discuss the implications of the DNAR orders perioperatively, clarify the patient's goals and preferences, reach agreement with the patient or surrogate, and document plans in the medical record. Similar considerations apply to DNAR orders during conscious sedation for procedures.

Emergency Medical Services

When emergency medical personnel are called to the home of a patient with serious illness, CPR might not be appropriate. Paramedic policies and protocols should include provisions for DNAR orders. Most states allow physicians to write DNAR orders on a POLST form or a computerized registry (30). A DNAR order should not automatically preclude other appropriate care, such as oxygen or transport to the hospital. Paramedics face dilemmas when a family member requests that CPR be withheld, but there is no formal DNAR order. Many family members report that they called 911 because they needed help with a frightening complication, wanted someone to confirm death, or did not know what else to do (31). Although it is compassionate to withhold CPR in this situation, it is also ethically problematic because the first responders cannot verify the patient's medical condition or rule out problems such as elder abuse (30).

Family Presence During Resuscitation Efforts

Many family members would like to be present during resuscitation. A critical evidence-based literature review found that family presence during resuscitation in the emergency department setting does not affect patient mortality or resuscitation quality (32). Moreover, offering family presence during resuscitation may reduce subsequent symptoms of anxiety and depression in family members. The overwhelming majority of relatives who observe resuscitation attempts believed it helped them accept the patient's death and prevented prolonged grief. Some physicians and nurses fear that the presence of family during resuscitation will cause stress in caregivers, or even interfere with care. Hospitals should offer them the opportunity to be present (33), provided that educational preparation and emotional support are available.

SUMMARY

1. CPR is not appropriate for many patients, especially when cardiac arrest is expected.
2. Physicians should elicit patients' preferences about CPR and write DNAR orders in the medical record.
3. The question is not whether physicians should discuss DNAR orders with their patients, but how to do so with compassion and caring.

References

1. Fendler TJ, Spertus JA, Kennedy KF, et al. Alignment of do-not-resuscitate status with patients' likelihood of favorable neurological survival after in-hospital cardiac arrest. *JAMA* 2015;314:1264-1271.
2. Kalkman S, Hooft L, Meijerman JM, et al. Survival after perioperative cardiopulmonary resuscitation: providing an evidence base for ethical management of do-not-resuscitate orders. *Anesthesiology* 2016;124:723-729.
3. Peberdy MA, Kaye W, Ornato JP, et al. Cardiopulmonary resuscitation of adults in the hospital: a report of 14720 cardiac arrests from the National Registry of Cardiopulmonary Resuscitation. *Resuscitation* 2003;58:297-308.
4. Ebell MH, Afonso AM. Pre-arrest predictors of failure to survive after in-hospital cardiopulmonary resuscitation: a meta-analysis. *Fam Pract* 2011;28:505-515.
5. Mancini ME, Diekema DS, Hoadley TA, et al. Part 3: ethical issues: 2015 american heart association guidelines update for cardiopulmonary resuscitation and emergency cardiovascular care. *Circulation* 2015;132:S383-S396.
6. Bosslet GT, Lo B, White DB. Resolving family-clinician disputes in the context of contested definitions of futility. *Perspect Biol Med* 2018;60:314-318.

7. Ebell MH, Becker LA, Barry HC, et al. Survival analysis after in-hospital cardiopulmonary resuscitation. *J Gen Intern Med* 1998;13:805-816.

8. Curtis JR, park DR, Krone MR, et al. The use of the medical futility rationale in do not attempt resuscitation orders. *JAMA* 1995;273:124-128.

9. Schneiderman LJ, Jecker NS, Jonsen AR. Medical futility: its meaning and ethical implications. *Ann Intern Med* 1990;112:949-954.

10. Schneiderman LJ, Jecker NS, Jonsen AR. Medical futility: response to critiques. *Ann Intern Med* 1996;125:669-674.

11. Teno JM, Hakim RB, Knaus WA, et al. Preferences for cardiopulmonary resuscitation: physican–patient agreement and hospital resource use. *J Gen Intern Med* 1995;10:179-186.

12. Shmerling RH, Bedell SA, Lilienfeld A, et al. Discussing cardiopulmonary resuscitation: a study of elderly outpatients. *J Gen Intern Med* 1988;3:317-321.

13. Lo B, Mc Leod G, Saika G. Patient attitudes towards discussing life-sustaining treatment. *Arch Intern Med* 1986;146:1613-1615.

14. Reilly BM, Magnussen CR, Ross J, et al. Can we talk? Inpatient discussions about advance directives in a community hospital. Attending physicians' attitudes, their inpatients' wishes, and reported experience. *Arch Intern Med* 1994;154:2299-2308.

15. Hoffman JC, Wenger NS, Davis RH, et al. Patient preferences for communication with physicians about end-of-life decisions. *Ann Intern Med* 1997;127:1-12.

16. Fischer GS, Tulsky JA, Rose MR, et al. Patient knowledge and physician predications of treatment preferences after discussions of advance directives. *J Gen Intern Med* 1998;13:447-454.

17. Diem SJ, Lantos JD, Tulsky JA. Cardiopulmonary resuscitation on television. Miracles and misinformation. *N Engl J Med* 1996;334:1578-1582.

18. Murphy DJ, Burrows D, Santilli S, et al. The influence of the probability of survival on patients' preferences regarding cardiopulmonary resuscitation. *N Engl J Med* 1994;330:545-549.

19. O'Brien LA, Grisso JA, Maislin G, et al. Nursing home residents' preferences for life-sustaining treatments. *JAMA* 1995;254:1175-1179.

20. Lo B, Quill T, Tulsky J. Discussing palliative care with patients. *Ann Intern Med* 1999;130:744-749.

21. Tulsky JA, Chesney MA, Lo B. How do medical residents discuss resuscitation with patients? *J Gen Intern Med* 1995;10:436-442.

22. El-Jawahri A, Mitchell SL, Paasche-Orlow MK, et al. A randomized controlled trial of a cpr and intubation video decision support tool for hospitalized patients. *J Gen Intern Med* 2015;30:1071-1080.

23. Tulsky JA, Chesney MA, Lo B. "See one, do one, teach one?" Housestaff experience discussing do-not-resuscitate orders. *Arch Intern Med* 1996;156:1285-1289.

24. Back AL, Arnold RM, Quill TE. Hope for the best, and prepare for the worst. *Ann Intern Med* 2003;138:439-443.

25. Lynn J, Teno J, Phillips RS, et al. Perceptions by family members of the dying experience of older and seriously ill patients. *Ann Intern Med* 1997;126:97-106.

26. Curtis JR, Cook DJ, Sinuff T, et al. Noninvasive positive pressure ventilation in critical and palliative care settings: understanding the goals of therapy. *Crit Care Med* 2007;35:932-939.

27. Zapata JA, Widera E. Partial codes-a symptom of a larger problem. *JAMA Internal Medicine* 2016;176:1058-1059.

28. Morrison W, Feudtner C. Quick and limited is better than slow, sloppy, or sly. *Am J Bioeth* 2011;11:15-16.

29. Kon AA. Informed non-dissent: a better option than slow codes when families cannot bear to say "let her die." *Am J Bioeth* 2011;11:22-23.

30. Kellermann A, Lynn J. Withholding resuscitation in prehospital care. *Ann Intern Med* 2006;144:692-693.

31. Feder S, Matheny RL, Loveless RS, Jr., et al. Withholding resuscitation: a new approach to prehospital end-of-life decisions. *Ann Intern Med* 2006;144:634-640.

32. Oczkowski SJ, Mazzetti I, Cupido C, et al. Family presence during resuscitation: a Canadian Critical Care Society position paper. *Canadian Respir J* 2015;22:201-205.

33. Morrison LJ, Kierzek G, Diekema DS, et al. Part 3: ethics: 2010 American Heart Association Guidelines for Cardiopulmonary Resuscitation and Emergency Cardiovascular Care. *Circulation* 2010;122:S665-S675.

ANNOTATED BIBLIOGRAPHY

1. Tulsky JA, Chesney MA, Lo B. How do medical residents discuss resuscitation with patients? *J Gen Intern Med* 1995;10:436–442.
   Shows how, in discussions with patients regarding CPR, residents failed to provide key information about CPR and missed opportunities to discuss the patient's values and goals.
2. Curtis JR, Park DR, Krone MR. The use of the medical futility rationale in do not attempt resuscitation orders. *JAMA* 1995;273:124–128.
   Empirical study documenting problems and mistakes that occur when physicians claim that CPR would be futile.
3. Mancini ME, Diekema DS, Hoadley TA, et al. Part 3: Ethical Issues: 2015 American Heart Association Guidelines Update for Cardiopulmonary Resuscitation and Emergency Cardiovascular Care. *Circulation* 2015;132:S383-S396.
   Consensus ethical guidelines presented in CPR certification courses.
4. Zapata JA, Widera E. Partial codes-a symptom of a larger problem. *JAMA Internal Medicine* 2016;176:1058-1059.
   Advice to physicians on clarifying how a partial code might achieve the patient's goals of care.
5. Morrison W, Feudtner C. Quick and limited is better than slow, sloppy, or sly. *Am J Bioeth* 2011;11:15-16. Kon AA. Informed non-dissent: a better option than slow codes when families cannot bear to say "let her die". *Am J Bioeth* 2011;11:22-23.
   Two thoughtful articles on "slow" codes, offering practical advice on how physicians might constructively speak with families in cases when "slow" codes are being considered.

Tube and Intravenous Feedings

INTRODUCTION

Tube and intravenous feedings can prolong life in patients with some conditions. Persons with unresponsive wakefulness can live for years with tube feedings. Patients with short bowel syndrome can lead active lives for many years with parenteral hyperalimentation. However, in a severe, progressive illness such as advanced dementia or metastatic cancer, tube feedings might merely prolong death and subject patients to indignity. Eighty-five percent of patients with advanced dementia develop feeding problems, and almost 50% die within 6 months (2). Rates of tube feeding vary widely across states and nursing homes that are larger, without dementia care units. Organizational, cultural, and fiscal features of the nursing home or hospital are related to rates of feeding tubes (1, 3, 4).

CASE 18.1   **Tube feedings in a patient with severe dementia (5)**

Mrs. F's daughter reports that she has eaten almost nothing all weekend. A 70-year-old woman with advanced dementia, Mrs. F rarely speaks, is confined to a wheelchair, and requires diapers for incontinence. She has been kept out of a nursing home by the efforts of a devoted family and a geriatric day care center. During the past year, her social actions have decreased and her food intake has become increasingly erratic. First she stopped feeding herself. Now, although her family feeds her by hand, her intake continues to decline. Once she required overnight hospitalization for dehydration. During the past week, she has been clamping her mouth shut, pushing the spoon away with her hand, and spitting out food. Over the weekend, her intake declined despite coaxing with her favorite foods. If hand feedings continue to decline, should she be fed through a feeding tube? The patient's sister says, "We can't let her starve to death!" The daughter, however, says, "She's telling us to stop. We're just torturing her." Mrs. F had never indicated what she would want done in this situation.

REASONS TO PROVIDE TUBE FEEDINGS

Allow Reversal of Causes of Feeding Problems

Decreased oral intake might result from reversible medical problems, such as intercurrent illness, mouth lesions, side effects of medications, or psychosocial problems, such as a desire for more control, depression, or a change of caregivers. Sometimes, hand feedings can be made more acceptable to the patient, for example, by slowing the pace of feeding, offering smaller bites, altering the taste or consistency, reminding the demented patient to swallow, or gently touching him or her (5).

Temporary use of tube or intravenous feedings might resolve the crisis and allow the underlying problem to be identified and treated.

Provide Ordinary Basic Care

Many people regard tube feedings as basic humane care. In this view, feeding is an essential part of caring for the helpless, just like providing a warm, clean bed (6, 7). Recent Roman Catholic teaching considers artificial nutrition to be ordinary care in principle, although traditional Catholic doctrine allows tube feedings to be refused if excessively burdensome (7, 8).

Prolong Life

Many advocates of tube feedings believe that they prolong life in persons with advanced, progressive dementia and reduced oral intake. However, the weight of clinical evidence is that tube feedings do not prolong life compared with continued offering of food and drink by hand (2). Even with tube feedings, such patients die from other complications of advanced dementia.

Prevent Distressing Symptoms

Everyone has temporarily experienced thirst or hunger and can imagine how agonizing it must be to starve to death. Similarly, everyone appreciates how upset infants become when they are not fed. By analogy, some people believe that adult patients with terminal illness or advanced dementia suffer when tube feedings are withheld. However, if patients continue to receive hand feedings and sips of fluids as they wish, they can maintain sufficient oral intake to alleviate hunger and thirst.

REASONS TO WITHHOLD TUBE FEEDINGS

Caregivers who would withhold tube feedings from patients with severe, progressive illness frame the issues differently. They agree that it is morally obligatory to give bottles to infants, provide groceries to homebound persons, and offer spoonfuls of food to persons with dementia. However, opponents offer several reasons for withholding tube feedings when patients such as Mrs. F refuse oral intake.

Burdens of Tube and Intravenous Feedings Outweigh Benefits

Like all interventions, tube and intravenous feedings have burdens, as well as benefits. For patients with severe dementia or metastatic cancer, the benefits of tube feedings are limited, compared with continued offerings of food by hand. Treatable reasons for decreased oral intake are identified and corrected in few such patients. Fifty percent of patients with severe dementia who receive tube feedings die within 6 months, and there is little evidence that tube feedings prolong life, decrease aspiration pneumonia, or improve functional status or comfort in patients with severe dementia, compared with continued offerings of food by hand (2).

Tube feeding has significant burdens and complications and is associated with agitation, greater use of physical and chemical restraints, tube-related complications, and development of new pressure ulcers (2). Patients who pull out feeding tubes might be communicating refusal, expressing discomfort or anger, seeking attention or control, or acting in a purely reflexive manner. Caregivers tend to ascribe motivations to such patients on the basis of their own attitudes toward feeding tubes (9).

Over one third of patients with dementia who have feeding tubes require physical or pharmacologic restraints (10). Restraining demented patients to prevent them from pulling out tubes compromises their independence and dignity, particularly because they cannot appreciate how the feeding tube will help them (5). Restraints also increase patient agitation. Many patients would not want to be restrained. In a study of nursing home residents, 33% said they wanted tube feedings if they were unable to eat because of permanent brain damage that also left them unable to recognize people.

However, after learning that physical restraints are sometimes applied to patients receiving tube feedings, 25% of residents who initially wanted tube feedings or were not sure changed their minds and preferred not to have them (11). Sedation or "chemical restraint," which might appear to be more acceptable, also compromises patient dignity.

The American Geriatrics Society position paper on feeding tubes states: "Hand feeding is at least as good as tube feeding for the outcomes of death, aspiration pneumonia, functional status, and comfort. Tube feeding is associated with agitation, greater use of physical and chemical restraints, greater healthcare use due to tube-related complications, and development of new pressure ulcers" (2).

Symptoms Can Be Effectively Treated as Oral Intake Declines

Patients with severe dementia or metastatic cancer seldom experience thirst or hunger if they continue to refuse oral intake. In a study from a comfort care unit, almost all lucid, terminally ill patients reduced intake of food and fluids to less than their nutritional needs. About two thirds never experienced hunger, and about one third experienced hunger only initially. Symptoms of thirst or dry mouth were more common, with 36% experiencing them until death. In all patients, small intake of food and fluids, ice chips, and meticulous mouth care relieved symptoms of hunger and dry mouth (12). In another study, hospice nurses rated quality of death of patients who refused food and water as 8 on a 9-point scale, where 9 was a very good death (13). With reduced oral intake, symptoms such as nausea, vomiting, edema, cough, and incontinence are reduced (14). Family members need to be reassured that any discomfort can and will be treated (15).

Caring Should Be Provided Directly, Not Through Symbols

The goal of providing comfort and compassion to patients with advanced dementia or terminal illness can be more effectively achieved directly than through symbolic actions (5), for example, holding the patient's hand, stroking his or her cheek, or giving a backrub.

Ironically, artificial feedings might be impersonal. With tube feedings, the caregiver might focus more attention on technical issues, such as positioning the feeding tube and checking the residual volume, than on the patient. If tube feedings proceed without complication, then social interaction between the caregiver and patient can be minimal. Moreover, the patient has no control over tube feedings except to pull out the tube. In contrast, with hand feedings patients determine the timing, pace, and even the content of feedings. Patients can turn away or clamp their mouths shut. Thus, hand feedings that provide inadequate nutrition might be more respectful of the patient's human needs than tube feedings that deliver adequate calories impersonally.

Tube Feedings Do Not Achieve Goals of Care

Many people believe that tube and intravenous feedings for patients with advanced dementia or other terminal illness do not achieve goals of care. As discussed above, there is no convincing evidence that they prolong life, and symptoms of hunger and thirst can be effectively relieved. Furthermore, having to restrain patients receiving tube feedings seem inhumane.

Tube and Intravenous Feedings Should Not Be Considered Ordinary Care

Labeling artificial feedings as "ordinary" care is questionable. Cessation of the desire for food and drink is part of the natural history of severe illnesses, such as severe dementia or metastatic cancer. In other Western societies, such as the United Kingdom and Sweden, tube feedings are rarely administered to patients with severe dementia. In addition, long-term intravenous or nasogastric tube feedings have become technically possible only in the past 30 years. The Food and Drug Administration regulates artificial feedings as drugs and medical devices, not as foods. Furthermore, feeding gastrostomy or jejunostomy tubes require a surgical or endoscopic procedure for insertion.

More fundamentally, two Presidential bioethics commissions and virtually all court decisions do not regard tube and intravenous feedings as "ordinary care" that is obligatory in all cases; instead, these interventions may be withheld or withdrawn if their burdens outweigh the benefits in the individual patient (16-18). As with other interventions, tube and intravenous feedings should not be provided simply because they are technically feasible.

The President's Council on Bioethics, while emphasizing the inherent dignity of persons with disabilities such as severe dementia, stated that if treatment "would require sedation, physical restraint, frequent re-locations, ... treatment itself adds to the un-consenting and un-comprehending patient's miseries, burdens, or degradations.... In cases such as this where patient resistance makes the very activity of getting treated a great burden—not simply physically in terms of pain, but humanly in terms of the patient's overall well-being—the decision to cease treatment and accept an earlier death seems morally permissible once other alternatives fail, and it may even be the best choice among a range of imperfect options" (17).

It is ethically problematic to say that withholding artificial feedings causes the patient's death. Determining *a single* cause of death when many factors are contributing to the patient's death is a controversial philosophical topic (19). Nonetheless, in such cases, death is legally attributed to the underlying dementia and not to foregoing medical interventions—provided that the reasons for withholding treatment are ethically acceptable. Chapter 14 discusses these distinctions in detail.

LEGAL ISSUES

According to court decisions, artificial feedings are similar to other medical interventions, which have benefits and burdens for the patient (18). The predominant judicial opinion is that artificial feedings are medical interventions that may be withheld under appropriate circumstances, not comfort measures that must always be given. In several states, courts have ruled that tube feedings may be withheld from a patient's persistent vegetative or minimally conscious state only if there is clear and convincing evidence that the patient would refuse. Some states set stricter standards for withholding or withdrawing tube feedings than for other medical interventions, when advance directives or surrogate decision-making is used (20).

CLINICAL RECOMMENDATIONS

When patients with conditions such as severe dementia stop eating and cannot be fed by hand, physicians and surrogates should discuss the goals of care and the benefits and burdens of tube feedings. Long-term tube feedings are appropriate if patients have expressed their informed wishes for this intervention under these circumstances and the surrogate concurs. Tube feedings, however, should not be the default choice.

Decisions about feeding tubes in patients with advanced dementia often fail to follow guidelines for shared decision-making and advance care planning (2). When families of patients who died from dementia and had feeding tubes were interviewed, 14% said that there had been no discussion of feeding tubes, and 42% reported a discussion that was less than 15 minutes (10). Over one half believed that the health care provider strongly favored the use of a feeding tube, and 13% felt pressured to use a feeding tube. Other studies show that the prevalence of feeding tubes is strongly associated with characteristics of the nursing home, such as lower staffing levels and institutional culture (2). Physicians should discuss the trajectory of advanced dementia with surrogates and put decreased oral intake and refusal of feedings by hand as part of the natural history of the condition (2). The order "comfort feedings only" has been proposed on Physicians Orders for Life Sustaining Medical Treatment forms to indicate that feedings and fluids should continue to be offered by hand, but not tube feedings (21). Institutions have an important role in encouraging surrogates to make informed decisions about feeding tubes and assuring that there is no pressure on them to institute tube feedings (2).

CASE 18.1 *Continued*

Mrs. F's physician first checked for mouth or gum problems and infections such as pneumonia and urinary tract infection. Finding none, the doctor then continued a discussion of goals of care. She expressed sadness over Mrs. F's decline and empathy with what the family were experiencing, She next explored the sister's concerns, and explained how declining oral intake was part of the natural history of Alzheimer's disease.

After responding to the family's questions, the physician discussed with the family goals of care and the known risks and unproven benefits of tube feeding. She discussed several options, pausing frequently to see if there were questions. One was continuing to offer food and fluids by hand. The physician explained that patients like Mrs. F generally live just as long with this "comfort feeding only" approach as with tube feedings. The doctor said that many families choose this approach, giving them permission to do so. The physician paused to ask if there were questions or concerns about this approach. A second option was a time-limited trial of tube feedings, with reassessment in 2 weeks. If Mrs. F repeatedly pulls out the nasogastric tube, the goals of care would be reconsidered. The physician recommended against restraints or sedation if she removed the tube. The physician said that tube feedings would not prolong her life. A third option was a feeding gastrostomy, which is less obtrusive and more difficult to remove than a nasogastric tube. The physician emphasized that these decisions are difficult, and no family could be more devoted. The physician suggested the family talk among themselves about what was best for Mrs. F and scheduled a time to continue discussions.

SUMMARY

1. Tube and intravenous feedings in patients with severe, progressive illness such as advanced Alzheimer's disease have risks and burdens, with only limited benefits compared with continuing to offer food and fluids by hand.
2. Such interventions may be withheld or withdrawn from patients with advanced dementia if they do not serve the goal of relieving distress and discomfort.

References

1. Gieniusz M, Sinvani L, Kozikowski A, et al. Percutaneous feeding tubes in individuals with advanced dementia: are physicians "choosing wisely"? *J Am Geriatr Soc* 2018;66:64-69.
2. American Geriatrics Society feeding tubes in advanced dementia position statement. *J Am Geriatr Soc* 2014;62:1590-1593.
3. Teno JM, Mitchell SL, Gozalo PL, et al. Hospital characteristics associated with feeding tube placement in nursing home residents with advanced cognitive impairment. *JAMA* 2010;303:544-550.
4. Mitchell SL, Teno JM, Roy J, et al. Clinical and organizational factors associated with feeding tube use among nursing home residents with advanced cognitive impairment. *JAMA* 2003;290:73-80.
5. Lo B, Dornbrand L. Guiding the hand that feeds: caring for the demented elderly. *N Engl J Med* 1984;311:402-404.
6. Pope John Paul II. On life-sustaining treatments and the vegetative state: scientific advances and ethical dilemmas. *Natl Cathol Bioeth Q* 2004;4:573-576.
7. Sulmasy DP. Terri Schiavo and the Roman Catholic tradition of forgoing extraordinary means of care. *J Law Med Ethics* 2005;33:359-362.
8. Bradley CT. Roman Catholic doctrine guiding end-of-life care: a summary of the recent discourse. *J Palliat Med* 2009;12:373-377.
9. Kuehlmeyer K, Schuler AF, Kolb C, et al. Evaluating nonverbal behavior of individuals with dementia during feeding: a survey of the nursing staff in residential care homes for elderly adults. *J Am Geriatr Soc* 2015;63:2544-2549.

10. Teno JM, Mitchell SL, Kuo SK, et al. Decision-making and outcomes of feeding tube insertion: a five-state study. *J Am Geriatr Soc* 2011;59:881-886.

11. O'Brien LA, Siegert EA, Grisso JA, et al. Tube feeding preferences among nursing home residents. *J Gen Intern Med* 1997;12:364-371.

12. McCann RM, Hall WJ, Groth-Juncker A. Comfort care for terminally ill patients: the appropriate use of nutrition and hydration. *JAMA* 1994;272:1263-1266.

13. Ganzini L, Goy ER, Miller LL, et al. Nurses' experiences with hospice patients who refuse food and fluids to hasten death. *N Engl J Med* 2003;349:359-365.

14. Billings JA. Comfort measures for the terminally ill: is dehydration painful? *J Am Geriat Soc* 1985;33:808-810.

15. Casarett D, Kapo J, Caplan A. Appropriate use of artificial nutrition and hydration—fundamental principles and recommendations. *N Engl J Med* 2005;353:2607-2612.

16. President's Commission for the Study of Ethical Problems in Medicine and Biomedical and Behavioral Research. *Deciding to Forego Life-sustaining Treatment*. Washington: U.S. Government Printing Office; 1983:82-89.

17. The President's Council on Bioethics. *Taking Care: Ethical Caregiving in Our Aging Society*. 2005. Available at: https://bioethicsarchive.georgetown.edu/pcbe/reports/taking_care/index.html

18. Meisel A, Cerminara KL, Pope TM. *The Right to Die*. 3rd ed. New York: Wolters Kluwer; 2014.

19. Brock D. Forgoing life-sustaining food and water: is it killing? In: Lynn J, ed. *By No Extraordinary Means*. Expanded edition ed. Bloomington: Indiana University Press; 1989:117-131.

20. Brody H, Hermer LD, Scott LD, et al. Artificial nutrition and hydration: the evolution of ethics, evidence, and policy. *J Gen Intern Med* 2011;26:1053-1058.

21. Palecek EJ, Teno JM, Casarett DJ, et al. Comfort feeding only: a proposal to bring clarity to decision-making regarding difficulty with eating for persons with advanced dementia. *J Am Geriatr Soc* 2010;58:580-584.

ANNOTATED BIBLIOGRAPHY

1. Lo B, Dornbrand L. Guiding the hand that feeds: caring for the demented elderly. *N Engl J Med* 1984;311:402-404.

   Argues that tube feedings might not be appropriate palliative care for patients with advanced Alzheimer's disease who refuse feedings by hand, particularly if patients require restraints to prevent them from pulling out the tubes.

2. The President's Council on Bioethics. *Taking Care: Ethical Caregiving in Our Aging Society*. Washington, DC: U.S. Executive Office of the President; 2005.

   Urges that when doctors and families must make hard choices for patients who lack decision-making capacity, they should try to benefit the life the patient still has, even when that life has been diminished by illness.

3. American Geriatrics Society feeding tubes in advanced dementia position statement. *J Am Ger Soc* 2014;62:1590-1593.

   Emphasizes that careful hand feedings have similar outcomes as tube feedings, which are a medial intervention that surrogates may decline. Summarizes evidence supporting these recommendations.

19

Physician-Assisted Suicide and Active Euthanasia

INTRODUCTION

As of July 2018, physician-assisted suicide for terminally ill patients is legal in seven states—California, Colorado, Hawaii, Montana, Oregon, Vermont, and Washington, besides the District of Columbia, which together comprise 18% of the US population. The Supreme Court has ruled that there is neither a constitutional right to physician-assisted suicide nor a constitutional barrier to states permitting it; hence its legal status is determined by each state. Current polls show that a majority of the population and of physicians now support physician-assisted suicide for terminally ill patients. Active euthanasia is illegal in all states.

DEFINING TERMS CLEARLY

Imprecise terminology and rhetorical slogans are common in discussions of assisted suicide and euthanasia. Several actions should be distinguished (*see* also Chapter 14).

Active Voluntary Euthanasia

In *active euthanasia*, the physician administers a lethal dose of medication, such as potassium chloride. The physician supplies the means of death and is the final human agent in the events leading to the patient's death. Active euthanasia is sometimes called *mercy killing*. Euthanasia is called *voluntary* when the patient requests it, *involuntary* when the patient opposes it, and *nonvoluntary* when the patient lacks decision-making capacity and cannot express a preference. There is general agreement that involuntary euthanasia is wrong because it violates a patient's right not to be killed. Nonvoluntary euthanasia is also generally considered unacceptable because it might be applied selectively to the disadvantaged and the vulnerable. As we later discuss, some people believe voluntary euthanasia may be justified in some circumstances.

Assisted Suicide

In *assisted suicide*, the patient swallows a lethal dose of drugs or activates a device to administer the drugs. Physicians might assist in a variety of ways. They might complete state-required processes and documentation and write a prescription for a lethal dose of medication.

Many people consider assisted suicide less ethically problematic than active euthanasia. Although the physician provides the means of death, the patient must carry out an independent act. This fact might have several important ethical implications. The patient's subsequent intervening action might lessen the physician's moral responsibility. Patients have free will and are morally responsible for their acts. Although other people might influence the patient, they are not regarded as the cause of the patient's actions unless there is coercion. Moreover, there might be less danger of abuse with assisted suicide than active euthanasia because patients can change their minds and not simply take the relevant pills.

Physicians, however, must not underestimate their moral responsibility if they assist a patient in committing suicide. The motive, intent, justification, and outcome are the same as in active euthanasia. In other situations, people may be held morally responsible for assisting or encouraging another person to commit an immoral act.

Some physicians who prescribe a lethal dose of medications might claim that they did not know that the patient planned to commit suicide. For example, some doctors might prescribe secobarbital at the request of a patient with serious chronic illness without discussing suicide. It would be disingenuous to abjure responsibility in this situation. Doctors almost never prescribe secobarbital except as a means for suicide. More important, discussions of the patient's interest in suicide present opportunities for the physician to identify and address palliative care needs so that the patient no longer feels that suicide is the best option.

Recently, the terms *physician-assisted death* or *physician aid-in-dying* have been used because they are more neutral and less emotionally charged. This book uses the term *aid-in-dying* to refer to Oregon and Washington, which use it in state laws. California uses the term *physician-assisted death*. However, this book does not adopt aid-in-dying generally because it is not used consistently to refer only to giving a prescription for a lethal dose of medication to a terminally ill patient. Indeed, in recent debates in Britain, the terms *assisted death*, *assisted dying*, and *medical assistance to die* were used to refer to both active euthanasia and physician-assisted suicide. Our concern is that a term that is used in inconsistent and ambiguous ways may worsen existing confusion over ethically distinct actions.

Withholding or Withdrawing Medical Interventions

Active euthanasia and assisted suicide are ethically different from withholding or withdrawing interventions, which are also termed *allowing to die* or *passive euthanasia*. Ethically and legally, medical interventions may be withheld or withdrawn if a competent patient or an appropriate surrogate refuses them (*see* Chapter 14). A patient's refusal of life-sustaining treatment is honored because patients have a right to be free of unwanted bodily invasions and medical interventions. Under such circumstances, the underlying illness, not the physician's action or inaction, is considered the cause of death. This is the case even though some patients who refuse life-prolonging interventions in fact want to hasten their death, not just be free of unwanted medical interventions. Therefore, physicians who object to assisted suicide or active euthanasia should not impose interventions that the patient does not want.

This distinction between killing and allowing to die may provide practical guidance, but it is logically problematic (1, 2). Many philosophers have rejected the distinction between acting and refraining from action, pointing out that withholding effective treatment would be condemned if done against the patient's wishes or for malicious motives.

Administering Appropriate Doses of Opioids or Sedatives

Active euthanasia and assisted suicide can be distinguished from high doses of opioids or sedatives to relieve severe pain in patients with terminal illness or to relieve dyspnea when patients forego mechanical ventilation (*see* Chapter 14). In these situations, the goal of care is to relieve suffering. In rare cases, the dose required to relieve refractory symptoms might hasten death if lower doses have not relieved the patient's symptoms (3). Objections to active euthanasia and assisted suicide should not deter physicians from providing aggressive palliative care and proportionate palliative sedation (4). Indeed, fear that terminal symptoms will not be relieved leads some patients to seek assisted suicide or active euthanasia (4).

REASONS IN FAVOR OF ASSISTED SUICIDE AND ACTIVE EUTHANASIA

Respect for Patient Autonomy

The prospect of a long, debilitating illness that would destroy their sense of identity and dignity horrifies many people, who fear increased dependence on others for basic needs such as feeding, bathing, and toilet use. They might not want their family and friends to remember them as progressively debilitated. Proponents contend that competent patients with terminal illness should have control over the time and manner of their death. In this view, it is inconsistent to permit patients to end their lives by refusing medical interventions after a complication occurs but not to end it more directly beforehand.

Compassion for Patients Who Are Suffering

Some argue that assisted suicide and active euthanasia show compassion for patients in the final stages of a terminal illness. Many people regard it as inhumane to require such patients to suffer a downhill course while waiting to die of complications. As one author puts it, "People who want an early peaceful death for themselves or their relatives are not rejecting or denigrating the sanctity of life; on the contrary, they believe that a quicker death shows more respect for life than a protracted one" (5). In some circumstances, terminally ill patients have refractory symptoms despite optimal palliative care. For example, some patients with cancer of the esophagus or head and neck cannot swallow their secretions, and some cancer patients experience intractable massive hemoptysis, hematemesis, or hematochezia (4). Such patients can be sedated so that they are no longer conscious of their symptoms, but their death will not be dignified or peaceful.

Proponents also argue that physicians cannot prevent people from killing themselves but only alter the means by which they do so. When lethal drugs are not available, some patients resort to hanging or guns. Such gruesome means of death distress family members and friends. Advocates contend that terminally ill patients should have a more humane means of ending their lives.

REASONS AGAINST ASSISTED SUICIDE AND ACTIVE EUTHANASIA

The Sanctity of Life

Many people assert that these acts demean the sacredness of human life and violate fundamental moral prohibitions against killing human beings (6).

Suffering Can Almost Always Be Relieved

Palliative care is often inadequate in terminally ill patients. Opponents fear that assisted suicide and active euthanasia will allow physicians to avoid the difficult task of providing physical and spiritual comfort to dying patients. Furthermore, some people suggest that suffering can be redemptive and that patients have a duty to endure it or cope courageously (7).

The Physician's Role

Opponents argue that active euthanasia and assisted suicide are incompatible with the physician's role as healer (6). In this view, patients would lose trust in physicians if these practices were permitted. In one study, 19% of oncology patients said they would change physicians if told their physician had provided active euthanasia or physician-assisted suicide for other patients (8).

Requests for Assisted Suicide Are Not Autonomous

Most terminally ill patients change their minds on suicide after receiving better palliative care or treatment for depression. Thus, their initial requests may not be truly autonomous. Patients requesting assisted suicide are commonly in a zone between clinical depression and the sadness of anticipating their death (9).

Fears of Abuse

A slippery slope might occur; if physician-assisted suicide is permitted for competent terminally ill patients, it would be logically inconsistent to deny it to patients who have previously requested it but have lost decision-making capacity (10). A patient with mild Alzheimer disease might not want to live if he or she could no longer recognize his or her family. At that stage, however, the patient would no longer be capable of making an informed request. Thus, if the patient is not permitted to request physician-assisted suicide or active euthanasia through an advance directive, the patient would face a cruel dilemma: to end life when it is still meaningful or to live in an unacceptably dehumanized condition later. Furthermore, some patients with severe amyotrophic lateral sclerosis (ALS) might want to hasten their death to avoid mechanical ventilation and feeding tubes and to relieve their suffering. However, such patients might lack the physical ability to ingest medication without assistance. Thus, respecting their wishes to hasten death might require active euthanasia.

A second type of slippery slope is empirical rather than logical (10). At first, physicians who participate in assisted suicide might carefully ensure that every case is appropriate, but over time they might become less diligent in providing palliative care or checking that the patient's request is voluntary. Eventually, assisted suicide might occur when palliative care was grossly inadequate or major depression was unaddressed. In Oregon and Washington, however, these concerns have not materialized (11).

Active euthanasia raises particular fears about abuse. Euthanasia for competent patients logically leads to euthanasia of patients who lack decision-making capacity. Furthermore, relief of unbearable suffering might be used to justify active euthanasia in mentally incapacitated patients who had never requested it. Another fear is that pressures to control health care costs will result in nonvoluntary euthanasia of persons whose care is regarded as too burdensome or too expensive (12). Patients with chronic illness or disability might feel pressured by family members or physicians into terminating their lives.

LEGALIZATION OF PHYSICIAN AID-IN-DYING

Oregon and Washington have the longest experience with aid-in-dying and the most detailed annual reports. In these states, terminally ill, competent adults may request medication to end their life (13). The patient must make a written request that is witnessed by two people who attest that the patient is competent, acting voluntarily, and not coerced. Fifteen days after this written request, the patient must repeat the request orally. An additional 48 hours must elapse before the prescription can be filled. The patient may rescind the request at any time. Physicians must ensure that patients are informed about their diagnosis, prognosis, and therapeutic alternatives, such as palliative care. A consultant must confirm that the patient has a terminal disease, is capable of making health care decisions, is informed, and is acting voluntarily. Patients with a psychiatric disorder that impairs judgment must be referred for counseling. Physicians who comply with the provisions of the law are granted legal immunity from criminal, civil, and professional disciplinary actions. Their actions are termed *physician aid-in-dying* because giving a patient a prescription for a dose of medication to end his or her life remains illegal in other circumstances. Physicians and other health care workers may refuse to participate. If a patient ingests a lethal dose of medication under this law, life insurance policies are not voided.

The law sets several important limits. The law specifically prohibits active euthanasia, mercy killing, and lethal injection. Physicians are not allowed to provide assistance to patients who are too incapacitated to take lethal medication themselves. Patients are excluded if they suffer from nonterminal illnesses, lack decision-making capacity, or are too sick to survive the waiting periods. Patients may not request aid-in-dying through advance directives or surrogate decision makers.

THE PRACTICE OF PHYSICIAN AID-IN-DYING IN THE UNITED STATES

Current Practice in States That Legalized Aid-In-Dying

Official state reports on aid-in-dying in Oregon do not confirm concerns that legalizing physician-assisted suicide would harm vulnerable patients or undermine palliative care (14). Almost all patients receiving aid-in-dying have health insurance, and the vast majority were enrolled in hospice. Compared with other terminal patients, patients who died after ingesting a lethal dose of medication were younger and more highly educated. Almost all are white and non-Hispanic. Cancer is the most common diagnosis. Poverty, lack of education or health insurance, or poor quality of care did not play a major role in patients' requests. The number of reported deaths occurring through aid-in-dying was 0.4% and has not increased over time. Patients from other states have not migrated to Oregon to request such assistance. The most common reasons for seeking aid-in-dying were inability to carry out activities that made life enjoyable, loss of autonomy, and loss of dignity. Only a minority had inadequate pain control or concerns about it. Reports from other states that have legalized aid-in-dying, which are less extensive or span fewer years, similarly do not substantiate concerns about harming vulnerable patients or undermining palliative care.

About 1 in 6 terminally ill patients talks about aid-in-dying with their families, 1 in 50 talks with their physician, and about 1 in 500 requests a lethal prescription (15). Those who make such a request are more concerned about independence and control over their lives than intractable physical suffering. Between 16% and 26% of patients who receive a lethal prescription from physicians do not use it (4).

Family members of patients who requested aid-in-dying did not report more depression, grief, or mental health services use following the patient's death compared with other bereaved families, but felt more prepared and accepting of the death (16). Physicians who have participated in aid-in-dying report that it is emotionally intense and time-consuming (17).

Practice Where Aid-In-Dying Is Not Legal

Requests Occur Although the Practice Is Not Legal

Even if prohibited, physician-assisted suicide and active euthanasia are practiced in the United States. In a 1998 study, 18% of physicians in a national sample said that in their careers they had received a request for physician-assisted suicide, and 11% had received a request for active euthanasia (18). In a 1996 study, more than 50% of oncologists had received a request for physician-assisted suicide, and 38% had received a request for active euthanasia (19). Twelve percent of cancer patients said they had serious discussions about active euthanasia or physician-assisted suicide with their family or physician, and 3.4% said they hoarded drugs (19).

Physicians Provide Requested Assistance Even When Illegal

Despite prohibitions, 3.3% of physicians report that they have written a prescription to be used to hasten death, and 4.7% have administered a lethal injection (18). Among oncologists, 13% have assisted suicide and 1.8% have performed active euthanasia (19).

Physicians Are Confused About These Practices

In older reports, some cases that physicians characterized as physician-assisted suicide or active euthanasia would be accurately described differently. For example, in 13% of cases, physicians actually provided high doses of opioids for pain relief; such palliation of symptoms is ethically distinct from assisted suicide or active euthanasia (8). In another 9% of cases, patients overdosed without asking the physician for a prescription for a lethal dose, which cannot be described as physician-assisted suicide or active euthanasia (8). Furthermore, 12% of physicians who said that they had assisted suicide actually ordered a nurse to inject medications to end the patient's life; this action is active euthanasia (8).

ASSISTED SUICIDE AND ACTIVE EUTHANASIA IN THE NETHERLANDS

In the Netherlands, both active euthanasia and assisted suicide have been legal in certain situations since 2002. A competent patient with a terminal illness must make a voluntary and persistent request for active euthanasia or assisted suicide, and two physicians must certify that the patient is terminally ill. Because the Netherlands periodically conducts careful studies of a sample of all deaths, they have the most thorough empirical information on the practice of active euthanasia and assisted suicide. In the Netherlands, active euthanasia occurs in 2.8% of deaths and assisted suicide occurs in 0.1% (20). The rate of active euthanasia has increased slightly since 2002 (20).

Evidence Does Not Support Concerns About Abuse

Abuse has not been widespread, and there is no apparent disproportionate use in vulnerable populations. Physicians do not substitute hastening death for the provision of palliative care. Instead, they intensify the alleviation of symptoms much more often than they undertake euthanasia or physician-assisted suicide, and the increase in the alleviation of symptoms is also much steeper than the increase in euthanasia. Physicians grant fewer than half of euthanasia requests from patients (21).

Confusion Between Active Euthanasia and Palliative Sedation

The line between euthanasia and the less controversial, much more common practice of palliative sedation can be blurred in practice. In about 20% of cases that the investigators classified as euthanasia or physician-assisted suicide, the treating physicians viewed the case as alleviation of symptoms or palliative or terminal sedation. Thus in the Netherlands, some physicians who say they are undertaking palliative sedation actually carry out euthanasia (21).

Procedural Safeguards Are Sometimes Violated

In 0.2% of deaths, Dutch physicians ended the patient's life without the patient's explicit, concurrent request (20). In more than one half of these cases, the patient had discussed these decisions previously with the physician. In about one quarter of these cases, however, the physician did not discuss these actions with anyone, including relatives or colleagues (21). Furthermore, physicians in the Netherlands fail to report 20% of cases of assisted suicide and euthanasia, as required by law (21). These cases in which procedural safeguards are violated raise concerns about the adequacy of official reports on physician assisted suicide in the United States, which are far less detailed than the Dutch studies of a sample of all deaths.

Unintended Adverse Events

When patients attempted physician-assisted suicide, technical problems occurred in 10% of cases, most commonly difficulty swallowing the pills. Adverse effects occurred in 7%, most commonly nausea and vomiting. In 18% of cases, a physician later administered a lethal drug, most commonly because the patient did not die or did not die as soon as expected. These adverse events are a reason why active euthanasia is more common than assisted suicide in the Netherlands. When physicians attempted active euthanasia, technical problems occurred in 5% of cases, most commonly difficulty finding a vein. Adverse effects occurred in 3% of cases, most commonly spasm and myoclonus. In 5% of cases, death did not occur or took longer than expected (22).

Outcomes for Survivors

Family and friends of patients who died by euthanasia do not appear to have worse outcomes. In one study, survivors of such cancer patients had fewer symptoms of traumatic grief and fewer posttraumatic stress reactions than family and friends of patients who died of natural causes (23).

HOW SHOULD PHYSICIANS RESPOND TO REQUESTS FOR ASSISTED SUICIDE?

Physicians must be prepared for questions from patients on assisted suicide or active euthanasia. Like the general public, doctors disagree over the morality of these controversial actions. Regardless of their personal views, physicians should respond in certain ways (Table 19-1) (9).

Clarify the Reasons for the Request

Why is the patient asking a question or making a request at this time? Because of improvements in palliative care, currently most requests are triggered not by unrelieved pain and physical symptoms, but by loss of dignity, independence, or a wish to control the timing and manner of their death (4). Requests might also result from psychosocial problems, a spiritual crisis, or a fear of abandonment (24, 25). Physicians need to screen patients for major depression, which can be treated even in terminally ill patients.

Fears that talking about assisted suicide or active euthanasia will encourage patients to carry out these acts are unfounded. Most terminally ill patients have already thought about these issues and feel relieved that physicians are willing to discuss them. Suicidal patients with terminal illness deserve the same careful evaluation and mobilization of resources as suicidal patients who are not terminally ill.

Address the Patient's Palliative Care Needs

After their suffering and concerns are addressed, almost one half of patients who requested aid-in-dying change their minds (4). Pain relief can be improved through using higher and more frequent doses of opioids, administering them on a regular schedule rather than as needed, and giving patients more control over dosage. In addition to alleviating physical suffering, physicians can help patients come to terms with their mortality and to find meaning in the final stage of their lives. Instead of trying to resolve problems or reassure patients, doctors should explore the patient's suffering using open-ended questions and empathic comments: "That sounds very distressing. Can you tell me more?" (26). Attentive listening validates the patient's emotions and shows the patient that he or she has been understood. The physician should consult with palliative care specialists, psychiatrists or psychologists, social workers, and chaplains as needed. Physicians also can arrange home hospice, mobilize family members and friends, and be available to patients.

Questions for Supporters of Physician Aid-in-Dying

Which Patients to Assist?

Physicians in states where physician aid-in-dying is legal need to decide whether to assist any patient who meets the legal requirements, or only participate in certain circumstances. Physicians are most likely to support physician aid-in-dying in cases of unremitting pain (19). Many physicians who support the legalization of physician aid-in-dying may have cases of refractory physical suffering in

TABLE 19-1.   Responding to Requests for Assisted Suicide or Active Euthanasia
Clarify the reasons for the request.
Address the patient's palliative care needs.
Supporters of physician aid-in-dying need to decide which patients to assist and how to address complications.
Opponents of physician aid-in-dying need to decide what ongoing care to provide and how to maintain their integrity.
Respect patients with different views on physician aid-in-dying.
Consult a trusted and wise colleague.

mind. But perceived loss of autonomy and dignity is now a more common reason for requesting physician aid-in-dying than inadequate pain control (11). Some physicians may decide not assist in a patient's death in such circumstances (4).

Supporters of physician aid-in-dying may be more willing to assist their own patients, with whom they have an ongoing relationship that facilitates discussion of concerns and assessment of decision-making capacity (4). Supporters may also be willing to assist patients of close colleagues, who can help identify and alleviate the patient's distress but might be opposed to physician aid-in-dying themselves, or willing to participate but inexperienced in doing so. However, many physicians may hesitate to make physician aid-in-dying a prominent part of their practice because of the intense emotional and time commitment required.

How to Address Complications of Physician Aid-in-Dying?

Physicians who support physician aid-in-dying need to consider how to address the potential for rare but distressing adverse outcomes, including longer time to death than expected (up to 24 hours or more), awakening from unconsciousness, nausea, vomiting, and gasping (11). Physicians who participate in physician aid-in-dying can help patients and their families plan for worst-case scenarios, such as whether to call 911 if distressing symptoms develop after lethal medications are ingested. Physicians should clarify whether they or another professional, such as a hospice nurse, is willing and permitted to be present during medication ingestion (4).

Questions for Opponents of Physician Aid-in-Dying

What Ongoing Care to Provide After Patients Request Aid-in-Dying?

Physicians who oppose physician aid-in-dying should continue to care for patients who ask about or request it. The physician's professional obligation to address a patient's suffering is particularly strong when they have a long-term relationship. Relief from suffering may allow the patient to find reasons to continue to live, as previously discussed. Some patients want to see their current physician for ongoing care, even knowing the doctor respectfully opposes physician aid-in-dying.

How to Maintain the Physician's Integrity?

Physicians who oppose physician aid-in-dying understandably do not want to compromise their moral integrity or violate their conscience. Some might fear that even discussing physician aid-in-dying with patients signifies support or approval and therefore makes them complicit. Complicity in physician aid-in-dying, however, requires clearly expressing approval, completing and documenting legal requirements, or writing a prescription for a lethal dose of medication. However, physicians who explore patients' needs and concerns, try to alleviate pain and distress, and clearly state their opposition to assisted suicide should not consider themselves complicit in physician aid-in-dying (4). Even continuing to care for a patient who has obtained a prescription from another physician need not make a physician complicit. On the contrary, by trying to address the patient's concerns and reasons for requesting physician aid-in-dying, the physician might help the patient find reasons to continue living.

Respect Patients with Different Views on Physician Aid-in-Dying

Patients, like physicians, commonly base their support or opposition to aid-in-dying on intensely private moral and religious beliefs as well as their values and goals. Physicians should respect the highly personal nature of these decisions and not unduly influence patients, or be perceived as doing so.

Physicians should not participate in assisted suicide or active euthanasia against their conscience or religious beliefs. When communicating their refusal, physicians also need to also address the patient's concerns and show empathy for the patient's plight. The physician might say, "I hear that you are deeply distressed by your illness. I'll try my best to relieve your suffering. But I can't write a prescription for medicine you can use to kill yourself. My conscience won't allow me to do that." Such physicians need to emphasize their commitment to provide ongoing palliative care.

Some patients may want a new physician if they learn that their current physician's views on aid-in-dying differ from their own (19, 27). Patients who oppose physician aid-in-dying might fear that a physician who supports it might encourage them to consider it. Conversely, patients who are open to physician aid-in-dying might want to choose a supportive physician early in their illness rather than potentially changing physicians later in their illness.

Consult a Trusted and Wise Colleague

Most physicians find patient requests for assisted suicide or active euthanasia to be highly stressful. As with any other difficult case, a second opinion or discussion with a colleague is generally helpful. Often, a colleague can suggest how to improve palliative care or how to talk with the patient.

Situations in Which Assisted Suicide Might Be Justified

Many physicians can conceive of a case in which they would consider assisted suicide morally permissible (28). The combination of all of the following circumstances would constitute the strongest case for agreeing to a patient's request (29, 30).

- *The patient has a terminal illness* or a progressive, incurable condition causing unrelenting suffering, such as ALS.
- *The patient is experiencing intractable symptoms* despite optimal comprehensive palliative care. Even the best palliative care cannot relieve intractable bleeding or inability to swallow secretions. Actual distress is more compelling than anticipated future symptoms. Many physicians are more sympathetic to patients with physical distress than to patients with mental distress. The distinction between physical and mental suffering might be philosophically untenable, but it is helpful for pragmatic reasons because mistakes and suboptimal treatment may be more likely with psychological and existential suffering.
- *The patient's request is voluntary, informed, and repeated.* Ideally, the patient raises the issue and is willing to discuss it with family members, friends, or clergy.
- *The physician has a long-term relationship with the patient* that started before the patient requested assistance with suicide.
- *The physician has consulted experts in* palliative care and depression.

In cases in which these conditions are present, it is not unethical for physicians to assist in suicide. Active euthanasia is more problematic because it presents greater potential for abuse, particularly with patients who lack decision-making capacity. Although requests by surrogates for active euthanasia are usually motivated by compassion, the risk of projection, misinterpretation, and abuse are great. Surrogates might interpret a gesture or a look as an unspoken request to hasten death, saying, for example, "I looked into his eyes and I just knew what he was asking me to do." Prohibiting active euthanasia for patients who lack decision-making capacity is sound public policy and clinical ethics.

Physicians may be confused as to whether they are providing palliative sedation, terminal sedation, or euthanasia. Doctors must be careful to keep clearly in mind the line between proportional palliative sedation and active euthanasia (*see* Chapter 15).

SUMMARY

1. Whether physicians support or oppose legalization of physician aid-in-dying, they will face difficult questions when patients request assistance.
2. It should never be easy for a physician to respond to a request for assisted suicide from a patient who is dying in great suffering despite excellent palliative care.
3. Regardless of the physician's decision, patients deserve an honest answer to their questions or request, as well as efforts to understand their distress and alleviate it through more intensive palliative care.

References

1. Brock D. Forgoing life-sustaining food and water: is it killing? In: Lynn J, ed. *By No Extraordinary Means.* Expanded edition ed. Bloomington: Indiana University Press; 1989:117-131.
2. Alpers A, Lo B. Does it make clinical sense to equate terminally ill patients who require life-sustaining interventions with those who do not? *JAMA* 1997;277:1705-1708.
3. Lo B, Rubenfeld G. Palliative sedation in dying patients: "we turn to it when everything else hasn't worked." *JAMA* 2005;294:1810-1816.
4. Lo B. Beyond legalization—dilemmas physicians confront regarding aid in dying. *N Engl J Med* 2018;378:2060-2062.
5. Dworkin R. *Life's Dominion.* New York: Alfred A. Knopf; 1993.
6. Yang YT, Curlin FA. Why physicians should oppose assisted suicide. *JAMA* 2016;315:247-248.
7. Pellegrino ED. Doctors must not kill. *J Clin Ethics* 1992;3:95-102.
8. Emanuel EJ, Daniels ER, Fairclough DL, et al. The practice of euthanasia and physician-assisted suicide in the United States: adherence to proposed safeguards and effects on physicians. *JAMA* 1998;280:507-513.
9. Quill TE, Back AL, Block SD. Responding to patients requesting physician-assisted death: physician involvement at the very end of life. *JAMA* 2016;315:245-246.
10. Lewis P. The empirical slippery slope from voluntary to involuntary euthanasia. *J Law Med Ethics* 2007;35:197-210.
11. Emanuel EJ, Onwuteaka-Philipsen BD, Urwin JW, et al. Attitudes and practices of euthanasia and physician-assisted suicide in the United States, Canada, and Europe. *JAMA* 2016;316:79-90.
12. Sulmasy DP. Managed care and managed death. *Arch Intern Med* 1995;155:133-136.
13. Gostin LO, Roberts AE. Physician-assisted dying: a turning point? *JAMA* 2016;315:249-250.
14. Oregon Health Authority. *Death with Dignity Act Annual Reports.* 2018. Available at: http://www.oregon.gov/oha/PH/PROVIDERPARTNERRESOURCES/EVALUATIONRESEARCH/DEATHWITHDIG-NITYACT/Pages/ar-index.aspx. Accessed March 24, 2018.
15. Quill TE, Arnold R, Back AL. Discussing treatment preferences with patients who want "everything." *Ann Intern Med* 2009;151:345-349.
16. Ganzini L, Goy ER, Dobscha SK, et al. Mental health outcomes of family members of Oregonians who request physician aid in dying. *J Pain Symptom Manage* 2009;38:807-815.
17. Dobscha SK, Heintz RT, Press N, et al. Oregon physicians' responses to requests for assisted suicide: a qualitative study. *J Palliat Med* 2004;7:451-61.
18. Meier DE, Emmons CA, Wallenstein S, et al. Physician-assisted death in the United States: a national prevalence survey. *N Engl J Med* 1998;338:1193-1201.
19. Emanuel EJ, Fairclough DL, Daniels ER, et al. Euthanasia and physician-assisted suicide: attitudes and experiences among oncology patients, oncologists, and the general public. *Lancet* 1996;347:1805-1810.
20. Onwuteaka-Philipsen BD, Brinkman-Stoppelenburg A, Penning C, et al. Trends in end-of-life practices before and after the enactment of the euthanasia law in the Netherlands from 1990 to 2010: a repeated cross-sectional survey. *Lancet* 2012;380:908-915.
21. Lo B. Euthanasia in the Netherlands: what lessons for elsewhere? *Lancet* 2012;380:569-570.
22. Groenewoud JH, van der Heide A, Onwuteaka-Philipsen BD, et al. Clinical problems with the performance of euthanasia and physician-assisted suicide in The Netherlands. *N Engl J Med* 2000;342:551-556.
23. Swarte NB, van der Lee ML, van der Bom JG, et al. Effects of euthanasia on the bereaved family and friends: a cross sectional study. *BMJ* 2003;327:189.
24. Quill TE. Doctor, I want to die. Will you help me? *JAMA* 1993;270:870-873.
25. Muskin PR. The request to die: role for a psychodynamic perspective on physician-assisted suicide. *JAMA* 1998;279:323-328.
26. Lo B, Quill T, Tulsky J. Discussing palliative care with patients. *Ann Intern Med* 1999;130:744-749.
27. Ganzini L, Nelson HD, Lee MA, et al. Oregon physicians' attitudes about and experiences with end-of-life care since passage of the Oregon Death with Dignity Act. *JAMA* 2001;285:2363-2369.
28. Bachman JG, Alcser KH, Doukas DJ, et al. Attitudes of Michigan physicians and the public toward legalizing physician-assisted suicide and voluntary euthanasia. *N Engl J Med* 1996;334:303-309.
29. Quill TE, Cassel CK, Meier DE. Care of the terminally ill: proposed clinical criteria for physician-assisted suicide. *N Engl J Med* 1992;327:1380-1384.
30. Miller FG, Quill TE, Brody H, et al. Regulating physician-assisted death. *N Engl J Med* 1994;331:119-123.

ANNOTATED BIBLIOGRAPHY

1. Gostin LO, Roberts AE. Physician-assisted dying: a turning point? *JAMA* 2016;315:249-250.
   Summarizes recent legislation and considers evidence on concerns about the practice.
2. Yang YT, Curlin FA. Why physicians should oppose assisted suicide. *JAMA* 2016;315:247-248.
   Forceful summary of reasons for opposing assisted suicide.
3. Quill TE, Back AL, Block SD. Responding to patients requesting physician-assisted death: physician involvement at the very end of life. *JAMA* 2016;315:245.
   Suggestions on how doctors can respond when terminally ill patients request physicians to hasten their death, with emphasis on intensifying palliative care and the physician-patient relationship.
4. Lo B. Beyond legalization—dilemmas physicians confront regarding aid in dying. *N Engl J Med* 2018;378:2060-2062.
   Discusses ethical issues physicians face when patients request aid-in-dying. Both supporters and opponents of legalization of physician aid-in-dying will encounter dilemmas in patient care.
5. Lo B. Euthanasia in the Netherlands: what lessons for elsewhere? *Lancet* 2012;380:569-570.
   The absence of widespread abuse of euthanasia the Netherlands is unlikely to settle controversies over euthanasia in other countries. However, cases that raise ethical concerns have important implications for other countries, particularly that physicians may be confused as to whether they are providing palliative sedation, terminal sedation, or euthanasia.

Unresponsive Wakefulness and the Minimally Conscious State

INTRODUCTION

Patients such as Karen Ann Quinlan, Nancy Cruzan, and Theresa Schiavo (*see* Chapter 22), who were diagnosed as being in a persistent vegetative state (PVS), have dramatized fundamental ethical questions about the goals of medicine, the definition of being a person, and appropriate withholding life-sustaining interventions. Important advances in neurology have led to a new conceptual framework and terminology for such patients and raised additional dilemmas regarding decisions for their care.

This chapter discusses two severe disorders of consciousness, unresponsive wakefulness (UW) and the minimally conscious state (MCS), and analyzes the philosophical quandaries they present and how to make decisions for patients in these conditions.

DEFINITIONS AND CLINICAL FEATURES

Conditions That Must Be Distinguished

Several catastrophic neurologic conditions need to be carefully distinguished.

Patients who meet criteria for *brain death* have neither cortical nor brainstem function (*see* Chapter 21). They are comatose, without spontaneous breathing. Their eyes are closed, and there is no facial expression or vocalization.

Patients in a *coma* are alive but unconscious and have no sleep–wake cycles. They do not respond to pain except through reflex movements.

Patients in the *locked-in syndrome* are conscious but have no motor function except for eye movements. Such patients might be able to communicate by blinking their eyes.

Patients with *severe dementia* might be virtually unresponsive, but they are conscious and might have some motor function.

Unresponsive Wakefulness

The term unresponsive wakefulness, or UW, is now preferred instead of vegetative state, which has negative connotations.

Definition and Clinical Features

Patients with UW are unresponsive and unconscious, with no awareness of their environment (1, 2). However, they retain sleep–wake cycles and therefore are not comatose. When awake, patients with UW may open their eyes, blink, and have roving eye movements and unsustained visual pursuit. They may have facial movements and expressions and may grunt, grimace, smile, and produce tears.

Patients might withdraw or posture in response to noxious stimuli and turn in the direction of sudden loud noises. Reflexes such as sucking, chewing, and swallowing might also be present. However, such patients show no purposeful activity and cannot obey verbal commands. These patients have brainstem function but no cortical function.

Some observers, particularly family members, believe that a patient diagnosed as having UW is aware of surroundings or has responded to them, for example, by watching them cross the room or crying when talked to. The crucial issue is whether such responses to external stimuli can be replicated.

Treatment

Amantadine is commonly given to patients after severe brain injury on the basis of the results of a short-term randomized trial and relatively few adverse effects. However, the clinical significance of resulting improvement in assessment scales in unclear. Transcranial direct current stimulation of the brain, which is noninvasive, has shown promise. A variety of other pharmacologic and neurostimulatory approaches have been reported; without well-designed controlled trials it is impossible to evaluate their effectiveness.

Neurorehabilitation in a specialized unit may be beneficial. However, insurance coverage is a challenge in the United States.

Patients with UW generally require tube feedings because they cannot swallow or protect their airway. They are incontinent and require total nursing care. Common complications are decubitus ulcers, aspiration pneumonia, and urosepsis.

Prognosis in Unresponsive Wakefulness

Prognosis for recovery of consciousness can be established only after prolonged observation. Previously it was thought that patients in UW for 3 months after nontraumatic injury, such as anoxic brain damage during a cardiac arrest, or for 12 months after traumatic brain injury, only rarely regain consciousness (3). However, older studies of prognosis are flawed because poor prognosis is a self-fulfilling prophecy if life-sustaining interventions are withdrawn and neurorehabilitation is not offered.

Prognosis is better in patients who begin to improve by 7 weeks after the brain injury (4). Recent studies document that some patients who are discharged from months–long neurorehabilitation in UW may regain consciousness years later (5). However, methodological flaws in follow-up studies make quantitative prognostication impossible. As in all clinical medicine, uncertainty must be acknowledged. The mean survival of patients in UW is 2 to 5 years. A few US patients have been reported to survive longer than 15 years.

Minimally Conscious State

Patients with wakefulness and some awareness and purposeful motor response to external stimuli or verbal requests are said to be in an MCS. They might respond to a moving object with their eyes, respond yes or no to questions, follow simple commands, show purposeful behavior in manipulating objects, or verbalize intelligibly. These findings, although reproducible, may be partial, fluctuating, and inconsistent. Patients with MCS are dependent on others for all activities of daily living and have very limited means to communicate.

Diagnosis of Minimally Conscious State

Standardized, careful neurobehavioral testing by experienced observers is considered the best way to diagnose the MCS. As many as 37% to 43% of patients who were believed to have UW on the basis of routine clinical evaluation were found on repeated standardized assessments to have purposeful responses and thus be in MCS (6). Such neurobehavioral testing is challenging because behavioral responses by a patient may be observed at some times but not others (7).

Between 10% and 24% patients who are diagnosed clinically in referral centers as having UW may have evidence of willful brain activity on sophisticated diagnostic testing (6). For example, patients undergo functional magnetic resonance imaging (fMRI) while being asked to imagine doing tasks, for example, swinging the arm back and forth as if playing tennis and visualizing walking through familiar surroundings. In some patients believed to be in UW, fMRI activity in some brain areas was similar to activity in normal subjects imagining these tasks, even though no clinical movement was detected (8). Quantitative electroencephalography (EEG) may similarly reveal responses to simple commands to squeeze a hand or wriggle toes. However, these tests have methodological problems, including the lack of a gold standard for defining consciousness, and carrying out the tests and interpreting findings are technically challenging. The needed expertise is available only in specialized referral centers.

Prognosis in the Minimally Conscious State

Patients in MCS have a better prognosis than those in UW. In a study of patients admitted in MCS after traumatic brain injury to a neurorehabilitation center, 37% of patients had regained consciousness by discharge, and about half of these had no more than moderate disability (9). Discharge occurred a mean of about 4 months after the brain injury but could be as long as a year. Long-term improvement in consciousness years after the brain injury is also possible, but such patients often remain severely disabled (5).

CLINICAL DECISIONS FOR PATIENTS WITH DISORDERS OF CONSCIOUSNESS

For several reasons, decisions for patients with disorders of consciousness are even more difficult than decisions for other patients who lack decision-making capacity.

- The event causing the devastating disorders of consciousness was unanticipated and sudden.
- Advance care planning is unusual and limited. Even when people have previously made pertinent statements, they may be challenging to interpret. For instance, if a patient said that he or she "wouldn't want to live like a vegetable," did he or she understand that some return of consciousness is possible?
- Medical information about these conditions is evolving.
- Diagnosis is difficult to establish and understand.
- Prognosis is difficult to determine, particularly early after onset. Reports of poor prognosis may be biased if life-sustaining interventions are withdrawn prematurely in many patients. Assessments of prognosis are probabilistic and cannot predict the outcome in an individual patient. The trajectory of the patient's course is helpful. If a patient continues to show functional improvement beginning several weeks after acute brain injury, many families decide to continue rehabilitation, hoping for continued improvement.
- The effectiveness of treatments is uncertain.
- Misunderstandings are common. For example, movies commonly depict recovery from disorders of consciousness as sudden and complete, but in reality recovery is slow and gradual (10).
- People disagree sharply over goals of care and their willingness to continue rehabilitation and life-sustaining interventions when potential outcomes include severe functional limitations and very limited ability to express their wishes and emotions.

Goals of Care

People differ sharply in how they view UW and MCS and the goals of care. On the one hand, some patients and families want to continue life-sustaining interventions because they believe that life is precious and worth continuing, no matter what the degree of neurologic and functional impairment. Some would want no effort and time spared to try to improve outcomes, even if those outcomes involved severe disability and a small probability of living independently. Some relatives consider a patient who responds only in rudimentary ways a full member of the family.

On the other hand, other patients and families view UW and MCS as states worse than death because of severely limited awareness, motor function, and communication; continued loss of dignity, independence, and privacy; and dependence on others for daily care. Some may believe that MCS is even worse than UW because patients have some awareness of their cognitive, functional, and communication limitations.

Communication with Families

In communicating with families of patients with UW and MCS, physicians should follow guidelines for making decisions for patients who lack decision-making capacity (*see* Chapters 11-13). In particular, physicians and other health care workers should provide emotional support for families facing a difficult, unexpected situation, acknowledge the probabilistic nature of prognostic predictions and the limitations of evidence, and be aware of their own biases.

Medical Interventions May Be Withheld or Withdrawn

A time-limited trial of intensive care for at least 3 days is appropriate unless the patient has additional severe diseases, injuries, or complications that predict a poor outcome or the patient has previously indicated that he or she would limit interventions in such a situation (10, 11). Many families will choose to continue rehabilitative care as long as the patient continues to improve meaningfully over an appropriate time course (11).

As Chapter 13 discussed, when patients lack decision-making capacity, interventions, including life-sustaining interventions in intensive care, cardiopulmonary resuscitation, and antibiotics for infection, may be withheld on the basis of advance directives or decisions by appropriate surrogates. If life-sustaining interventions are withdrawn, physicians must be alert for symptoms of discomfort and distress, which may manifest only as tachycardia or tachypnea (10). It is better to err on the side of interpreting ambiguous findings as distress that needs to be treated with aggressive palliative care.

Tube Feedings Are a Medical Intervention That May Be Withheld or Withdrawn

Some people consider feeding tubes "ordinary" nursing care that must always be provided. Feeding tubes, however, have benefits and burdens that must be assessed for the individual patient. As discussed in Chapter 15, it is permissible to withhold or withdraw tube feedings from persons in UW or MCS, in accordance with the patient's prior directives, values, goals of care, or best interests as interpreted by family members. In practice, many people are ambivalent about tube feedings in this situation.

Supporting Family Requests for Interventions

Some families will ask about or request that physicians order tests to better ascertain diagnosis or prognosis or to decide on interventions intended to improve outcomes (7). As with any questions or requests by relatives, physicians should respond with empathy, addressing both the substantive questions and the underlying emotions. Physicians can serve as patient advocates for requests that are medically appropriate, for example, to obtain access to and coverage for neurorehabilitation (12). In addition, physicians can help patients gain access to research studies of new diagnostic or therapeutic interventions.

SUMMARY

1. The prognosis of patients with UW and MCS treated with neurocritical care and neurorehabilitation is better than outcomes reported in the older literature.
2. Clinical decisions are complicated because of emerging information about diagnosis and prognosis, the slow and gradual nature of improvement, and divergent interpretations of the patient's clinical condition. Most important, patients and families have different values and goals regarding their care.
3. In addressing ethical dilemmas regarding UW and MCS, guidelines for decision-making in patients who lack decision-making capacity should be followed.
4. It is permissible to withdraw feeding tubes and other medical interventions from patients in UW and MCS in accordance with the patient's values, goals, or advance directives or decisions by appropriate surrogates.

References

1. Monti MM, Laureys S, Owen AM. The vegetative state. *BMJ* 2010;341:c3765.
2. Bernat JL. Current controversies in states of chronic unconsciousness. *Neurology* 2010;75:S33-S38.
3. The Multi-Society Task Force on PVS. Medical aspects of the persistent vegetative state. *N Engl J Med* 1994;330:1499-1508,1572-1579.
4. Steppacher I, Kaps M, Kissler J. Will time heal? A long-term follow-up of severe disorders of consciousness. *Ann Clin Transl Neurol* 2014;1:401-1408.
5. Yelden K, Duport S, James LM, et al. Late recovery of awareness in prolonged disorders of consciousness—a cross-sectional cohort study. *Disabil Rehabil* 2017:1-6.
6. Bender A, Jox RJ, Grill E, et al. Persistent vegetative state and minimally conscious state: a systematic review and meta-analysis of diagnostic procedures. *Dtsch Arztebl Int* 2015;112:235-242.
7. Jox RJ, Bernat JL, Laureys S, et al. Disorders of consciousness: responding to requests for novel diagnostic and therapeutic interventions. *Lancet Neurol* 2012;11:732-738.
8. Monti MM, Vanhaudenhuyse A, Coleman MR, et al. Willful modulation of brain activity in disorders of consciousness. *N Engl J Med* 2010;362:579-589.
9. Klein AM, Howell K, Vogler J, et al. Rehabilitation outcome of unconscious traumatic brain injury patients. *J Neurotrauma* 2013;30:1476-1483.
10. Frontera JA, Curtis JR, Nelson JE, et al. Integrating palliative care into the care of neurocritically ill patients: a report from the improving palliative care in the ICU project advisory board and the center to advance palliative care. *Crit Care Med* 2015;43:1964-1977.
11. Souter MJ, Blissitt PA, Blosser S, et al. Recommendations for the critical care management of devastating brain injury: prognostication, psychosocial, and ethical management: a position statement for healthcare professionals from the neurocritical care society. *Neurocrit Care* 2015;23:4-13.
12. Fins JJ. Neuroethics and disorders of consciousness: discerning brain states in clinical practice and research. *AMA J Ethics* 2016;18:1182-1191.

ANNOTATED BIBLIOGRAPHY

1. Souter MJ, Blissitt PA, Blosser S, et al. Recommendations for the critical care management of devastating brain injury: prognostication, psychosocial, and ethical management: a position statement for healthcare professionals from the neurocritical care society. *Neurocrit Care* 2015;23:4-13.
   Frontera JA, Curtis JR, Nelson JE, et al. Integrating palliative care into the care of neurocritically ill patients: a report from the improving palliative care in the icu project advisory board and the center to advance palliative care. *Crit Care Med* 2015;43:1964-77.
   Thoughtful recommendations for ethical and clinical aspects of caring for patients in coma, UW, and MCS, taking into account recent scientific and clinical knowledge

Determination of Death

INTRODUCTION

Accurate and consistent determinations of death are essential because declaring a patient dead has profound consequences: mourning begins, and funeral services, burial, or cremation are held. Pensions and health insurance coverage are terminated, properties pass on to heirs, life insurance policies are paid, and spouses may remarry.

Traditional cardiopulmonary criteria for death are problematic if a patient's breathing and circulation are sustained on life support after all cerebral functions have irreversibly ceased. Organ transplantation has raised unprecedented ethical issues about the declaration of death. Transplant teams want to retrieve organs as soon as possible. However, relatives and the public want assurance that organs are not harvested prematurely from persons who are not truly dead. Criteria for brain death have been developed to.

Defining death is controversial because it involves cultural, social, and religious values, as well as scientific judgment. This chapter discusses ethical issues regarding cardiopulmonary, whole-brain, and higher brain criteria for death.

CARDIOPULMONARY CRITERIA FOR DEATH

Traditionally, physicians declare patients dead using cardiopulmonary criteria: the irreversible cessation of circulatory and respiratory functions. After cessation of heartbeat and breathing, brain functions cease permanently within minutes unless artificial life support is instituted.

With the development of intensive care units, circulation and breathing can be sustained for months or longer after the brain has irreversibly ceased to function. Disputes about cardiopulmonary criteria for death also arise when persons are killed by criminal acts. Some defendants in murder trials contended that the victim's death was caused by removal of vital organs for transplantation, not by their actions. Because of these problems with cardiopulmonary criteria for death, the definition of death was revised to include the irreversible cessation of brain function.

Determination of death using cardiopulmonary criteria has become more complicated with recent interest in retrieving organs for transplantation from persons declared dead by cardiopulmonary criteria (*see* also Chapter 41) (1). Patients or surrogates decide that life-sustaining interventions will be withdrawn, resuscitation will not be initiated, and organs may be removed for transplantation. These donors are transported to the operating room, where life support is withdrawn, death is declared using cardiorespiratory criteria, and organs are promptly retrieved.

Cases have been reported of autoresuscitation, the spontaneous return of circulation after cardiac arrest without resuscitative procedures (2). In adults, resuscitation has been reported 10 minutes after failed CPR and 3 minutes after withdrawal of life-sustaining interventions.

Several ethical concerns have been raised about this practice (1). First, are these donors really dead? The time from the development of asystole to declaration of death is typically about 2 to 5 minutes, a cut point beyond which spontaneousy return of circulation is thought to be very low. Setting a longer waiting period would increase the likelihood that ischemia would compromise the donated organ. Second, cardiac transplantation presents several ethical concerns. Successful pediatric heart transplants have been carried out after only 75 seconds of asystole, shorter than the time that is believed to preclude autoresuscitation. Moreover, if the heart is transplanted and functions in the donor provide circulation, has the cessation of cardiac function been negated? Third, to achieve better outcomes after transplantation, some centers use extracorporeal membrane oxygenation to perfuse organs before organs are recovered. Large-bore catheters are inserted before death is declared. The dying patient receives invasive procedures solely to benefit the transplant recipient. Finally, the family's experience of the patient's death may seem rushed and impersonal when death occurs in the operating room. If organs cannot be retrieved because of prolonged hypotension, grieving can be more difficult for survivors.

In response to these concerns, a consensus panel recommended that the term *donation* after cardiac death not be used, as the statutory standards for death by cardiopulmonary criteria require irreversible cessation of circulation, not death of the heart itself (1). This panel also argued that *permanent* cessation of circulatory and respiratory functions (because a decision has been made not to initiate resuscitation) is equivalent to *irreversible* loss of such function (it is impossible to be restored).

In rebuttal, other scholars have argued that this justification is a legal fiction that will confuse physicians, nurses, and the public and undermine trust in transplantation. In their view, it would be more accurate to overturn the "dead donor rule" and say that these donors are not really dead but that it is morally acceptable to remove their organs for transplantation (3, 4).

BRAIN CRITERIA FOR DEATH

Patients who have irreversibly lost all brain function are considered dead, even though medical technology can support their circulation and breathing. Brain death in the United States is defined as irreversible loss of functioning in the entire brain, both the cortex and the brainstem. This is also called *whole-brain death*. Destruction of the brain ultimately leads to cessation of spontaneous cardiac function.

Currently, the clinical tests for brain death include coma, absence of brainstem function, and apnea (5, 6). Potentially reversible causes of coma, such as drug overdose or hypothermia, must be ruled out. Circulation and spinal cord reflexes might be intact in brain death. Confirmatory testing with an electroencephalogram (EEG) and imaging studies of intracranial blood flow may be helpful but are not mandatory. The determination of brain death in children involves separate guidelines and procedures (7).

Recently, brain criteria for death have been questioned (8). In some patients declared dead by brain criteria, there might be persistence of some cerebral blood flow, oxygen and glucose metabolism, EEG activity, brainstem-evoked potentials, secretion of antidiuretic hormone, and temperature regulation (3, 9). Moreover, some patients diagnosed as dead by brain criteria mount a febrile response to infections and a stress response to surgical incisions. Thus, the body system may continue to function as a whole organism.

In exceptional cases, there might be a substantial discrepancy between determinations of death using brain criteria and cardiopulmonary criteria. Several pregnant women meeting brain criteria had their vital functions sustained for months until the fetus could be delivered (3, 9).

The President's Council on Bioethics rejected integrated functioning as the key criterion characterizing a living organism and instead proposed that an organism is alive if it is receptive to its environment, is able to act upon the world to obtain what it needs, and has a drive to obtain what it needs, including air and nutrients. In their view, a person who has irreversibly lost consciousness and spontaneous breathing is dead (3, 9).

Death determined by brain criteria needs to be carefully distinguished from unresponsive wakefulness, formerly called the vegetative state (*see* Chapter 20). In death by brain criteria, there is no cortical or brainstem function. In contrast, patients in unresponsive wakefulness have intact brainstem function and spontaneous breathing and circulation.

Misunderstandings Over Brain Criteria for Death

US neurologists do not have a consistent rationale for accepting brain death as death, nor a clear understanding of diagnostic tests for brain criteria for death (10). In an earlier survey, only 35% of physicians who were responsible for declaring death were able to identify irreversible loss of all brain function as the criterion for determining death and apply it to simple case vignettes of death (11). Among other health care workers involved in the care of persons declared brain dead, more than 70% were unable to identify brain criteria for death. When asked to explain their personal opinions about two case vignettes, 58% of all respondents did not consistently use a coherent concept of death. Thirty-six percent believed that it is appropriate to retrieve organs from a patient in a vegetative state who does not meet whole-brain criteria for death.

Higher Brain Criteria for Death

Some writers argue that a person who has irreversible loss of higher brain function in the cerebral cortex, rather than loss of whole-brain function, should be considered dead because consciousness, self-awareness, the potential for thought, and interactions with others are essential for being a person (12). In this view, persons with unresponsive wakefulness would be considered dead. However, a "higher brain" or neocortical definition of death, has been rejected as public policy in the United States (13). The higher brain criteria for death confuse what it means to be a person with what it means to be alive. It might be appropriate to say that individuals without cortical function are no longer persons in the philosophic sense of having rights and interests. It does not follow logically, however, that they should be considered dead. Finally, burying or cremating individuals with unresponsive wakefulness, who have spontaneous breathing and pulse, seems intuitively wrong.

Disagreement on Brain Criteria for Death

Some persons reject the concept of brain criteria for death for religious or philosophic reasons (14, 15). For example, some orthodox Jews, Native Americans, and Japanese believe that a person is alive until he or she literally stops breathing (16, 17). No distinction is made between mechanical ventilation and spontaneous breathing. In this view, a person on a ventilator who meets the brain criteria for death is not dead.

Legal Status of Brain Criteria for Death

Most states have adopted the Uniform Determination of Death Act, which declares, "Any individual who has sustained either (1) irreversible cessation of circulatory and respiratory functions, or (2) irreversible cessation of all functions of the entire brain, including the brainstem, is dead. A determination of death must be made in accordance with accepted medical standards" (3). Thus, a person may be declared dead if he or she meets either cardiopulmonary criteria (absence of breathing and pulse) or brain-death criteria. For most patients who are not on life support, these two criteria are equivalent. Courts have upheld determinations of death made by physicians according to brain criteria in accordance with state law (19).

Four states require physicians to accommodate families who object to determination of death by brain criteria (18, 19). New Jersey authorizes the declaration of brain death, except in cases in which the physician has "reason to believe" that "such a declaration would violate the personal religious beliefs of the individual." For such individuals, death must be declared according to traditional cardiorespiratory criteria. Similarly, New York requires "reasonable accommodation of the individual's religious or moral objection" to brain criteria for death. When such cases occur, the physician and staff should try to negotiate a compromise, respecting the patient's religious beliefs while allowing sufficient limitation of care to allow asystole to occur soon (14).

PRACTICAL SUGGESTIONS

An experienced neurologist should be consulted before a patient is declared dead by brain criteria for death. Explaining brain criteria for death to relatives requires sensitivity and patience. Some family members might believe the patient will regain consciousness, particularly if the death was sudden or unexpected. In almost all cases, compassionate explanations and emotional support from health care workers help the family accept the situation.

If organ transplantation is feasible, a physician not associated with the transplantation team should declare death to avoid any conflict of interest.

After a patient has been declared dead by brain-death criteria, all life-sustaining interventions should be discontinued, with certain exceptions. Maintaining life support might be appropriate until family members can come to the hospital, until organs for transplantation can be harvested or, under exceptional circumstances, until a fetus can be delivered.

SUMMARY

1. Patients may be declared dead using either whole brain or cardiopulmonary criteria.
2. Confusion over brain criteria for death is common; many physicians do not understand that irreversible loss of all brain function is required.

References

1. Bernat JL, Capron AM, Bleck TP, et al. The circulatory–respiratory determination of death in organ donation. *Crit Care Med* 2010;38:963-70.
2. Hornby L, Dhanani S, Shemie SD. Update of a systematic review of autoresuscitation after cardiac arrest. *Crit Care Med* 2018;46:e268-e272.
3. Miller FG, Truog RD. *Death, Dying, and Organ Transplantation*. New York: Oxford University Press; 2012.
4. Shah SK, Truog RD, Miller FG. Death and legal fictions. *J Med Ethics* 2011.
5. Wijdicks EFM. The diagnosis of brain death. *N Engl J Med* 2001;344:1215-1221.
6. Wijdicks EF, Varelas PN, Gronseth GS, et al. Evidence-based guideline update: determining brain death in adults: report of the Quality Standards Subcommittee of the American Academy of Neurology. *Neurology* 2010;74:1911-1918.
7. Nakagawa TA, Ashwal S, Mathur M, et al. Guidelines for the determination of brain death in infants and children: an update of the 1987 Task Force recommendations. *Crit Care Med* 2011;39:2139-2155.
8. Lewis A, Bernat JL, Blosser S, et al. An interdisciplinary response to contemporary concerns about brain death determination. *Neurology* 2018;90:423-426.
9. President's Council on Bioethics. *Controversies in the Determination of Death 2008*. Available from: http://bioethics.georgetown.edu/pcbe/reports/death/index.html
10. Joffe AR, Anton NR, Duff JP, et al. A survey of American neurologists about brain death: understanding the conceptual basis and diagnostic tests for brain death. *Ann Inten Care* 2012;2:4.
11. Youngner SJ, Landefeld CS, Coulton CJ, et al. "Brain death" and organ retrieval: a cross-sectional survey of knowledge and concepts among health professionals. *JAMA* 1989;261:2205-2210.
12. Capron AM. Brain death—well settled yet still unresolved. *N Engl J Med* 2001;344:1244-1246.
13. Bernat JL. The whole-brain concept of death remains optimum public policy. *J Law Med Ethics* 2006;34:35-43, 3.
14. Inwald D, Jakobovits I, Petros A. Brain stem death: managing care when accepted medical guidelines and religious beliefs are in conflict. Consideration and compromise are possible. *BMJ* 2000;320:1266-1267.
15. Olick RS. Brain death, religious freedom, and public policy: New Jersey's land ark legislative initiative. *Kennedy Instit Ethics J* 1991;1:275-288.
16. Bagheri A. Individual choice in the definition of death. *J Med Ethics* 2007;33:146-149.
17. Dorff EN. Applying traditional Jewish law to PVS. *NeuroRehabilitation* 2004;19:277-283.
18. Pope TM. Brain death rejected: expanding legal duties to accommodate religious objections. In: Cohen G, ed. *Law, Religion and Health in the US*. Cambridge University Press; 2016.
19. Lewis A, Pope TM. Physician power to declare death by neurologic criteria threatened. *Neurocrit Care* 2017;26:446-449.

ANNOTATED BIBLIOGRAPHY

1. Lewis A, Bernat JL, Blosser S, et al. An interdisciplinary response to contemporary concerns about brain death determination. *Neurology* 2018;90:423-426.

Consensus statement defending concept of determination of death by brain criteria.

2. Capron AM. Brain death—Well settled yet still unresolved. *N Engl J Med* 2001;344:1244-1246.

President's Council on Bioethics. Controversies in the Determination of Death. Washington, DC: President's Council on Bioethics; 2008. http://bioethics.georgetown.edu/pcbe/reports/death/index.html. Accessed November 11, 2011.

Miller FG, Truog RD. *Death, Dying, and Organ Transplantation*. New York, NY: Oxford University Press; 2012.

Bernat JL, Capron AM, Bleck TP, et al. The circulatory-respiratory determination of death in organ donation. *Crit Care Med* 2010;38:963-970.

Analyses of philosophic debates over the cardiopulmonary and whole-brain criteria for determining death.

3. Lewis A, Pope TM. Physician power to declare death by neurologic criteria threatened. *Neurocrit Care* 2017;26:446-449.

Discusses cases in which families opposed declaration of death by brain criteria.

Legal Rulings on Life-Sustaining Interventions

INTRODUCTION

Dramatic legal cases regarding life-sustaining interventions have captured public attention, shaped clinical practice, and motivated people to discuss their preferences for such interventions.

THE QUINLAN CASE

In 1976, the Karen Ann Quinlan case dramatized dilemmas regarding the withdrawal of life support when there is no prospect of regaining consciousness (1).

The Case

Karen Ann Quinlan was a 22-year-old woman in a persistent vegetative state or PVS (now called unresponsive wakefulness, *see* Chapter 20) because of an unknown illness. Her physicians agreed that she would never regain consciousness. She was on mechanical ventilation, and her physicians believed that she would die if the ventilator were withdrawn. Her father, after consulting with his priest and the hospital chaplain, asked that the ventilator be withdrawn. When the physicians refused, her father asked the courts to appoint him Karen's legal guardian with the authority to terminate the ventilator. The Catholic bishops of New Jersey supported his request.

The Court Ruling

The New Jersey Supreme Court ruled that Karen Ann Quinlan's right to privacy included a right to decline medical treatment and that her father as guardian could exercise this right on her behalf, giving his "best judgment" as to whether she would have declined treatment herself.

The court held unanimously that if Karen's guardian and family, her attending physician, and a hospital "ethics committee" agreed that "there is no reasonable possibility" of recovering a "cognitive and sapient state," the ventilator may be withdrawn. In advocating hospital ethics committees, the court wrote, "In the real world and in relationship to the momentous decision contemplated, the value of additional views and diverse knowledge is apparent" (1). No party would face any civil or criminal liability for discontinuing the ventilator. The court also declared that generally such decisions need not be brought to court "not only because that would be a gratuitous encroachment upon the medical profession's field of competence, but because it would be impossibly cumbersome."

Implications of the Case

As the first "right to die" case, the Quinlan case stimulated wide public discussion about life-sustaining interventions. The ruling legitimized the idea that life-sustaining interventions might be inappropriate in some situations. The Quinlan court case supported decision-making by patients, families, and physicians without routine involvement of the courts. The Quinlan decision also encouraged the development of hospital ethics committees. In hindsight, the Quinlan case also illustrates how medical prognostication is fallible. Although Ms. Quinlan's physicians expected her to die after the ventilator was discontinued, she survived for 10 years in unresponsive wakefulness without ventilatory support. Physicians now realize that patients in unresponsive wakefulness have intact brainstem function and breathe without assistance.

THE CRUZAN CASE

In the Cruzan case, the US Supreme Court issued its first decision on the "right to die" (2–5). The ruling sparked state and federal legislation to encourage the use of advance directives.

The Case

Nancy Cruzan was a 33-year-old woman who was in a PVS following an automobile accident in 1983. A month after the accident, a feeding gastrostomy tube was inserted. In 1987, realizing that her condition would not improve, her parents asked that the tube feedings be discontinued. Because the state hospital caring for Cruzan insisted on a court order, the case entered the legal system.

A year before her accident, Cruzan told her housemate that she "didn't want to live" as a "vegetable." If she "couldn't do for herself things alone even halfway, or not at all, she wouldn't want to live that way and she hoped that her family would know that" (6). Cruzan's parents asked that tube feedings be discontinued because they knew "in our hearts" that she would not want to continue living in her condition (6).

The Missouri Ruling

The 1988 Missouri Supreme Court ruling in the case severely restricted family decision-making on behalf of incompetent patients (7). Life-sustaining interventions could be withheld only with "the most rigid of formalities," such as a living will or a clear and convincing statement that the patient would not want the specific intervention in that situation. The court found no reliable evidence that Nancy Cruzan would have specifically refused artificial feedings. It asserted that Missouri's "unqualified" interest in preserving life, regardless of the patient's prognosis, outweighed any rights an incompetent patient might have to refuse treatment.

The U.S. Supreme Court Ruling

By a 5-to-4 vote, the US Supreme Court affirmed the Missouri ruling in 1990 (8). Although competent patients might have a "constitutionally protected liberty interest in refusing unwanted medical treatment," the Court declared that incompetent patients do not have the same right because they cannot exercise it directly. Thus, states may establish "procedural safeguards" governing medical decisions for incompetent patients that are more stringent than requirements for competent patients. The majority opinion declared that the individual's right to refuse treatment must be balanced against relevant state interests. The Court held that the Constitution allows states to assert an unqualified interest in "the protection and preservation of human life." It ruled that the Constitution also allows states to establish procedures to prevent abuses, to exclude quality of life as a consideration in treatment decisions, and to err on the side of continuing life-sustaining treatment. In short, states may require life-sustaining interventions when there is no clear and convincing evidence that the incompetent patient would refuse it. Although the Constitution permits states to rely on family decision making for incompetent patients, it does not mandate that they do so.

In dissent, Justice Brennan, joined by Justices Marshall and Blackmun, declared that being free of unwanted medical treatment is a fundamental constitutional right that extends to incompetent and competent patients and includes refusal of artificial fluid and nutrition. Families or patient-designated surrogates should generally make decisions for incompetent patients. In a separate dissent, Justice

Stevens went further, declaring that the Constitution requires that the best interests of the incompetent patient be followed.

The Death of Nancy Cruzan

After the Supreme Court ruling, the Cruzans petitioned the trial court in Missouri to rehear the case because new witnesses had come forward. One woman who worked with Cruzan testified that Cruzan had said that if she were a "vegetable," she would not want to be fed by force or kept alive by machines. Cruzan's attending physician changed his mind and was now in favor of stopping her feedings. The state of Missouri withdrew from further court proceedings, and in December 1990 the judge authorized removal of Cruzan's tube feedings (9).

Implications of the Cruzan Case

The Cruzan ruling spurred legislation to facilitate the use of advance directives. Many states adopted or revised laws specifically allowing patients to appoint health care proxies. The federal Patient Self Determination Act was enacted and took effect in December 1991. Under this law, virtually all hospitals, nursing homes, and health maintenance organizations must, at the time of admission, give patients written information about their right to provide advance directives.

The Cruzan case stimulated patients to think about their preferences for life-sustaining interventions and to name a surrogate decision maker if they were to lose decision-making capacity. Currently, advance care planning discussions regarding the patient's values and goals are the preferred approach because written documents do not completely relieve surrogates of the need to make difficult decisions regarding patients who have lost decision-making capacity (see Chapters 11 and 12).

THE PHYSICIAN-ASSISTED SUICIDE CASES

The Cases

Competent, terminally ill patients who wanted to end their lives by taking a lethal dose of medications, along with physicians who were willing to write such a prescription, brought court cases in New York and Washington State. These patients had various terminal illnesses, such as cancer, AIDS, and emphysema. The plaintiffs asserted that New York and Washington's prohibitions on physician-assisted suicide were unconstitutional.

The Lower Court Rulings

Two federal appellate courts declared a constitutional right to physician-assisted suicide. The Second Circuit ruled that New York State violated the 14th Amendment's guarantee of equal protection by allowing some terminally ill patients to hasten death by foregoing life-sustaining treatments, while forbidding other terminally ill patients to hasten death using a prescription for a lethal dose of medication (10). In the Washington case, the Ninth Circuit declared that the 14th Amendment's guarantee of liberty included the right to determine the time and manner of one's death through physician-assisted suicide (11).

The US Supreme Court Rulings

In 1997, the Supreme Court issued a pair of unanimous rulings that held that there is no constitutional right to physician-assisted suicide (12,13). Thus, the Washington and New York laws prohibiting physician-assisted suicide did not violate the Constitution. The Supreme Court rejected the claim that terminally ill patients had a "fundamental liberty interest" in obtaining physician-assisted suicide. According to the Court, states have legitimate reasons for prohibiting assisted suicide (12), including preserving human life, preventing suicide, protecting vulnerable groups, protecting the integrity of the medical profession, and avoiding a slippery slope to euthanasia. The Court also ruled that under the Constitution states may permit patients to forego life-sustaining treatment while prohibiting physician-assisted suicide (13). The court declared that the distinction between physician-assisted suicide and withdrawal of life-sustaining treatment is important and logical. When physicians withdraw treatment, they intend only to respect the patient's wishes, not to end the patient's life. Moreover, the cause of death is the underlying fatal disease, not the physician's action.

The Court further declared that the Constitution allows states to prohibit physician-assisted suicide, which intentionally hastens death, while permitting palliative care that might hasten death, but is intended to relieve pain (13). According to the Court, the rationale of double effect distinguished the use of high-dose narcotics from euthanasia or assisted suicide. The Court noted that "painkilling drugs may hasten a patient's death, but the physician's purpose and intent is, or may be, only to ease his patient's pain. . . . The law has long used actors' intent or purpose to distinguish between two acts that may have the same result" (13).

Implications of the Cases

By ruling that there is no constitutional right to physician-assisted suicide, these rulings shifted the attention of advocates for physician-assisted suicide (now called physician aid-in-dying) to working to have states legalize the practice. In 2018, almost 20% of the US population resides in states where it is legal.

The justices suggested that the double-effect doctrine provides a rational and constitutional basis for states to allow high-dose narcotics for pain relief in terminally ill patients while prohibiting assisted suicide (14–16). Thus, the majority opinion suggests a justification for aggressive palliative care. Three concurring justices went further, suggesting that the Constitution obligates states to permit physicians to provide adequate pain relief at the end of life, even if such care leads to unconsciousness or hastens death. The opinions therefore provide physicians legal reassurance regarding aggressive palliative care generally and proportionate palliative sedation in particular (*see* Chapter 15).

THE SCHIAVO CASE

The Case

Theresa Schiavo, a 27-year-old woman, suffered a cardiac arrest in 1990 because of potassium abnormalities and never regained consciousness. In 1998, as the legally appointed guardian, her husband asked the court to discontinue tube feedings. Her parents opposed the withdrawal of tube feedings.

The Court Rulings and the Florida Law

The trial court ruled that there was clear and convincing evidence that she would want the feedings discontinued. A long, complicated series of legal disputes ensued. The parents filed various appeals, contending that there was new evidence about her wishes, that she was not in PVS, and that her condition might improve. In 2002, the trial court held a new hearing on her current condition and on whether any new treatments might be effective. That court ruled "the credible evidence overwhelmingly supports that Terri Schiavo remains in a persistent vegetative state" (17). The court also held that the preponderance of the evidence was that no treatment would significantly improve her quality of life. The parents also claimed that new witnesses would testify that Terri's husband lied about her wishes. The court ruled that this new evidence, even if it were accepted as credible, would not meet the legal requirement that the original decision was "no longer equitable" (18). The state appellate court ruled against the parents' appeals in four separate rulings (19). The Florida Supreme Court declined to hear the case.

Prolife advocates, the Florida legislature, and Governor Jeb Bush then became involved in the case. In 2003, a law called "Terri's law" authorized the governor to issue a stay to prevent the withholding of nutrition and hydration from a patient in PVS who has no written advance directive when a member of the patient's family challenges the withholding of nutrition and hydration. In October

2003, Gov. Bush issued such a stay for Ms. Schiavo. In 2004, a Florida court ruled the law was unconstitutional, and the Florida Supreme Court affirmed that decision.

In 2005, Congress passed a law to give federal courts jurisdiction over this case. A federal district court refused to grant an injunction to halt the withdrawal of Ms. Schiavo's feeding tube, and a federal appeals court declared the law unconstitutional. The Supreme Court declined to hear the case.

Implications of the Case

Disagreements Among Family Members

The Schiavo case illustrates how intractable and bitter disputes might arise among family members of patients who lack decision-making capacity. Both the husband and the parents accused each other of acting in bad faith. The courts emphasized the desirability of having a final decision that closed the case and urged the family to end the dispute and to move forward. This case shows, however, that the legal system might not be able to resolve disputes when families are so sharply divided.

Involvement of Third Parties and the Courts

The Schiavo case is unique because of the involvement of prolife advocacy groups, the Florida legislature, the governor, and the US Congress. The involvement of third-party groups who have no direct connection with the patient raises several concerns. One is intrusion into the patient's liberty and privacy. Ordinarily, decisions about end-of-life care are delegated to families without interference by third parties. In polls, the overwhelming majority of persons say that they would want decisions to be made by their families rather than by government officials. Patients, however, might not anticipate that their family might disagree so sharply over their care. In addition, the court challenges by government officials and "Terri's law" raise fundamental questions about the appropriate role of the executive and legislative branches of government in cases that have been decided by the courts and when appeals have been exhausted.

Role of Medical Expertise and Evidence

In Internet discussions about the case and in court proceedings, some parties asserted that Ms. Schiavo was not in a PVS and that novel treatments might allow her to recover consciousness. The Florida appellate court emphasized that the legal system allowed both sides to examine the evidence on these points and to cross-examine witnesses (19). The court explained the reasoning that led it to agree with the guardianship court's ruling, that there was no evidence of a treatment that offered such promise of restoring Ms. Schiavo's cortical function or that she would choose to accept such a treatment. The high quality of medical evidence in the legal proceedings and the analysis of the credibility of that evidence contrasts sharply with Internet discussions in which claims are asserted without any evidence or without assessment of the credibility of the offered evidence.

Importance of Appointing a Proxy Decision-Maker

Terri Schiavo did not complete an advance directive designating a proxy to make decisions for her. Had she done so, the disputes between the parents and husband would likely have been resolved sooner. It is unrealistic to expect a young healthy woman to anticipate the situation that Ms. Schiavo experienced and to make informed judgments about what she would want done in a catastrophic illness. However, it is not asking too much for a healthy person to appoint a proxy whom she trusts to make decisions for her in such a situation.

SUMMARY

1. Landmark court cases have helped shape public policy regarding life-sustaining interventions.
2. Physicians need to know enough about these court rulings to correct misunderstandings by patients and colleagues or be willing to seek legal expertise.

References

1. *In the Matter of Karen Quinlan.* 70 N.J. 10, 335 A. 2d 647 (1976).
2. Angell M. Prisoners of technology: the case of Nancy Cruzan. *N Engl J Med* 1990;322:1226-1228.
3. Annas GJ. Nancy Cruzan and the right to die. *N Engl J Med* 1990;323:670-673.
4. Orentlicher D. From the office of the general counsel. The right to die after Cruzan. *JAMA* 1990;264:2444-2447.
5. Lo B, Steinbrook R. Beyond the Cruzan case: the U.S. Supreme Court and medical practice. *Ann Intern Med* 1991;114:895-901.
6. Brief for petitioners. Cruzan v. Missouri Department of Health (No. 89-1503).
7. *Cruzan v. Harmon,* 760 S.W. 2d 408.
8. *Cruzan v. Missouri, Department of Health,* 497 U.S. 261, 110 S. Ct. 2841 (1990).
9. *Cruzan v. Harmon,* No. CV384-9P, Circuit court of Missouri (Mo. Cir. Ct. Jasper County Dec. 14, 1990) (Teel, J.).
10. *Quill v. Vacco,* 830 F3d 716 (2nd Cir. 1966).
11. *Compassion in Dying v. Washington,* 79 F3d 790 (9th Cir. 1966) (en banc).
12. *Washington v. Glucksberg,* 117 S. Ct. 2258 (1997).
13. *Vacco v. Quill,* 117 S. Ct. 2293 (1997).
14. Alpers A, Lo B. The Supreme Court addresses physician-assisted suicide: can its decisions improve palliative care? *Arch Fam Pract* 1999;8:200-205.
15. Burt RA. The Supreme Court speaks: not assisted suicide but a constitutional right to palliative care. *N Engl J Med* 1997;337:1234-1236.
16. Gostin LO. Deciding life and death in the courtroom. *JAMA* 1997;278:1523-1528.
17. *In re Guardianship of Theresa Marie Schiavo,* No. 90-2908-GB-003 (Fla. Cir. Ct. 2002).
18. *In re Guardianship of Theresa Marie Schiavo,* 792 So. 2d 551 (Fla. 2001).
19. *In re Guardianship of Theresa Marie Schiavo,* 851 So. 2d 182 (Fla. 2003).

ANNOTATED BIBLIOGRAPHY

1. Burt RA. The Supreme Court speaks: not assisted suicide but a constitutional right to palliative care. *N Engl J Med* 1997;337:1234-1236.
   Alpers A, Lo B. The Supreme Court addresses physician-assisted suicide: can its decisions improve palliative care? *Arch Fam Pract* 1999;8:200-205.
   Two articles that discuss the important Supreme Court rulings in the two 1997 physician-assisted suicide cases.
2. Annas GJ. "Culture of life" politics at the bedside—The case of Schiavo. *N Engl J Med* 2005;352:1710-1715.
   Analysis of the Schiavo case.

The Doctor–Patient Relationship

Overview of the Doctor–Patient Relationship

INTRODUCTION

A strong doctor–patient relationship has many dimensions, as previous chapters have discussed. Physicians have a fiduciary obligation to act in their patients' best interests, which requires up-to-date medical knowledge, an understanding of the patient's values, goals, and preferences, and sound clinical judgment. Physicians should also help patients make informed decisions about their care, maintain confidentiality, avoid misrepresentation, and keep promises. Beyond that, patients also want caregivers who are compassionate and caring. In addition, patients want a physician who is available, coordinates their care, and guides them through the complicated health care system.

DIFFERENT DOCTOR–PATIENT RELATIONSHIPS

In broad terms, several distinct types of doctor–patient relationships have been described. Such variation raises the question of what kind of doctor–patient relationship is most appropriate for a particular physician, patient, and clinical situation.

Models of the Doctor–Patient Relationship

Several models of the doctor–patient relationship have been described: paternalism, informed choice, and shared decision-making.

Paternalism

Physicians make treatment decisions with little input from the patient, on the basis of what they believe to be the patient's best interests. Patients who prefer this decision-making style value the physician's expertise and believe that clear recommendations protect them from harm (1). Physicians' recommendations, however, might be unduly influenced by their personal values, which often differ from those of patients.

Informed Choice

Patients make the decisions about their own health care. Physicians provide relevant medical information but withhold their opinion. This is also known as the consumerist model. Physicians might decline to give a recommendation, even if a patient explicitly requests them to do so.

Shared Decision-Making

Both the physician and patient play active roles (*see* also Chapter 3). The physician gives information to the patient on treatment benefits and risks, the patient gives information to the physician about his or her values, the patient and physician discuss treatment options, and both work together to develop a plan of care that reflects the patient's informed preferences, needs, goals, and values (2-4). Shared decision-making respects patients as persons and may have a positive impact on health outcomes (5). It is commonly associated with a patient-centered approach to the medical interview, in which physicians ascertain and incorporate patients' expectations, feelings, and illness beliefs.

Several variations of shared decision-making have been described. The physician may act as a teacher or friend: encouraging patients to think about health-related values, helping them deliberate about their options, and trying to persuade them to accept recommendations (6). This interaction requires more effort and engagement than simply giving a recommendation. In another variation, physicians serve as facilitators or coaches, helping the patient think through how his or her values apply to the decision at hand (7). In this approach, physicians go beyond the role of providing information, but do not make a recommendation unless asked to do so.

What Decision-Making Style Do Patients Prefer?

Although most patients now prefer shared decision-making, others prefer different decision-making styles. In one study, 62% of respondents preferred shared decision-making, 28% preferred consumerism, and 9% preferred paternalism (5). Seventy percent usually experienced their preferred style of clinical decision-making. In another survey, 96% of respondents preferred to be offered choices and to be asked their opinions, whereas 52% preferred to leave final decisions to their physicians and 44% preferred to rely on physicians for medical information rather than seeking out information themselves (8). Thus, although almost all patients in this study wanted to be involved in decision-making, many wanted the physician to make the final decision. Women, more educated people, and healthier people were more likely to prefer an active role in decision-making. African American, Hispanic, and elderly respondents were more likely to prefer that physicians make the decisions. Patient preferences for decision-making might vary across clinical scenarios. For example, patients with problems like a fracture or appendicitis, where one option is stronger preferred, might prefer a more directive decision-making style. In contrast, for management of chronic disease, patients might be more likely to prefer shared decision-making. Recently, a number of developments indicate that some patients want more control over their medical care. The Internet allows patients to seek information from sources other than physicians and to order some services, such as genomic testing, directly. Mobile devices allow patients to gather information about their medical condition, exercise, and diet without consulting a health care professional.

Looking at what decision-making style patients actually experience, physicians commonly used a more directive, or paternalistic, style with older, less educated, and sicker patients and a more patient-centered style with younger, better educated, and more socioeconomically advantaged patients (5).

What Decision-Making Style Should Physicians Adopt?

Given this variation in preferred decision-making style, it makes sense to try to match patient preferences with the physician's actual style. Such matching respects patient autonomy and might enhance patient satisfaction with and trust in their doctors. Congruence might occur if patients choose physicians with compatible decision-making styles or if physicians modify their decision-making style to accommodate the patient's preferences. For example, physicians who generally refrain from giving explicit recommendations might do so for patients whom they know prefer a directive style.

Physicians and Entrepreneurism

Modern medicine encourages physicians to adopt an entrepreneurial approach to their work. Many standard business practices, however, might conflict with the goals and ideals of medicine (9). Business people can greatly increase their net income through targeting profitable markets, dropping unprofitable services, and using advertising to increase the demand for their product (10). These practices are considered acceptable for businesspeople who are selling computers or running a restaurant. However, should physicians or health care organizations offer services only to well-insured patients (11); drop unprofitable services, such as primary care; or increase demand for profitable services that offer little or no benefit to patients? To the extent that health care is considered a basic need or a right rather than a commodity, a predominantly commercial approach is disturbing. Moreover, medicine as a profession defines itself as putting the patient's interests first (12).

Concierge Medicine

In this arrangement, also called direct patient contracting practices, patients pay a monthly or annual fee to the primary physician (13). Arrangements vary; some physicians accept insurance payments, whereas others require patients to pay for all services. Tests, specialist care, and hospitalization require insurance coverage. Patients may be promised longer visits and improved access, continuity, and coordination of care. Physicians have smaller panels, reduced administrative burdens, less stress, greater work satisfaction, and higher income per hour of clinical practice.

Critics charge that retainer medicine increases existing health disparities and poor access to primary care for patients who cannot afford such arrangements. Defenders argue that individual physicians, including those practicing retainer medicine, have no ethical obligation to address issues of access and cost of care. Access is society's problem to be solved by legislators, government officials, and insurers. A few concierge practices serve less wealthy patients, charging lower fees and encouraging patients to have low-cost, high deductible hospital insurance. There are no good studies on the outcomes, quality of care, or costs of concierge practices (13).

However, claiming, as individual physicians or as a profession, that access to care and health disparities are someone else's problem to fix presents a thin view of moral responsibility (14). Retainer medicine physicians, who especially know the value of better access to care and longer visits, should advocate for a health care system that provides them for all patients, not just those who can pay for it (14). Furthermore, all physicians should provide some medical care to patients who have poor access to care—for example, by regularly volunteering to provide care for underserved patients.

The chapters in this section of the book discuss specific situations in which the doctor–patient relationship is problematic or difficult. Chapter 24 discusses situations in which physicians decline to care for patients because they fear that their own health or safety is jeopardized or consider a patient difficult or obnoxious. Chapter 25 discusses the ethical issues that might arise when patients give gifts to their physicians. Chapter 26 analyzes sexual relationships between physicians and patients and discusses how such contact might harm patients. Chapter 27 suggests secret information from family members or friends about a patient. Chapter 28 analyzes how clinical research, which is essential for medical progress, presents risks to patients who participate in studies.

References

1. Swenson SL, Zettler P, Lo B. "She gave it her best shot right away": Patient experiences of biomedical and patient-centered communication. *Patient Educ Couns* 2006;61:200-211.
2. Elwyn G, Durand MA, Song J, et al. A three-talk model for shared decision making: multistage consultation process. *BMJ* 2017;359:j4891.
3. Murray E, Charles C, Gafni A. Shared decision-making in primary care: tailoring the Charles et al. model to fit the context of general practice. *Patient Educ Couns* 2006;62:205-211.
4. Charles CA, Whelan T, Gafni A, et al. Shared treatment decision making: what does it mean to physicians? *J Clin Oncol* 2003;21:932-936.
5. Murray E, Pollack L, White M, et al. Clinical decision-making: Patients' preferences and experiences. *Patient Educ Couns* 2007;65:189-196.
6. Emanuel EJ, Emanuel LL. Four models of the physician–patient relationship. *JAMA* 1992;267:2221-2226.
7. White DB, Malvar G, Karr J, et al. Expanding the paradigm of the physician's role in surrogate decision-making: an empirically derived framework. *Crit Care Med* 2010;38:743-750.
8. Levinson W, Kao A, Kuby A, et al. Not all patients want to participate in decision making. A national study of public preferences. *J Gen Intern Med* 2005;20:531-535.

9. Kassirer JP. Managed care and the morality of the marketplace. *N Engl J Med* 1995;333:50-52.

10. Jonsen AR. Ethics remain at the heart of medicine: physicians and entrepreneurship. *West J Med* 1986;144:480-483.

11. Brennan TA. Concierge care and the future of general internal medicine. *J Gen Intern Med* 2005;20:1190.

12. Medical professionalism in the new millennium: a physician charter. *Ann Intern Med* 2002;136:243-246.

13. Doherty R. Assessing the patient care implications of "concierge" and other direct patient contracting practices: a policy position paper from the american college of physicians. *Ann Intern Med* 2015;163:949-952.

14. Lo B. Retainer medicine: why not for all? *Ann Intern Med* 2011;155:641-642.

Refusal to Care for Patients

INTRODUCTION

Physicians might refuse to care for persons for a variety of reasons, including an unacceptable threat to their personal safety, their personal moral objections to providing care, or a counterproductive or adversarial doctor–patient relationship. Such refusal to provide care raises ethical dilemmas because the patient's medical needs and best interests might be compromised by the physician's refusal. Although the law generally permits physicians to decide whether to accept new patients, it seems inhumane for physicians to refuse crucial medical care to sick persons in need. The following case illustrates such a refusal to care for a patient.

CASE 24.1 **Surgery in an HIV-infected patient**

Mr. N is a 43-year-old man with asymptomatic HIV infection. While crossing a street, he is struck by a car running a red light. He suffers a comminuted fracture of the proximal femoral shaft. The surgeons decline to operate because the patient's viral titer has not been checked recently, saying that this fracture can be managed without surgery. Moreover, in orthopedics operations, sharp bone fragments from seropositive patients may penetrate gloves and subject health care workers to an unacceptable risk of lethal illness.

In Case 24.1, the surgeon fears contracting a fatal blood-borne infection. Standard treatment for this fracture is operative fixation with an intramedullary rod. Closed treatment requires several months of traction and has poorer outcomes. Early in the HIV epidemic, HIV infection was a fatal illness with no effective treatment. Similarly, during the severe acute respiratory syndrome (SARS) epidemic of 2002 and the Ebola virus outbreak of 2014 some health care workers refused to care for infected patients. Indeed, throughout history physicians have often abandoned their patients during deadly epidemics, such as plague, smallpox, and yellow fever (1). Thus it is important to acknowledge the tension between the ethical ideal that physicians should care for patients even at some personal risk and the reality of fears of dying from a fatal infection. As we discuss later, institutional responsibilities to provide protective equipment is a necessary adjust to responsibility of individual physicians.

THE CONTEXT OF THE DOCTOR–PATIENT RELATIONSHIP

Ethical Obligations to Care for Patients

Physicians present themselves to the public as helpers of the sick and needy, who use their expertise for the benefit of patients. The ethical ideal is that patients will receive needed care, even in cases in which the physician might find it risky, difficult, or inconvenient. At the beginning of the HIV epidemic, the Surgeon General declared, "Health care in this country has always been predicated on the assumption that somehow, everyone will be cared for, and no one will be turned away. As a physician and an American, I'm proud to be part of a tradition of care that will not abandon the sick or disabled, whoever they are."

In the doctor–patient relationship, the patient's best interests should take priority over the doctor's self-interest (*see* Chapter 4). Physicians should not refuse care to patients whom they personally dislike or whose actions, such as smoking, alcohol and substance abuse, or nonadherence to medications, make treatment more difficult.

Furthermore, physicians are exhorted to provide needed medical care even to patients whose actions are morally reprehensible. Doctors are expected to provide care to the perpetrator of a violent assault, as well as to the victim. Even in war, physicians are expected to attend to the sick and injured, regardless of which side they are on.

Legal Definition of the Doctor–Patient Relationship

Society as a whole and the medical profession have a moral obligation to care for sick persons, yet individual doctors generally have no legal duty to provide care. The law generally characterizes the doctor–patient relationship as a contract between autonomous individuals who are free to enter into or break off the relationship, provided that the patient is not abandoned (2). Courts have ruled that physicians have no legal duty to treat new patients who seek care in the absence of an agreement to provide medical care, such as a contract with a health maintenance organization (HMO). For example, it is legal for physicians to schedule new patient appointments only for people with adequate health insurance. Similarly, physicians may restrict the scope of their practice to a particular specialty or range of problems. Thus, an internist would not be expected to perform surgery, just as a psychiatrist would not be expected to treat meningitis.

The legal right to decline to care for patients, however, is limited in many important ways. The Americans with Disabilities Act also forbids physicians from declining to care for patients on the basis of race, sex, national origin, religion, or disability (3).

Employment contracts, as with hospitals or HMOs, may oblige physicians to care for all qualified persons who seek treatment. Similarly, physicians who are on call for a hospital may be required as a condition of staff privileges to provide care to persons who present there. As discussed later in this chapter, emergency departments are required to provide indicated emergency care to patients who seek it.

Physicians and hospitals, however, are not required to provide care when an "individual poses a direct threat to the health or safety of others that cannot be eliminated or reduced by reasonable accommodation" (4). Direct threat refers to "a significant risk of substantial harm," not risks that are "slightly increased," "speculative," or "remote." This determination of risk must be made according to objective, scientific evidence, not simply the health care worker's subjective judgment. Caring for HIV-infected persons is not considered a "direct threat" to health care workers (5).

OCCUPATIONAL RISKS TO PHYSICIANS

Emerging infections, such as HIV infection, SARS, and Ebola, have several characteristics that heighten fears of health care workers: the threat is new and potentially lethal, important information about risk and transmission is unknown or emerging, effective treatments and preventive equipment are lacking, and messages from public officials may be inconsistent or unsupported by evidence. Even if the probability of transmission is low, the infection is or may be fatal.

Serious Occupational Risks

Nearly one in 10 US health care workers has a needlestick injury each year (6). Surgeons and operating room staff are at higher risk for occupational blood-borne infections than office-based physicians.

The risk of seroconversion after a percutaneous exposure to the blood of a seropositive patient is 0.3%, and after mucocutaneous exposure the risk is 0.09% (7). Postexposure prophylaxis with combination antiretroviral therapies can reduce the incidence of occupational HIV infection. The risk of occupational hepatitis B after parenteral exposure to the blood of an infected patient with e antigen is between 19% and 37%. The risk of contracting hepatitis C after parenteral exposure to the blood of an infected patient is 1.9%.

Concern about occupational HIV infection has led to important improvements in hospital inflectional control (6). Standard precautions are now required to prevent exposure to blood or other bodily fluids. Operating room techniques have been changed to decrease the likelihood of sharps injuries through "no touch" techniques. Alternatives to needles and other sharp implements have been introduced. Instead of sutures, wounds are now closed with tape, staples, and tissue glue. Laparoscopic and robotic surgery reduce risk compared with open procedures. Of note, these improvements in infection control were developed only after health care workers contracted occupational HIV infection early in the epidemic. Similarly, adequate protective gear had not been developed early in the Ebola epidemic.

In addition to infections risks, angry or psychotic patients might physically threaten or harm health care workers. About one quarter of emergency department physicians reported being physically assaulted during the previous year (8). Nurses and nurses' aides suffer even higher rates of physical violence.

Responding to Occupational Risks

The risk of serious occupational illness is often framed as the responsibility of individual health care worker to provide care even at personal risk. However, hospitals and clinics have ethical and legal obligations to mitigate risks.

Acknowledge and Address Fears

Physicians and health officials must acknowledge their human fears and limitations; only then are reflection, discussion, and constructive action possible. Fears about safety need to be acknowledged as an understandable human reaction, rather than condemned as hysteria. In previous epidemics, many physicians, including Galen and Sydenham, fled from patients with fatal contagious diseases (1). Health care workers need their concerns addressed in a nonjudgmental way.

Some techniques for encouraging health care workers to accept occupational risks are usually ineffective. Moral exhortations to provide care might go unheeded. Indeed, health care workers might be outraged at the suggestion that it is unethical to worry about their safety. Reassurance that a risk is low or comparable to other risks generally is counterproductive. People reject the suggestion that because they accept risks of greater magnitude, such as the risk of automobile accidents, they should also accept the risk in question (9).

Reduce Occupational Risks

Hospitals and clinics must provide a safe working environment, which includes protective equipment such as masks, gowns, and gloves. At the onset of an emerging infectious epidemic, however, the best protective measures might not be known, or standard protective measures may be ineffective. New equipment might need to be developed and made available, for example, retractable needles and other safety-engineered devices to reduce the risk of sharps injuries and blood-borne infections.

Support Health Care Workers Who Are Exposed to Contagious Diseases

Health care institutions should support health care workers who put themselves at risk, for example, through prompt, compassionate, confidential occupational health services that provide both clinical services and emotional support. The general public also should acknowledge the work of health care workers and not fear them as vectors of contagion.

Balance Risks to Health Care Workers and Benefits to Patients

Health care workers should provide care if the medical benefit to the patient is clearly established, substantial, and highly probable, provided that appropriate precautions have been taken to reduce risk. On the other hand, severe risks to health care workers might justify delaying or postponing interventions whose benefits are unproved, uncertain, or marginal.

Judgments about the benefits and risks of treatment need to be scientifically sound. In Case 24.1, it would be misleading for physicians to say that operative reduction for this condition is not indicated in seropositive persons. Such surgery is routinely performed for this indication in patients who have other diseases, such as cancer, with poor prognoses. If physicians bias their medical judgments to avoid caring for seropositive persons, patients and the public will justifiably question their recommendations on other issues.

CONSCIENTIOUS OBJECTION BY PHYSICIANS

This ethical ideal of providing needed care may conflict with a health care worker's core moral and religious beliefs. Physicians may decline to provide such care to maintain their moral integrity. For example, Catholic physicians who consider abortions or contraception immoral do not provide or prescribe such care. Moreover, such physicians may decline to discuss these options with patients or refer them to other physicians who would provide them because they believe that such actions would be complicity with an immoral action (10, 11).

On the one hand, there are strong reasons to honor claims of conscience, even if one disagrees with the beliefs animating those claims (*see* also Chap 1) (11-13). All people, including health care professionals, should be free to act on sincerely, deeply held religious and moral beliefs, which are essential to who they are as individual persons. Respecting conscientious objections promotes moral reflection, religious freedom, and tolerance. In the United States, these have traditionally been important social values. Historically, many founding settlers in the United States were seeking refuge from religious persecution in Europe.

On the other hand, there are also strong countervailing reasons to ensure that patients in need receive medically appropriate care (12, 14). When patients present for medical care, the expectation is that they should be informed of the medically feasible options for care and have access to medically appropriate care delivered in a timely manner. Under the doctrine of informed consent, physicians should not withhold information about accepted options for care even if they personally disagree with them and would not personally provide them. If a standard intervention is beyond the scope of the physician's or institution's practice, the patient should be referred to a provider who can provide the care. Thus, when physicians decline to offer patients information about options, they are restricting patients' ability to make informed choices about their care.

These conflicting ethical guidelines may be reconciled by placing the duty to provide care that a patient needs on the health care institution where the patient seeks care, rather than on the individual health care professional (14). The clinic, hospital, or pharmacy should have an obligation to assure that patients receive needed care. Institutions should make reasonable accommodation to their employees' personal beliefs by arranging staffing so that another professional provides the service (15). Timely access to a willing physician is particularly important for services that must be provided on an emergency basis or within a narrow window of opportunity. Health care workers who raise a conscientious objection should not obstruct the patient from receiving care from others or provide misinformation to the patient (16). That is, the health care worker seeking to maintain his or her moral integrity and follow his or her conscience should not, in his or her professional role, try to prevent patients from obtaining medical care that he or she morally objects to but that other providers would provide as appropriate care (17).

Additional dilemmas arise if a health care organization declares that certain services violate their institutional mission, as when Catholic hospitals do not provide family planning or abortion services. Although there are strong reasons to respect an institutional policy that is based on religious beliefs, it is also essential to inform patients when they select a provider, establish care, schedule appointments, or present for care that certain interventions will not be provided. It cannot be assumed that a woman seeking care at a Catholic-affiliated hospital knows that some reproductive services will not be provided (18, 19). In fact, when a Catholic hospital merges with or acquires other hospitals and requires other hospitals not to provide certain services, the other hospital may retain its original name, with no indication of its new Catholic affiliation. Many patients who seek care at an institution may not accept the moral beliefs that animate the institution. Because of geography, insurance restrictions, or ambulance policies, however, patients may have no alternative provider.

If health care professionals or institutions decide that for reasons of conscience they cannot provide certain services, they should inform patients, preferably before the services are actually needed, so that patients can decide whether to seek care elsewhere (20). Many patients have to select a provider for insurance purposes, and it would be highly burdensome or even impossible for them to switch providers when they need the specific service. Thus, at a woman's first visit for reproductive or obstetrical care, she should be told if the physician or practice does not prescribe contraception or provide abortions.

Further dilemmas arise when hospitals forbid physicians who work there from providing information to patients about services such as family planning or referring patients for such services. These restrictions may impinge on physicians' conscience, freedom of religion, free speech, and medical judgment. Restricting such communication also denies important medical information to patients and imposes the institution's views on them. In the Internet era, such institutions can refer patients to balanced and medically accurate websites for information.

Although conscientious objections should be reasonably accommodated, there are important limits. First, refraining from providing an intervention must be distinguished from insisting on providing interventions that an informed patient has refused. As Chapter 5 discusses, patients have a right to be free of unwanted medical interventions. Thus, providers may not insist that a patient receive CPR, tube feedings, or other life-sustaining interventions over their objections, even if their insistence is based on deeply held moral values. Second, claims of conscience should not justify refusing needed treatment to patients because of their race, ethnicity, national origin, religion, gender, or sexual orientation. Such discrimination violates the physician's ethical duty to respect patients as persons and to care for those in need, and may also violate antidiscrimination laws and regulations.

DIFFICULT DOCTOR–PATIENT RELATIONSHIPS

Ideally, the doctor–patient relationship is a partnership whose goal is the patient's well-being. In some cases, however, the relationship might be unproductive or adversarial and the physician might consider the patient a "problem" or "difficult" patient, as in the following case (21).

CASE 24.2 | Disruptive and uncooperative patient

Ms. W is a 35-year-old woman with end-stage renal disease who repeatedly misses dialysis appointments and requires emergency dialysis. She also does not take her medications regularly or follow her diet, is frequently intoxicated, and disrupts the dialysis unit with her obscene and insulting language and attempts to strike health care workers who are connecting her to the dialysis machine. Other patients request to change the time of their dialysis, and nurses try to avoid shifts when she is scheduled. When she presents to the emergency department with shortness of breath and is found to have congestive heart failure and hyperkalemia, the nephrologist considers refusing dialysis.

In Case 24.2, Ms. W repeatedly misses appointments, fails to take her medications, and requires emergency care after missing scheduled appointments. Furthermore, she is disruptive, angry, and violent. Physicians commonly view such patients as "bad" patients who have broken the implicit rules of the doctor–patient relationship (22). Health care workers are understandably frustrated when the patient's own actions bring about or exacerbate medical problems. Some patient behaviors go beyond undermining their own health. Missing scheduled dialysis times disrupts the dialysis team's schedules and inconveniences staff. The patient may provoke such strong negative reactions in health care workers that a therapeutic relationship no longer exists (22). Doctors resent spending so much time and energy on such a patient that the care of other patients is compromised. Finally, physical threats or actual violence make it impossible for the dialysis staff to provide care and for other patients to receive care (23). Health care workers and other patients have a right to be free of abuse, threats, and violence.

Responding to Difficult Doctor–Patient Relationships

In most cases, physicians can find ways to improve a difficult doctor–patient relationship (Table 24-1).

Acknowledge that Problems Exist

The first step is for both physicians and patients to acknowledge problems. The physician might say, "I sense that both of us are disappointed with how your care is turning out."

Try to Understand the Patient's Perspective

Physicians might feel that some patients intentionally vex them, making their work more difficult. The patient, however, might have sound reasons for missing appointments, such as difficulties with insurance coverage, transportation, or childcare. Illness might cause patients to feel angry, frustrated, helpless, or out of control. Also, patients might not have control over some behaviors because of psychiatric conditions.

Physicians can elicit patients' perspectives through open-ended questions about the impact of their illness, other demands in their life, and barriers to care. Acknowledging a patient's emotions also encourages further discussion. Once their problems and frustration are acknowledged, patients might be better able to appreciate how their behavior is disrupting their care or the care of other patients.

Try to Understand Your Own Responses

Health care workers need to understand how their actions might exacerbate the patient's behavior. Physicians and nurses who are frustrated and angry might vent their anger on the patient or treat him or her curtly. Differences in ethnic background, social class, and lifestyle might exacerbate tensions.

Try to Negotiate Mutually Acceptable Plans for Continued Care

Physicians can try to set limits on disruptive behaviors and find mutually acceptable conditions for the doctor–patient relationship (24). A psychiatric or social work consultation can often be helpful. Physicians can give patients notice that certain behaviors will lead to termination of the doctor–patient relationship. Doctors can negotiate a formal "contract" that explicitly sets conditions under which the patient and physician will continue the relationship.

TABLE 24-1.   Improving Difficult Doctor–Patient Relationships
Acknowledge that problems exist.
Try to understand the patient's perspective.
Try to understand your own responses.
Try to negotiate mutually acceptable plans for continued care.

CASE 24.2 | *Continued*

In response to the physician's open-ended questions, Ms. W said she was frustrated at having to come to dialysis on a rigid schedule and admitted that when she drank heavily she missed sessions. Her physician said, "We're trying our best to help you, but it's hard for us if you take a swing at us and don't keep appointments." To set limits on her abusive and violent behavior, the doctor might say, "I'm willing to try to find a way that we can work together. But if you want to get care here, you cannot make obscene or abusive comments or swing at anyone." The doctor negotiated an agreement that the unit would continue to provide dialysis provided that a family member would accompany Ms. W to dialysis sessions and that she accept treatment for substance abuse and counseling (21). Ms. W and several relatives signed the contract.

When Ms. W did not change her behavior, her doctor notified her that he would no longer provide chronic dialysis and gave her a list of nephrologists in the area. However, Ms. W continued to present to the emergency department with congestive heart failure and uremia.

Terminating the Doctor–Patient Relationship

The patient and physician may agree to transfer the care of the patient to another physician. Physicians may also terminate the doctor–patient relationship in certain situations—for example, when a patient breaks his or her agreement about disruptive and violent behavior. Because termination is a drastic measure, it should be used only as a last resort after attempts to find common ground for ongoing care have failed.

Patient Abandonment

Legally and ethically, physicians may not abandon patients with whom they have established a doctor–patient relationship (21). When terminating a relationship, physicians need to give patients reasonable written notice, so that they can find a new physician and obtain needed timely care for ongoing medical problems. To help patients find another physician, doctors can give patients a list of other qualified physicians in the area or refer them to the county medical society.

Obligation to Provide Emergency Care

An emergency department must provide emergency care to patients who seek it. The public relies on emergency departments and physicians to provide proper emergency treatment and expects them to do so. Delays in emergency care might seriously harm patients.

The federal Emergency Medical Treatment and Labor Act prohibits emergency departments from transferring patients in unstable condition who need emergency care, as well as pregnant women in active labor. Every person seeking treatment in an emergency department must receive a screening examination. If the patient is found to have an emergency condition, the hospital must provide treatment to stabilize the patient's condition, within the constraints of the available staff and facilities.

CASE 24.2 | *Continued*

When Ms. W presents to the emergency department with life-threatening uremia and congestive heart failure, emergency dialysis must be provided (23), and a nephrologist and dialysis nurse must be called in. Therefore, the health care workers who have terminated her from providing chronic dialysis might still have to perform emergency dialysis. Sometimes, it is possible to make arrangements for different individuals or institutions to share the emergency care of such patients.

SUMMARY

1. Physicians have an ethical obligation to care for patients even at some personal risk or inconvenience.
2. Before unilaterally terminating a difficult doctor–patient relationship, physicians should try to understand the patient's perspective and to find some mutually acceptable arrangement for continuing care.
3. Conscience-based objections to providing services should be respected, but patients also should have access to information on options for care and access to medically indicated services.

References

1. Markel H. Ebola fever and global health responsibilities. *Milbank Q* 2014;92:633-639.
2. Annas GJ. Not saints, but healers: the legal duties of health care professionals in the AIDS epidemic. *Am J Public Health* 1988;78:844-849.
3. Americans with Disabilities Act of 1990. 42 USC §§12181,12182.
4. Americans with Disabilities Act Public Accommodation Regulations. 28 CFR § 36.201.
5. Gostin LO, Feldbaum C, Webber DW. Disability discrimination in America: HIV/AIDS and other health conditions. *JAMA* 1999;281:745-752.
6. Henderson DK. Management of needlestick injuries: a house officer who has a needlestick. *JAMA* 2012;307:75-84.
7. Panlilio AL, Cardo DM, Grohskopf LA, et al. Updated U.S. Public Health Service guidelines for the management of occupational exposures to HIV and recommendations for postexposure prophylaxis. *MMWR Recomm Rep* 2005;54:1-17.
8. Phillips JP. Workplace Violence against health care workers in the United States. *N Engl J Med* 2016;374:1661-1669.
9. Rosenbaum L. Communicating uncertainty—Ebola, public health, and the scientific process. *N Engl J Med* 2015;372:7-9.
10. Kaveny MC. Complicity with evil. *Criterion* 2003;42:20-29.
11. Sulmasy DP. What is conscience and why is respect for it so important? *Theor Med Bioeth* 2008;29:135-149.
12. Brock DW. Conscientious refusal by physicians and pharmacists: who is obligated to do what, and why? *Theor Med Bioeth* 2008;29:187-200.
13. Wicclair MR. *Conscientious Objection in Health Care*. Cambridge University Press; 2011.
14. Lewis-Newby M, Wicclair M, Pope T, et al. An official American Thoracic Society policy statement: managing conscientious objections in intensive care medicine. *Am J Respir Crit Care Med* 2015;191:219-227.
15. Cantor J, Baum K. The limits of conscientious objection—may pharmacists refuse to fill prescriptions for emergency contraception? *N Engl J Med* 2004;351:2008-2012.
16. Greenberger MD, Vogelstein R. Public health. Pharmacist refusals: a threat to women's health. *Science* 2005;308:1557-1558.
17. White DB, Brody B. Would accommodating some conscientious objections by physicians promote quality in medical care? *JAMA* 2011;305:1804-1805.
18. Freedman LR, Hebert LE, Battistelli MF, et al. Religious hospital policies on reproductive care: what do patients want to know? *Am J Obstet Gynecol* 2018;218:251.e1-.e9.
19. Guiahi M. Catholic health care and women's health. *Obstet Gynecol* 2018;131:534-537.
20. Stahl RY, Emanuel EJ. Physicians, not conscripts—conscientious objection in health care. *N Engl J Med* 2017;376:1380-1385.
21. Orentlicher D. Denying treatment to the noncompliant patient. *JAMA* 1991;265:1579-1582.
22. Stokes T, Dixon-Woods M, McKinley RK. Breaking up is never easy: GPs' accounts of removing patients from their lists. *Fam Pract* 2003;20:628-634.
23. Friedman EA. Must we treat noncompliant ESRD patients? *Semin Dial* 2001;14:23-27.
24. Quill TE. Partnerships in patient care: a contractual approach. *Ann Intern Med* 1983;98:228-234.

ANNOTATED BIBLIOGRAPHY

1. Annas GJ. Not saints, but healers: the legal duties of health care professionals in the AIDS epidemic. *Am J Public Health* 1988;78:844-849.

   Discusses how physicians have no legal duty to treat patients in most situations, despite a strong moral duty to do so.

2. Stahl RY, Emanuel EJ. Physicians, not conscripts—conscientious objection in health care. *N Engl J Med* 2017;376:1380-1385.

   Article on health care workers' conscientious refusals to provide care, arguing that patients needing the service should be referred to other providers or facilities that will provide needed care.

3. Sulmasy DP. What is conscience and why is respect for it so important? *Theoret Med Bioeth* 2008;29:135-149.

   Brock DW. Conscientious refusal by physicians and pharmacists: who is obligated to do what, and why? *Theoret Med Bioeth* 2008;29:187-200.

   Wicclair MR. *Conscientious Objection in Health Care*. Cambridge University Press; 2011.

   Thoughtful conceptual and normative analyses of conscience.

4. Friedman EA. Must we treat noncompliant ESRD patients? *Semin Dial* 2001;14:23-27.

   Discusses legal, ethical, and clinical aspects of denying treatment to noncompliant, abusive, violent dialysis patients.

5. Gostin LO, Feldbaum C, Webber DW. Disability discrimination in America: HIV/AIDS and other health conditions. *JAMA* 1999;281:745-752.

   Summary of disability law that explains that physicians may decline to care for infectious patients only if there is a significant risk of substantial harm.

Gifts from Patients to Physicians

INTRODUCTION

Modest gifts from patients, such as cookies, candy, flowers, and toys for children, gratify physicians and allow patients to express their appreciation. Other gifts, however, are problematic. Expensive gifts might compromise the physician's judgment. Very personal gifts imply more than a professional relationship. Physicians who feel uncomfortable about a gift might be uncertain how to respond.

Gifts from patients are often considered simply matters of social convention and etiquette, not ethics. This chapter points out how gifts from patients might raise ethical issues because they might change the doctor–patient relationship, impair clinical judgment, or erode public trust. Because physicians often find it embarrassing to discuss gifts, this chapter also suggests how to respond to problematic gifts from patients.

REASONS PATIENTS GIVE GIFTS TO PHYSICIANS

Because gifts may have multiple meanings, physicians should consider why a patient is giving a specific gift at a particular time (1, 2).

To Thank Physicians

Patients commonly send gifts to express appreciation to physicians for their care. Patients who have recovered from serious illness are understandably grateful to their physicians, particularly if the diagnosis was difficult, the treatment was complicated, or the physician was particularly supportive or involved. The gift is similar to a tip for outstanding service.

To Satisfy Their Own Needs

Gifts might also reflect the patient's psychological needs.

CASE 25.1	Cookies from a lonely elderly patient

A 74-year-old widow has hypertension, osteoarthritis, and mild depression. She has no surviving relatives, few friends, and few social activities. A new resident takes over her care. She talks about her sadness and emptiness, and he encourages her to attend a senior center. On the next visit she brings him a box of home-baked cookies.

To Enhance Future Care

Gifts might represent expectations for future care rather than thanks for past efforts. Patients might believe that a gift will gain them special consideration. For instance, some patients might want to have the last appointment of the day because of difficulties getting off from work. Other patients might hope that gifts will gain them more timely appointments or faster responses to phone calls. In rare cases, patients who give gifts might subsequently ask physicians to do something that is ethically questionable.

CASE 25.2 | Request for disability certification

A patient with mild asthma gives his physician a toy for his son at Christmas. The next month he asks the physician to complete a form for a disability parking sticker. The patient does not meet the objective criteria for hypoxemia or dyspnea listed on the form.

In Case 25.2, the timing of the gift and the request are disturbing. The physician might feel manipulated because an apparently thoughtful gift probably had strings attached. Deceiving third parties about a patient's condition is ethically problematic (*see* Chapter 6). To do so after receiving a gift would appear like accepting a bribe.

To Meet Cultural Expectations

In some cultures, gifts to physicians or other healers are routinely expected. Such gifts might show respect or be considered an essential aspect of the healing process. In some societies, bribery might be necessary to ensure access to care. Physicians need to consider whether gifts might have special cultural significance for patients and correct any misconceptions about the US medical care system.

PROBLEMS WITH GIFTS

It is human nature for patients who have given gifts to expect some consideration in return, either consciously or unconsciously (3); however, some gifts might lead to inappropriate expectations by patients.

Expectations for Special Treatment

Some patients might believe that gifts entitle them to special treatment. Beyond more convenient or prompter appointments, some patients might feel entitled to call the physician at home for routine issues. Even apparently small gifts are problematic if such expectations become burdensome to physicians. For example, physicians want to limit add-on appointments and after-hours phone calls to reduce personal stress and to protect their family life, yet they might find it difficult to refuse a request from a patient who has given a gift.

Changes in the Doctor–Patient Relationship

Some gifts might change the doctor–patient relationship inappropriately.

CASE 25.1 | *Continued.*

The lonely, elderly patient starts to bring gifts of food at every visit. Moreover, visits now focus on the physician rather than on the patient. The patient inquires about what foods the physician likes so that she can plan her next gift. She also expresses concern about whether he is getting enough sleep and has enough time off.

In Case 25.1, an overworked and underappreciated house officer might be delighted that someone takes a personal interest in him, but it is problematic if the physician assumes the role of a surrogate grandchild. Patient visits should focus on the patient's problems, not the physician's. The physician might miss opportunities to encourage and reinforce the patient's efforts to become more socially active in the community. In the long run, it is problematic for lonely patients to depend on the medical system for their emotional and social needs.

Other gifts violate the boundaries of the professional relationship. An extreme example might be the gift of lingerie or other intimate apparel, which implies a romantic relationship, not a professional one. Patients who overstep the boundaries of a professional relationship are acting out their own needs or fantasies. Not only should such gifts be refused, but also appropriate boundaries need to be promptly and firmly reestablished. After such a gift, a physician might need to transfer care to another physician.

For isolated patients, their physician might listen or pay attention to them more than anyone else. Bringing a gift might give them a sense of purpose or alleviate their loneliness. Taking initiative and showing concern for other people might be therapeutic. For other patients, giving a physician small gifts provides a personal connection to an impersonal medical system.

Impairment of Clinical Judgment

Gifts can create or strengthen personal ties, but too close a relationship might be undesirable. It is difficult to provide care to a close relative because emotional ties might cloud clinical judgment (2). In a similar way, gifts that establish or imply a very close personal relationship might compromise the physician's judgment. Expectations of special treatment might compromise care, as when a patient expects the physician to manage a complicated problem on the basis of a telephone call rather than an office visit. Psychologically, it may be difficult to say no to patients who have given gifts, even if they request interventions that are unsound medical practice. Similarly, a gift from a seriously ill patient might be problematic if it leads the physician to misrepresent bad news or causes the patient to develop unrealistic expectations.

Erosion of Public Trust

The doctor–patient relationship might be weakened if other patients believe that they will receive second-class care unless they offer gifts. Physicians serve as gatekeepers, allocating appointments, their time and attention, and health care resources. Generally, phone calls or appointments are allocated primarily on the basis of patient need. It would damage both the individual physician and the profession as a whole if patients believed that the best way to get the physician's attention is through a gift. Even a perception that physicians are allocating their efforts on the basis of favoritism might erode public trust.

Soliciting Gifts

Although this chapter has focused on gifts that patients offer to physicians, solicitation of gifts by physicians also merits attention. It is unethical for physicians to solicit personal gifts in return for services rendered because physicians' fees should be adequate compensation for their services. It might also be problematic for physicians to solicit contributions for some cause, such as a hospital or a political movement. Such solicitations might seem a natural way for physicians to work for causes they believe in, but patients might not feel free to decline the solicitation if their physician solicits it personally and knows whether they have responded. They might fear that the physician will not render prompt or meticulous care in the future if they refuse.

Physicians are increasingly asked to help hospitals and medical schools solicit donations from "grateful" patients, for example introducing staff from the development office or directly talking to their patients about donating. Most physicians are concerned that these actions could interfere with the doctor–patient relationship (4).

HOW TO RESPOND TO GIFTS FROM PATIENTS

In responding to gifts, physicians need to take into account the nature of the gift and the circumstances.

Accept Appropriate Gifts Graciously

Most small gifts from patients are well intentioned and appropriate and should be accepted graciously. Indeed, many patients would feel insulted if physicians did not accept homemade cookies, toys for Christmas, or clothes for a new baby. Similarly, it would be unfeeling not to accept a small gift after the physician has devoted a great deal of effort in helping a patient recover from a difficult illness.

Do Not Let Gifts Go to Your Head

Physicians should not allow gifts from patients to give them an exaggerated sense of their importance or skill. Many patients, because they are sick and dependent, are extremely grateful for competent, humane care. It is gratifying that such qualities in physicians are recognized and reinforced, but physicians should appreciate that they might simply have provided the kind of care that every patient deserves.

Appreciate That Some Gifts Are Problematic

Some gifts might seem disproportionate to the care provided (5).

CASE 25.3	Tickets to an opera

A 52-year-old businessman establishes care with a new physician. At the first visit, they discuss preventive measures such as exercise and diet. The next week the businessman offers the physician orchestra tickets to the opera opening night gala.

Intuitively, some gifts seem out of proportion to what the physician has done. Most physicians would feel comfortable accepting gifts worth less than $50, but many would feel uncomfortable accepting opening night opera tickets, as in Case 25.3, after a routine new patient visit. Even if a wealthy patient considers this a small gift, it might give the wrong impression to other patients. Furthermore, the physician might wonder whether such a lavish gift reflects unrealistic expectations for care. Finally, many physicians feel uncomfortable accepting cash gifts because they seem associated with commerce and profits.

Get Advice About the Gift

Most physicians, even if they are uncomfortable about gifts, hesitate to discuss them with colleagues. Physicians might not appreciate that many colleagues also feel awkward and uncertain about gifts. Other people, however, can help the physician interpret the significance of gifts and understand the patient's possible expectations. In judging a gift's appropriateness, physicians can apply a practical rule of thumb: How would colleagues and other patients react if they knew about the gift? If others would question the gift, it is best not to accept it.

Decline Gifts Without Rejecting the Patient

Even when physicians believe that declining a gift is appropriate, they might find it awkward to do so. Several strategies might allow the physician to decline the gift, while respecting the patient's feelings. Physicians should start by saying that they are grateful and touched. One approach is to explain that accepting such a gift might compromise the physician's ability to give high-quality care in the future. Although this approach is straightforward, patients often protest that they would never ask for special consideration. A second approach is to decline the gift politely but firmly without giving more specific reasons. Physicians might simply say that they could not possibly accept the gift and that their policy is not to accept such gifts, even though they are touched by the thoughtfulness. Alternatively, the physician can resolve concerns about a large gift, as in Case 25.3, by sharing it with others, for example, by donating it to house staff.

If the physician suspects that gifts reflect the patient's social isolation or other needs, as in Case 25.1, these issues should be addressed separately during patient visits.

What If the Patient Later Requests Special Treatment?

After a gift, the patient might later request special treatment. A practical guideline is for physicians to do what they would have done if the same request had come from a patient who had not given a gift (5).

SUMMARY

1. Usually, gifts are thoughtful gestures of appreciation that should be accepted graciously.
2. Some gifts may be ethically problematic.
3. Discussing gifts with colleagues and considering how other patients would react might help physicians respond to them appropriately.

References

1. Caddell A, Hazelton L. Accepting gifts from patients. *Can Fam Physician* 2013;59:1259-1260, e523-5.
2. Spence SA. Patients bearing gifts: are there strings attached? *BMJ* 2005;331:1527-1529.
3. Murray TH. Gifts of the body and the needs of strangers. *Hastings Cent Rep* 1987;17:30-38.
4. Walter JK, Griffith KA, Jagsi R. Oncologists' experiences and attitudes about their role in philanthropy and soliciting donations from grateful patients. *J Clin Oncol* 2015;33:3796-3801.
5. Lyckholm LJ. Should physicians accept gifts from patients? *JAMA* 1998;280:1944-1946.

ANNOTATED BIBLIOGRAPHY

1. Caddell A, Hazelton L. Accepting gifts from patients. *Can Fam Physician* 2013;59:1259-1260, e523-5.
   Brief, thoughtful review of the topic.
2. Spence SA. Patients bearing gifts: are there strings attached? *BMJ* 2005;331:1527-1529.
   Emphasizes that gifts may have multiple meanings and encourages physicians to reflect on why the patient is giving a specific gift at a particular time.

Sexual Contact Between Physicians and Patients

INTRODUCTION

The Hippocratic Oath forbids sexual relationships between physicians and patients. In the past few decades, however, some people argued that this prohibition was archaic because sexual mores have changed and sex between consenting adults should be a private matter. Consequently, discussions of sexual contact between physicians and patients were then commonly framed in terms of mutually consenting relationships triggered by romantic attractions. In those cases in which physicians were disciplined by state medical boards for sexual misconduct, the boards' emphasis was often on rehabilitation rather than punishment so that the physician's medical expertise were still available to the public.

Recent reports have shifted the focus to physicians who were serial sexual predators and took advantage of their professional role to abuse patients. In 2016, The Atlanta Journal Constitution ran a five-part investigative series entitled "Doctors & Sex Abuse," depicting cases in which physicians found guilty of sexually violating patients were allowed to continue to practice, putting additional patients at risk. A study found that 70% of physicians who had a modification of clinical privileges or a report of a malpractice payment for sexual misconduct were not disciplined by state medical boards (1).

A dramatic 2018 case commanded national attention. An osteopathic physician, who had been a physician for the US gymnastics team and for university athletic teams, pleaded guilty to sexual assault of over 150 women and girls under the guise of medical therapy. The dean of the university medical school and the president of the university resigned under pressure as a result of their failure to investigate and act on allegations of the physician's misconduct, which had started over 20 years previously, and to protect future patients. In this physician's trial, 60 women testified how their trust, dependency, and vulnerability were taken advantage of and how their accusations were repeatedly disregarded for years. At least one other case has been reported of a university failing to respond appropriately to multiple cases of inappropriate sexual behavior toward patients by a physician. Thus professional and legal oversight has failed to protect the victims of sexual predators who are physicians.

JUSTIFICATIONS FOR SEXUAL CONTACT

In an older national survey, 9% of physicians reported at least one sexual contact with a patient or former patient (2). Most cases involved male physicians and female patients. This study excluded cases in which the sexual relationship preceded the medical care, such as the provision of medical care to a spouse. Twenty-three percent of respondents said that one or more of their patients had revealed sexual contact with a previous physician. In other studies, between 5% and 10% of mental health professionals admitted to sexual contact with patients (3).

Several justifications are commonly offered for relaxing the traditional prohibition on sexual contacts between physicians and patients (4).

Respect for Privacy

Generally, sexual relationships between consenting adults are considered private matters with which other people and society have no right to interfere. In this view, it is demeaning and unrealistic to view patients as so vulnerable that they cannot make their own decisions about their private lives. Restricting freedom to enter into sexual relationships would be paternalistic and intrusive.

Lack of Harm to Patients

Many people believe that patients are no more likely to be harmed in sexual relationships with their physicians than they are in other sexual relationships. In the United States, short-term relationships and divorces are common. Anecdotally, many people know of happy marriages between physicians and former patients. In this view, even if some sexual relationships with physicians harm patients, there is no reason to prohibit all such relationships.

Lack of Social Opportunities for Physicians

In small towns and rural areas, a physician might care for a large proportion of the community. Social opportunities for physicians would be very limited if romantic and sexual relationships with patients were barred.

OBJECTIONS TO SEXUAL CONTACT WITH CURRENT PATIENTS

Professional codes of ethics consider sexual relationships with current patients unethical. The American Medical Association (AMA) declared, "Sexual conduct or a romantic relationship with a patient concurrent with the physician–patient relationship is unethical" (3). Patients might feel "angry, abandoned, humiliated, mistreated, or exploited by their physicians. Victims have been reported to experience guilt, severe mistrust of their own judgment, and mistrust of both men and physicians" (3). There are several reasons for such role-specific restrictions on physicians (Table 26-1).

Physicians Should Not Take Advantage of the Doctor–Patient Relationship

It might be difficult for patients to make truly autonomous decisions on sexual relationships with physicians. The physician–patient relationship commonly arises during the patient's illness, which can cause patients to be vulnerable and dependent. Patients usually place great weight on their physicians' advice and judgment and naturally develop feelings of trust, gratitude, and admiration toward physicians (5). Unconsciously, both parties might mistake such feelings for romantic or sexual attraction. Patients and physicians might not appreciate how such positive feelings result from the

TABLE 26-1.   Objections to Sexual Relationships with Current Patients
Physicians should not take advantage of the doctor–patient relationship
Physicians have power over patients
Trust in the profession will be undermined
Some patients are particularly vulnerable

doctor's role and not from the doctor's personal attributes. Although such transference has been most clearly described in patients undergoing psychotherapy, similar feelings might occur in all physician–patient relationships. Physicians might also misinterpret their own feelings of caring and concern for patients, which are a natural part of the doctor–patient relationship, as romantic or sexual attraction.

CASE 26.1 | **Current patient receiving active therapy**

A 45-year-old male physician is treating a 32-year-old woman for depression and peptic ulcer disease. The woman reveals that she was sexually abused as a child. The physician, who is going through a divorce, finds her attractive and considers initiating a romantic and sexual relationship with her.

In Case 26.1, a depressed patient discloses intimate personal information, which she might not have told anyone else. Physicians might take a detailed sexual or mental health history. Patients might reveal their innermost fantasies and fears. Patients undress for examinations and allow physicians to touch them and even invade their bodies during medical or surgical procedures. Such intimacy within the doctor–patient relationship is one-sided. Physicians do not reveal their personal feelings, thoughts, or bodies to patients. Thus, physicians know much more personal information about patients than patients know about them. Physicians might betray the patient's trust if they take advantage of such intimate information, consciously or unconsciously, in pursuing sexual relationships with patients. Case 26.1 suggests how a physician's personal problems and need for support and understanding might compromise his judgment (5).

Physicians Have Power Over Patients

The power that physicians have over patients might make it difficult for patients to decline sexual relationships with them. In Case 26.1, the very framing of the issues implies unequal power: the physician considers initiating a sexual liaison, as if it were inconceivable that the patient would refuse. Because physicians order tests and treatments and schedule appointments, they control patients' access to medical care. There might be an implied or inferred threat that if the patient does not agree to sexual contact, the patient's care will suffer (6). Some physicians might falsely reassure patients that an effective therapeutic relationship can continue after a sexual liaison (4). In egregious cases, the physician might portray sexual contact or a sexual liaison as part of medical therapy.

Trust in the Profession Will Be Undermined

If the medical profession were to condone sexual relationships with patients, the public might begin to believe that physicians are motivated by self-interest and are willing to take advantage of patients. Patients might become reluctant to visit physicians or discuss intimate matters, particularly psychiatric or gynecologic problems.

Some Patients Are Particularly Vulnerable

In Case 26.1, the patient's depression might compromise her ability to consent freely to a sexual relationship. Patients who have previously suffered assault, incest, or rape might find it difficult to refuse sexual relationships with authority figures and might feel particularly betrayed if the current relationship repeats previous traumatic experiences. Such persons might not even be aware that they are repeating a previous pattern of behavior.

The Patient's Medical Care Might Be Compromised

When physicians provide care to a spouse or intimate partner, they might not be thorough in taking a history, conducting an examination, or ordering diagnostic tests. When physicians are providing medical care to a sexual partner, their clinical judgment is likely to be compromised (7).

Legal Issues

Sexual relationships between physicians and current patients might lead to criminal charges or to disciplinary action by licensing boards (1). Physicians might also face civil suits for malpractice. Malpractice insurers might exclude coverage for civil claims relating to sexual misconduct because such behavior is not part of providing medical care.

Comparisons with Other Professions

In other professions, sexual relationships with clients are condemned. Churches are strongly criticized for covering up sexual relationships between clergy and parishioners and transferring offending priests or ministers without appropriate disciplinary action. Similarly, lawyers have been criticized for sexual relationships with clients, particularly in divorce cases. As in medicine, the concern is abuse of trust and power by professionals.

SEXUAL RELATIONSHIPS WITH FORMER PATIENTS

Although sexual relationships with current patients are generally considered inappropriate, there is less agreement about relationships with previous patients. In the previously cited survey, although 94% of physicians considered it unethical to have sexual relationships with current patients, only 36% of physicians considered it unethical to have sexual relationships with former patients (2).

CASE 26.2	Former patient, with no ongoing relationship

A female emergency physician treats a 28-year-old man who requires a tetanus shot for a foot wound. Several years later they meet again as single parents whose children attend the same school. They discover that they share many interests. The physician wonders if a romantic relationship would be unacceptable because of their previous professional relationship.

In Case 26.2, it is unlikely that the former patient feels dependent on the physician. Furthermore, the patient revealed little personal information during the doctor–patient relationship and is not particularly vulnerable on that basis. A relationship between equals seems as possible for them as for any other couple (5).

Feelings of dependency, however, might persist in other circumstances after care is terminated, as in the following case.

CASE 26.3	Recent surgical patient

A male surgeon performs an emergency laparotomy on a woman with appendicitis. During postoperative visits, he finds himself spending much more time with her than he usually does with patients. She is appreciative of his attention and solicitous about his long hours and fatigue. A month after her final postoperative visit, he invites her to dinner.

In Case 26.3, the patient might have strong feelings of gratitude and dependency soon after emergency surgery. Unlike Case 26.2, it might be more difficult for the patient to make an independent judgment about a relationship or to decline invitations from the surgeon, compared with other men she knows.

The AMA states, "Sexual or romantic relationships with former patients are also unethical if the physician uses or exploits trust, knowledge, emotions, or influence derived from the previous professional relationship" (3). Thus, it is important to identify situations in which dependency in doctor–patient relationship continues (5, 8). Several factors should be considered.

Termination of Medical Care

Termination of care and absence of contact should be complete, including cessation of office visits, telephone consultations, prescriptions, and reminder postcards about appointments or screening tests. In addition, a new physician should be identified so that the patient no longer regards the partner as his or her physician. An even stronger case would be if the former patient has already established care with another physician. The purpose of terminating care should not be the initiation of a sexual relationship.

Nature of the Doctor–Patient Relationship

Some types of medical care are so intimate that the doctor–patient relationship might never be completely ended. After counseling and therapy, patients might feel dependency and gratitude toward physician years after therapy has been terminated. The American Psychiatric Association considers any sexual contact with a former psychiatric patient as unethical. Some patients might be particularly vulnerable because of past victimization. In specialties that involve unique and intimate physical touching, such as surgery or gynecology, the patient might still regard the physician as being in that role years later. In contrast, in Case 26.2, a tetanus immunization is so routine (and administered by a nurse not the physician) that the patient's dependence on the physician might be similar to dependence on a librarian.

Time Since Last Medical Care

In Case 26.3, during the immediate postoperative period the patient's feelings of vulnerability and dependency undoubtedly continue. Amorous advances by the physician might take advantage of these feelings in the patient. The passage of time helps extinguish feelings of dependency toward physicians and reduces the risk that physicians will abuse their power in initiating sexual relationships with patients (6). The crucial issue, however, is not simply the amount of time but rather the lack of a continuous relationship and the "potential for misuse of emotions derived from the former professional relationship" (3).

Circumstances of Renewal of Contact

If the doctor and former patient renew their acquaintance in a medical context, the patient might resume his or her previous role as dependent patient. However, if the physician and former patient meet again in a nonmedical context, as in Case 26.2, it is less likely that the previous doctor–patient relationship has an impact.

SUGGESTIONS

Physicians who are considering sexual relationships with current or former patients might consider the following suggestions.

Recognize Early Signs of Romantic Interest

Rarely are sexual or romantic feelings so overwhelming that the physician is swept away by uncontrollable passion. Physicians should be alert to early signs of romantic feelings for a patient. For example, they might look forward to the next visit or pay particular attention to their appearance on the day of the patient's visit. Sexual misconduct often begins with seemingly minor violations of the boundaries of the doctor–patient relationship, such as talking about the physician's problems rather than the patient's or scheduling appointments outside office hours (7). Recognizing these early symptoms gives physicians time to act thoughtfully and to consider the potential problems (8).

Seek Advice

It is hard to think critically about romantic or sexual interests. The AMA recommends that "it would be advisable for a physician to seek consultation with a colleague before initiating a relationship with a former patient" (2). Confidential advice can provide an honest appraisal of the potential harm to the patient, the physician, and the medical profession. Such counsel might be a safeguard for physicians who might otherwise act impulsively. Although discussing such an intimate decision with other people might seem intrusive, sexual relationships are not completely private if they harm patients or undermine public trust in the medical profession.

Responding to Advances by Patients

In some cases, the patient takes the initiative in pursuing a romantic or sexual liaison. Physicians, however, may still be considered responsible because they are in a better position than patients to recognize the potential harms of such relationships. In medical decisions, physicians do not simply accede to a patient's requests or demands. Physicians have an ethical duty to act in patients' best interests, even if it clashes with their own self-interest.

SEXUAL ABUSE BY PHYSICIANS

Recent well-publicized cases have highlighted serial sexual predators who take advantage of their role as physicians. Although these cases may be rare or unusual, their impact is devastating to victims. Colleagues, leaders of health care organizations, and state licensing boards need to effectively address sexual contact with a patient that is not a mutually consenting, voluntary relationship between adults or that violates professional and ethical standards. As with other unprofessional conduct, a core responsibility for physicians is now "if you see something, say something." Colleagues are urged to intervene when they witness unprofessional behavior (*see* also Chapters 35 and 36). In addition, chiefs of service, department chairs, CEOs of hospitals and clinics, and deans of academic institutions need to put in place a system for receiving complaints of sexual misconduct by physicians and other health care workers that responds in a timely, respectful, and fair manner. Leaving allegations unaddressed for years, or allowing such physicians to continue to practice after being found guilty of seriously inappropriate sexual contact with patients is unacceptable as a matter of justice and harm to patients and is a responsibility for which institutional leaders are now held accountable.

SUMMARY

1. Patients naturally feel trust, dependency, and gratitude toward their physicians.
2. Sexual contact with current patients exploits such feelings and is unethical and, in some circumstances, may be illegal.
3. Sexual contact with former patients is also unethical if the physician takes advantage of emotions and influence deriving from the doctor–patient relationship.

References

1. AbuDagga A, Wolfe SM, Carome M, et al. Cross-sectional analysis of the 1039 U.S. physicians reported to the national practitioner data bank for sexual misconduct, 2003-2013. *Plos One*. 2016;11:e0147800.
2. Gartrell NG, Milliken N, Goodson WH, et al. Physician–patient sexual contact: prevalence and problems. *West J Med* 1992;157:139-143.
3. Council on Ethical and Judicial Affairs of the American Medical Association. Sexual misconduct and the practice of medicine. *JAMA* 1991;266:2741-2745.
4. Appelbaum PS, Jorgenson LM, Sutherland PK. Sexual contact between physicians and patients. *Arch Intern Med* 1994;154:2561-2565.
5. Collier R. When the doctor–patient relationship turns sexual. *CMAJ* 2016;188:247-248.

6. Appelbaum PS, Jorgenson L. Psychotherapist–patient sexual contact after termination of treatment: an analysis and proposal. *Am J Psychiatry* 1991;148:1466-1473.
7. Gabbard GO, Nadelson C. Professional boundaries in the physician–patient relationship. *JAMA* 1995;273:1445-1449.
8. Gutheil TG, Gabbard GO. Misuses and misunderstandings of boundary theory in clinical and regulatory settings. *Am J Psychiatry* 1998;155:409-414.

ANNOTATED BIBLIOGRAPHY

1. Council on Ethical and Judicial Affairs of the American Medical Association. Sexual misconduct and the practice of medicine. *JAMA* 1991;266:2741-2745.
   Thoughtful discussion of the topic, proposing that all sexual contact during the physician–patient relationship is unethical.
2. Gabbard GO, Nadelson C. Professional boundaries in the physician–patient relationship. *JAMA* 1995;273:1445-1449.
   Discusses how sexual misconduct with patients usually begins with apparently minor violations of the therapeutic relationship.
3. Collier R. When the doctor–patient relationship turns sexual. *CMAJ* 2016;188:247-248.
   Thoughtful recent review.

Secret Information About Patients

INTRODUCTION

Physicians might receive information about a patient from family members or friends who ask that their role be kept secret (1, 2). Doctors find such unsolicited information disconcerting. Telling the patient the secret or recording it in the medical record might pass on inaccurate or unhelpful information, while keeping the secret might involve the physician in deception. This chapter discusses the ethical issues posed by such secret information and how physicians can respond. The related issue of secrets that patients disclose confidentially to doctors is discussed in Chapter 5.

TYPES OF SECRETS FROM RELATIVES

Often a family member tells the doctor about the patient's deleterious personal habits, such as alcohol use or smoking (1, 2). The family member often tells a member of the physician's staff rather than the physician directly. The informer hopes that the physician will make the patient stop these unhealthy behaviors. Another type of secret involves mental or physical incapacity. The family member might tell the physician that the patient is demented, depressed, psychotic, or threatening others. Similarly, the family might be concerned that an elderly patient can no longer drive safely or live independently. The confider also might seek to draw the physician into family disputes over money, marital problems, or the lifestyles of grown children. Finally, family members might alert the physician to hidden physical symptoms, such as chest pain, that the patient might not discuss.

ETHICAL PROBLEMS WITH SUCH SECRETS

Secret information can be problematic in many ways. The information might be inaccurate. The informer might have ulterior motives, such as gaining an advantage in a family dispute. Secrets are disrespectful to the patient because they involve deception rather than open discussions. Finally, such secret disclosures trap the physician in a bind because both disclosing and keeping the secret are ethically problematic.

APPROACHES TO SECRETS

When presented with such a secret by the patient's family, the physician has several options, some of which involve deception or undermine patient trust.

Reveal the Secret to the Patient

There are several ethical objections to keeping such a secret. Patients might consider it a violation of trust and privacy if physicians talk to other people about them behind their backs (3). Patients might question the physician's allegiance. It is also deceptive for physicians to base their recommendations and plans on secret information from third parties rather than on the history obtained from the patient. Chapter 6 discusses why deception is ethically problematic for physicians.

Keeping secrets from patients is also impractical. Like all forms of deception, it might require additional, increasingly elaborate deception. Patients might ask why the physician is posing a particular question or ordering a particular test, in which case physicians will have to either reveal the secret information or deceive the patient.

Do Not Disclose to the Patient

One physician who was philosophically opposed to keeping such secrets found that in about one half of cases he did not tell the patient (1). First, there may be no point in doing so because the information is obvious or trivial. For example, a family member's report that the patient was a heavy smoker provides no new information if the patient smells of cigarettes. Second, the physician does not disclose the information because it is not relevant to the patient's medical care. For example, few physicians want to get involved in a parent's concerns about an adult patient's marriage. Third, disclosure might do more harm than good in the short run. Revealing the mother's objections to the patient's marriage might well precipitate or intensify a family argument. Fourth, the physician might intend to tell the patient, but finds no opportunity to bring it up naturally in the conversation. The right moment to disclose the secret may never occur.

In some cases, the physician might promise to keep the secret. The physician might later be caught between conflicting obligations to be forthright with patients and to keep promises. Physicians can avoid this dilemma and maintain their primary obligation to the patient by rejecting the informer's initial request to keep the information secret. Family members often preface their revelations with phrases such as, "I don't want my husband to know I told you, but. . .." It would be prudent for physicians to interrupt at this point, before the information is revealed, and explain their policy of disclosing such information and its source to patients.

Ask Informers to Disclose Their Role

Ethically, the best approach is for the physician to convince the informer to tell the patient about the information presented to the physician or to allow the physician to disclose the source of the information. If this is done, the physician can discuss the issue freely with the patient.

Disclose the Secret to Protect Third Parties

With increasing public concerns about mass shootings and other forms of violence against multiple victims, physicians have a duty to act to protect against imminent, severe risk to third parties who are not in a position to protect themselves (*see* also Chapter 5). For example, a family member might tell the physician that the patient is stockpiling weapons and having angry tirades. The physician should work with the family member to devise a plan that may involve, for example, contacting the police.

SUMMARY

1. Physicians face dilemmas when family members or friends give information about patients that they ask to be kept secret.
2. Acquiescence with such secrets, even if well intentioned, might undermine the patient's trust.
3. Telling the family member or friend that the information needs to be shared with the patient is the most effective way to prevent such an outcome.

References

1. Burnum JF. Secrets about patients. *N Engl J Med* 1991;324:1130-1133.
2. Reis S, Biderman A, Mitki R, et al. Secrets in primary care: a qualitative exploration and conceptual model. *J Gen Intern Med* 2007;22:1246-1253.
3. Bok S. *Secrets*. New York: Pantheon Books; 1982:116-135.

Clinical Research

INTRODUCTION

Research with human participants is essential to better understand the pathophysiology of illness and to improve clinical care. Participants in research accept risks and inconvenience primarily to advance scientific knowledge and to benefit others. Thus, there is an unavoidable ethical tension between protecting the well-being of research participants and gaining new knowledge that benefits future patients. Although clinical care also involves benefits and risks, the patient who undergoes the risks also derives the clinical benefits.

Physicians can be involved in research in various roles. Treating physicians may help refer and recruit participants in research. When patients consider entering a research project, they may ask their treating physician for advice. Furthermore, when researchers identify eligible participants from medical records, many institutional review boards (IRBs) require researchers to obtain the treating physician's permission before contacting patients with whom they have no previous relationship. Finally, treating physicians can also serve as investigators in research. Because clinical research might benefit society and future patients, physicians generally should encourage their patients to participate in well-designed studies, while also protecting the individual patient's interests.

This chapter takes the perspective of the physician in clinical practice.

ETHICAL PRINCIPLES FOR RESEARCH

Three ethical principles should guide research with human participants (1). The principle of *respect for persons* requires investigators to obtain informed and voluntary consent from research participants, to protect participants with impaired decision-making capacity, and to maintain confidentiality.

The principle of *beneficence* requires that the research design be scientifically sound and that the risks of the research be acceptable in relation to the likely benefits. Risks to participants include both physical harm from research interventions and also psychosocial harm, such as breaches of confidentiality, stigma, and discrimination. If the research question has already been settled or is trivial, or if the design of the study is so weak that valid conclusions are impossible, no risk to participants can be justified. The risks of participating in the study must be minimized, for example, by screening potential participants to exclude those very likely to suffer adverse effects and by monitoring participants for adverse effects.

Traditionally, clinical research has been regarded as risky, and potential participants were considered guinea pigs who needed to be protected from dangerous interventions. Increasingly, however, clinical research is regarded as beneficial rather than risky because it provides access to potentially life-saving new therapies in such conditions as cancer, HIV infection, and organ transplantation. Patients with such conditions might want increased access to clinical research, not greater protection.

Furthermore, research that compares standard therapies used in clinical practice offers the promise of improving the quality of ordinary care (2).

The principle of *justice* requires that the benefits and burdens of research be distributed fairly. Vulnerable populations lack the capacity to make informed and free choices about participating in a research project or are at increased risk for adverse events from the study. Vulnerable groups should be neither overrepresented in dangerous studies nor underrepresented in trials of promising new therapies. Justice also requires equitable access to the benefits of research. Rather than excluding from research vulnerable populations such as children and pregnant women, appropriate measures should be put in place to protect them and allow rigorous studies on the safety and efficacy of therapies in these groups to be carried out.

Overview of Research Ethics

Federal regulations require that many types of research with human participants be approved by an IRB. The IRB must ensure that the risks of the research are appropriate in light of the prospective benefits, the risks of research are minimized, and participants give informed consent.

Clinical research, which is intended to produce generalizable knowledge, must be distinguished from innovative clinical practice, in which a physician goes beyond usual practice to try to benefit a particular patient. For example, a physician might use a drug for an indication not approved by the Food and Drug Administration.

Risks and Benefits of Research

Even though a research study has been approved by an IRB, the balance of risks and benefits may not be appropriate for an individual patient.

CASE 28.1	Osteoporosis clinical trial

Mrs. L is a 70-year-old woman with a family history of osteoporosis. She is interested in entering a randomized placebo-controlled phase III clinical trial of a new preventive agent that is given by nasal spray once a month. Her current oral medication causes some gastrointestinal side effects, and she is unwilling to take medications by injection.

The use of placebo controls in clinical trials about osteoporosis is controversial (3). Measures to prevent osteoporotic fractures are only partially effective. Between 12 and 160 women need to be treated for a year to prevent a fracture (3). Many fractures will be clinically silent, diagnosed only by x-ray studies. To be adequately powered, a randomized trial will need at least 30 excess fractures in one arm. Some ethicists argue that the risk of foregoing standard effective preventive measures is small and that, therefore, a placebo control is acceptable. This concern could be addressed if the control arm received an effective current medication rather than a placebo; however, this would make the trial impractical. For some patients, however, the risks are higher and are unacceptable. For example, if Mrs. L has a very low bone density, previous painful compression fractures, or a history of falls, her risk of fracture is greater. She therefore would be at increased risk if she foregoes standard drugs. Her personal physician should ensure that Mrs. L understands these risks and recommend that she receive a drug that is known to be effective, rather than enrolling in the clinical trial and receive placebo or an unproven intervention. In other cases, a patient may be at unacceptable risk in a trial because he or she is more susceptible to adverse effects of a drug being tested—for example, because of preexisting impairment in an organ system in which adverse effects commonly occur.

In a randomized double-blind clinical trial, it sometimes becomes necessary to break the blinding to provide appropriate care to a patient. For example, in a serious emergency, the treating physician needs to know the patient's medications. In this situation, the individual patient's well-being is paramount, and the scientific goals of the research should be secondary.

Informed and Voluntary Consent

The ethical guideline of respect for persons and their autonomy requires that adult participants give informed and free consent to participate in research. The treating physician can play an important ethical and clinical role in helping the patient make an informed decision.

Table 28-1 lists pertinent issues that the prospective participant needs to be told and understand to give informed consent.

The Nature of the Research Project and Study Procedures

The prospective participant should understand that research is being conducted, what the purpose of the research is, how the study differs from standard care, and how the participants are being recruited. Participants need to know what they will be asked to do in the research project. On a practical level, they should be told how much time will be required and how often. Procedures that are not standard care should be identified as such. Alternative procedures or treatments that might be available outside the study should be discussed. If the study involves blinding or randomization, these concepts should be explained in terms that the patient can understand. Any financial interest of the investigators in the study intervention should be disclosed.

Risks and Potential Benefits of the Study

Medical, psychosocial, and economic risks and benefits should be described in lay terms. Economic risks might also be important. Participants should appreciate that insurance companies may deny reimbursement for procedures that are not standard clinical care.

Assurances That Participation in the Research Is Voluntary

Participants must appreciate that they may decline to participate in research, that declining will not compromise their medical care, and that they may withdraw from the project at any time.

Misconceptions About Research

A common misconception is that research will provide direct therapeutic benefits to the participants. This has been termed as the *therapeutic misconception* (4, 4a). Participants often do not understand how research differs from clinical care, often incorrectly believing that the study is designed to provide them a personal benefit and that the choice of interventions will be based on their individual needs, as in the case of clinical care. Moreover, they may not appreciate that the intervention is unproven and that they may not benefit. Most promising new interventions, despite encouraging preclinical results, fail to show significant advantages over standard therapy in rigorously designed clinical trials (5). In a randomized trial, participants may not receive the study intervention. Research participants commonly downplay the risks and are unrealistically optimistic about the benefits. Many research participants make statements that both support and are contrary to a therapeutic misconception; they may be motivated by the prospect of therapy to participate in a clinical trial, while understanding the scientific goal of the study (6).

Problems with the Consent Process

Consent forms for clinical research are too long and are not readable. These problems may be ameliorated by revisions to the federal regulations for research that have not gone into effect as of July

TABLE 28-1. Informed Consent in Research Projects
The nature of the research project study procedures
The risks and potential benefits of the study
Assurances that participation in the research is voluntary
Misconceptions about research

2018. Furthermore, discussions between investigators and participants, although providing details of study procedures, may not discuss the purpose of the research or the patient's expected prognosis (7).

Prospective participants in clinical trials should not underestimate the potential benefits. In clinical trials of cancer chemotherapy, patients randomized to the control group have better outcomes overall than patients who are eligible to participate, but choose not to (8). This might be due in part to collateral benefits of the trial, such as more intensive monitoring for adverse effects, greater attention to protocol details, and coordination of interventions by the research nurse.

The treating physician can often play a crucial role in helping the patient make an informed decision by eliciting and correcting any misunderstandings and encouraging the patient to ask questions. In some cases, the treating doctor may make a recommendation about participating in the research project that is tailored to the patient's individual circumstances.

Informed consent, in addition to allowing eligible participants to decide for themselves whether or not to participate, also fulfills a number of other roles, including providing transparency, gaining public trust, and promoting concordance with the patient's values. These functions may be achieved in other ways when informed consent is impossible, for example in research in acute illness and on standard medical practices (9).

Selection of Participants in Research

CASE 28.2	Research on patients with dementia

A new urinary catheter has been developed. A clinical trial is proposed to evaluate whether it is more effective and safer than the conventional catheter. Nursing home residents with Alzheimer disease and incontinence will be recruited as participants because enrollment and follow-up will be easier than in ambulatory patients.

Patients Who Lack Decision-Making Capacity

As in Case 28.2, patients who lack decision-making capacity cannot give informed consent to research studies and might not be able to protect themselves from harm. Research is essential, however, to improve therapies for their conditions. When prospective research participants lack such decision-making capacity, surrogates may give permission for them to participate in research. Ethical controversy occurs because surrogate decisions regarding research with mentally incapacitated persons often are not based on the patients' wishes or best interests. In one study, 31% of surrogates who believed that the patient would refuse to participate nonetheless gave consent, apparently contradicting the patient's preferences (10). Furthermore, 20% of surrogates who would not enroll in the study themselves nevertheless allowed the patient to participate in the research, perhaps acting contrary to the patient's best interests. Other studies have found that surrogates tend to base decisions about research participation on what would maximize the patient's well-being, rather than on the patient's values (11) or on what they would choose for themselves (12). Treating physicians can help assure the participation in research by persons who lack decision-making capacity is appropriate.

There are several approaches to consent for persons with dementia that treating physicians can facilitate. First, some patients who lack the capacity to make decisions about their research participation still retain the capacity to appoint a proxy to make such decisions. Second, research advance directives allow persons with early dementia to specify what kinds of research they would be willing to join later in their illness.

Patients Whose Consent Might Not Be Free

Some potential participants in research are vulnerable because their consent might be constrained. Participants might depend on physician-researchers for ongoing medical care, as in nursing homes, Veterans Affairs hospitals, or public hospitals and clinics. As in Case 28.2, such dependent populations are sometimes recruited as research participants because recruitment and follow-up are easier than with more autonomous individuals. Such patients, however, might not feel free to refuse to participate.

Fairness requires that vulnerable populations not be targeted as participants primarily for the convenience of investigators, if other populations would also be suitable participants for the study. In addition, researchers need to justify why they are not studying persons with unimpaired decision-making capacity, such as patients with spinal cord injuries who require catheters. The use of vulnerable participants for research is more justifiable if the research addresses the condition that makes the participants vulnerable, if it offers the prospect of direct therapeutic benefit, and if advocates for the vulnerable population have approved the project.

CONFLICTS OF INTEREST

Dual Roles for Clinician-Investigators

If an investigator is also the treating physician, eligible research participants may find it difficult to decline to participate in research. What is best for a particular patient's care might not be what is best for the research project. In some situations, it might be better for the patient to drop out of the study and receive individualized care. An investigator, however, wants study participants to enroll and continue in the trial so that the research question can be answered. Moreover, in some clinical trials physicians receive payments for each enrolled patient and study visit, with payments exceeding actual expenses of the study. The role of personal physician should take priority over the role of clinical researcher. The physician-investigator could separate these two roles, asking a colleague to obtain informed consent from his or her patients.

Responding to Conflicts of Interest

Treating physicians must address conflicts of interest regarding clinical research. Chapter 29 provides a broader discussion of conflicts of interest and discusses how financial incentives and intellectual commitments might lead to an unacceptable risk of bias.

Disclose Conflicting Interests

Treating physicians and investigators should disclose to patients any financial interest they have in a research project they discuss (13). Most participants would want to be informed of such financial conflicts (14). In one study, however, most participants in cancer clinical trials were not highly concerned about investigators' financial conflicts of interest (15). More than 70% of respondents would still have enrolled in the clinical trial even if the researcher had financial ties to the drug company sponsoring the trial or had received royalty payments. Only 31% wanted disclosure of the researcher's financial interests. However, other studies found that potential participants are concerned about a researcher holding a substantial equity interest in the company making the drug being tested (14, 16).

Manage Conflicts of Interest

Although disclosure is necessary to protect participants, in some situations treating physicians need to go further to manage or eliminate conflicts of interest. Payments for enrolling participants and study visits should be commensurate with the services provided.

Prohibit Unacceptable Conflicts of Interest

If an investigator holds a patent on the experimental intervention or has a management position or stock options in the company manufacturing it, he or she stands to gain or lose money personally depending on whether the study yields a positive or negative result. Such an investigator should not serve as principal investigator or other roles where the possibility of undue influence is high, such as determining endpoints, analyzing the data, or writing the first draft of a manuscript (17). However, such an investigator could continue to play an active role as co-investigator.

SUMMARY

1. Rigorous clinical research is essential to evaluate promising new therapies.
2. Treating physicians should also help assure that participants appreciate the key features of the research study and that there are no special considerations that would make it unduly risky for the patient to participate in the research.
3. Treating physicians can help patients with early-stage dementia articulate their values and preferences regarding participation in research.

References

1. National Commission for the Protection of Human Subjects of Biomedical and Behavioral Research. *The Belmont Report: Ethical Principles and Guidelines for the Protection of Human Subjects of Biomedical and Behavioral Research.* 1979. Available at: http://www.hhs.gov/ohrp/humansubjects/guidance/belmont.html. Accessed August 27, 2012.
2. Sugarman J, Califf RM. Ethics and regulatory complexities for pragmatic clinical trials. *JAMA* 2014;311:2381-2382.
3. Brody BA, Dickey N, Ellenberg SS, et al. Is the use of placebo controls ethically permissible in clinical trials of agents intended to reduce fractures in osteoporosis? *J Bone Miner Res* 2003;18:1105-1109.
4. Appelbaum PS, Lidz CW. Re-evaluating the therapeutic misconception: response to Miller and Joffe. *Kennedy Inst Ethics J* 2006;16:367-373.
4a. Miller FG, Joffe S. Evaluating the therapeutic misconception. *Kennedy Inst Ethics J* 2006;16:353-366.
5. Hwang TJ, Carpenter D, Lauffenburger JC, et al. Failure of investigational drugs in late-stage clinical development and publication of trial results. *JAMA Intern Med* 2016;176:1826-1833.
6. Kim SY, De Vries R, Holloway RG, et al. Understanding the "therapeutic misconception" from the research participant's perspective. *J Med Ethics* 2016;42:522-523.
7. Joffe S, Mack JW. Deliberation and the life cycle of informed consent. *Hastings Cent Rep* 2014;44:33-35.
8. Gross CP, Krumholz HM, Van Wye G, et al. Does random treatment assignment cause harm to research participants? *PLoS Med* 2006;2006:e188.
9. Dickert NW, Eyal N, Goldkind SF, et al. Reframing consent for clinical research: a function-based approach. *Am J Bioeth* 2017;17:3-11.
10. Warren JW, Sobal J, Tenney JH, et al. Informed consent by proxy. An issue in research with elderly patients. *N Engl J Med* 1986;315:1124-1128.
11. Karlawish J, Kim SYH, Knopman D, et al. The views of Alzheimer disease patients and their study partners on proxy consent for clinical trial enrollment. *Am J Ger Psych* 2008;16:240-247.
12. Muncie HL, Jr., Magaziner J, Hebel JR, et al. Proxies' decisions about clinical research participation for their charges. *J Am Geriatr Soc* 1997;45:929-933.
13. Moore v. Regents of University of California. 51 Cal.3d 120; Cal. Rptr. 146, 793 P.2d 479 (1990).
14. Kim SY, Millard RW, Nisbet P, et al. Potential research participants' views regarding researcher and institutional financial conflicts of interest. *J Med Ethics* 2004;30:73-79.
15. Hampson LA, Agrawal M, Joffe S, et al. Patients' views on financial conflicts of interest in cancer research trials. *N Engl J Med* 2006;355:2330-2337.
16. Weinfurt KP, Hall MA, Dinan MA, et al. Effects of disclosing financial interests on attitudes toward clinical research. *J Gen Intern Med* 2008;23:860-866.
17. Lo B, Field M. *Conflict of Interest in Medical Research, Education, and Practice.* 2009. Available at: http://www.nationalacademies.org/hmd/Reports/2009/Conflict-of-Interest-in-Medical-Research-Education-and-Practice.aspx. Accessed November 30, 2012.

ANNOTATED BIBLIOGRAPHY

1. Lo B. *Ethical Issues in Clinical Research: A Practical Guide.* Philadelphia, PA: Lippincott Williams & Wilkins; 2009.
   Comprehensive textbook of ethical issues in clinical research, with case discussions.
2. Emanuel E, Grady C, Crouch R, et al., eds. *The Oxford Textbook of Clinical Research Ethics.* New York, NY: Oxford University Press; 2008.
   Multiauthored book providing in-depth comprehensive discussion of research ethics.

SECTION V

CONFLICTS OF INTEREST

Overview of Conflicts of Interest

INTRODUCTION

In *The Doctor's Dilemma,* George Bernard Shaw questioned whether people can be impartial when they have strong financial interests in a decision. He wrote, "Nobody supposes that doctors are less virtuous than judges; but a judge whose salary and reputation depended on whether the verdict was for plaintiff or defendant, prosecutor or prisoner, should be as little trusted as a general in the pay of the enemy. To offer me a doctor as my judge, and then weight his decision with a bribe of a large sum of money . . . is to go wildly beyond . . .[what] human nature will bear" (1). Shaw's words have particular relevance to contemporary US medicine because of increasing concerns over conflicts of interest in medicine.

A conflict of interest is a situation that creates a risk that a person entrusted with the interests of a client, dependent, or the public will be unduly influenced by a secondary interest (2). A conflict of interest does not signify unethical, unprofessional, or illegal behavior. For physicians in clinical practice, the patient's health should be their primary interest and take precedence over secondary interests, such as their own financial or professional self-interest or the interests of a third party, such as a hospital. Financial conflicts of interest might result from, for example, reimbursement incentives, personal investments in medical facilities, gifts from drug companies, or grants, consulting positions, and ownership stakes with for-profit entities. Nonfinancial secondary interests might include physicians' personal or professional self-interest, which might be salient when physicians respond to mistakes, deal with impaired colleagues, or learn new invasive procedures. Conflicts of interest also occur when physicians conduct research or teach. When carrying out research, the physician's primary interest should be to obtain and present valid knowledge. In teaching, the physician's primary interest should be the accurate presentation of knowledge and a critical appraisal of the pertinent evidence.

Conflicts of interest might be ethically problematic for several reasons. Patients might suffer physical harm. Even if the patient suffers no clinical harm, the integrity of the physician's medical judgment might be compromised. Furthermore, conflicts of interest might undermine patients' trust that physicians are acting on their behalf.

Chapters 30 to 36 analyze specific conflicts of interest. This chapter discusses how to define conflicts of interest, who should decide what constitutes an unacceptable conflict of interest, and how physicians can manage conflicts of interest.

WHAT IS A CONFLICT OF INTEREST?

Conflicts of Interest in Nonmedical Situations

Conflicts of interest occur in all professions and in public service. A public official is entrusted with acting in the public interest. His or her role-specific primary interest is to serve the interests of the public; other interests, such as self-interest or the interest of a business or individual that contributed to his her campaign, should be secondary. He or she would violate that trust by allowing those secondary interests to unduly influence official decisions. In another example, a trustee has a role-specific primary interest in the welfare of the elderly person or child he or she represents. In the private sector, an employee responsible for purchasing for a company has a primary interest in fiscal responsibility and obtaining value when making purchases. In these situations, the primary interest would be subverted by accepting gifts, entertainment, or kickbacks from a company that the official oversees, a financial institution that a trustee works with, or a potential vendor to the company. The following case illustrates conflicts of interest in a nonmedical profession.

CASE 29.1 | **Conflicts of interest for a judge**

A judge is assigned to preside over several cases in which she has a personal connection:
- *A landlord–tenant case in which the landlord is her uncle*
- *A divorce case involving a former law partner*
- *A breach of contract dispute involving a company in which she owns stock*

A judge takes on the responsibility of deciding and managing cases fairly and respecting the law. This primary interest would be undermined if the judge presides over a case in which he or she has a personal interest or stake in the outcome (3). The judge's self-interest, or the interest of friends or colleagues, must be secondary. In Case 29.1, there are several concerns. The judge might decide the case in favor of the relative, the former partner, or her self-interest, even though the evidence did not support such a ruling. Even if the ruling is fair, the process by which the trial was conducted might be biased. For instance, the judge might take into account inappropriate factors or make rulings about motions and objections that an impartial decision maker would not make. These procedural errors would be disturbing even if the final ruling was appropriate. Moreover, conflicts of interest undermine public trust in the judicial system. This is an important consideration even if there is no indication that the particular case was managed improperly.

The judge facing a conflict of interest might honestly believe that he or she will be impartial and might even consciously try to compensate for having ties to a litigant. Nonetheless, the opposing party and the public might still suspect that another judge would have decided or managed the case differently. Thus, the judge is required to withdraw from cases that pose such a conflict of interest. Society sets rules that determine when judges or public officials must recuse themselves (3). The decision to withdraw is not up to the individual judge or official. There is no implication that the judge facing a conflict of interest is immoral or unprofessional. Simply put, it would be untenable to place any human being in such a situation, and the possibility that the primary interest will be compromised requires the judge to withdraw.

How Are Conflicts of Interest Defined?

People often use the term *conflict of interest* without defining it clearly.

Compromise of Physicians' Primary Interest

In clinical care, the narrowest definition of conflict of interest is that the patient's outcome is actually worse because the physician subordinated the patient's best interests. The physician might do so either intentionally or subconsciously. Analogously, in research the results in a project are biased, or the content of a continuing medical education is biased (4). Of note, conflicts of interest are only one source of bias in research or education; others might include lack of expertise, laziness, and poor judgment.

Compromise of Physicians' Judgment or the Decision-Making Process

More broadly, the physician's judgment or decision-making process might be compromised because of secondary interests, even though clinical outcomes are not worse. A secondary interest might cause bias or undue influence (4). For example, the physician more often prescribe a brand-name medication for diabetes or hypertension after attending a dinner symposium sponsored by a pharmaceutical company or after a discussion with a drug representative, without considering generic drugs of the same drug class. It is difficult to determine whether these problems in the decision-making process results from a conflict of interest or from poor judgment, incompetence, negligence, or a lapse of attention.

Potential for Detrimental Outcomes or Compromised Judgment

A still broader definition of conflict of interest, which we adopt, includes situations in which there is an unacceptable probability for secondary interests to unduly influence the primary interest. This definition does not require evidence of *actual* harm to patients or compromised judgment in the particular situation (2). Several arguments support this broader definition. First, it is usually very difficult, impractical, or impossible to determine whether harm occurred or decision procedures were inappropriate in a specific case. To make such a determination would require extensive data collection and review. As a matter of public policy, it would be prudent to ask physicians to avoid situations that offer a significant possibility of compromising patient care or research, even if no misbehavior can be proven in a particular case. Avoiding such situations also more effectively prevents patient harm, which is preferable to determining after the fact that harm occurred. This broader definition is consistent with how conflicts of interest are handled in other professions, as we discussed with judges and government officials.

The determination of whether the probability of undue influence is unacceptable or not should be made by independent, reasonable observers, not by the physician in the situation. This determination should take into account many factors, including the nature of the relationship and the likelihood and seriousness of the potential compromise of the primary interest (2). Furthermore, individual patients generally are not in position to determine whether clinical judgment and decision-making process were sound. However, patient advocacy groups or public interest groups play an important role in setting rules regarding conflicts of interest.

Misconceptions About Conflicts of Interest

Perceived or Apparent Conflicts of Interest

Certain situations sometimes are described as only *perceived* or *apparent* conflicts of interest, with the implication that there is no harm and even no potential for harm. For example, many physicians believe that accepting small gifts from drug companies, such as pens and writing pads, is harmless (*see* Chapter 33). However, there is some evidence that even such small gifts can impact on human behavior because gift giving induces feelings of reciprocity (2). Also, there is some evidence suggesting that such gifts affect prescribing behavior. Moreover, the perception of a conflict of interest might be damaging, even though the potential harm to patients is small. If the public believes that physicians are serving the interests of drug companies rather than those of their patients, trust in the individual doctor or the profession as a whole might be undermined. Recent commentators have argued that the concept of perceived or apparent conflicts of interest is misguided because all conflicts of interest represent a tendency for a secondary interest to unduly influence the primary interest (5); no actual bias or unacceptable consequences need to be demonstrated in any particular situation.

Competing Versus Conflicting Interests

The interests of the patient and physician never coincide completely. *Conflicting* interests, as we have defined them, should be prioritized in a certain way. The well-being of the patient should be regarded as primary, and the self-interest of the physician should be secondary. In contrast, in *competing* interests, both have claims to priority. For example, time devoted to patient care cannot be spent on the physician's important competing interests in continuing teaching, clinical research, or family activities. Such competing interests need to be accommodated and balanced. Priority of competing interests will depend on the individual physician and his or her values.

Implications About Unethical Behavior

Some physicians might be offended because concerns about potential or perceived conflicts of interest apparently impugn their integrity and imply they are acting unethically. Doctors need to understand that the public is not singling them out for censure, but simply treating them as human and therefore fallible. It is the situation that is problematic, not the person.

Situations that Are Not Conflicts of Interest

The term *conflict of interest* is often used loosely. A conflict of interest, in the sense defined previously, needs to be distinguished from conflicts between ethical guidelines, disagreements among health care professionals, or disagreements between patients and physicians.

A conflict of interest should be judged by a reasonable person in light of past experience and available facts about the situation. Thus, a situation is not a conflict of interest if a person has no decision-making authority or if the secondary interest is unrelated to primary interest. For example, it is not conflict of interest if a physician's receptionist owns stock in a drug company because he or she exercises no discretion over prescribing decisions. Nor is it conflict of interest for a physician to invest in a mutual fund involving drug companies, as the doctor has no control over the purchase or sale of stocks in the fund.

Financial Conflicts of Interest

Medicine is regarded as an altruistic profession because its primary goal is to benefit the patient, not to maximize physicians' income; however, no one expects physicians to work for free or begrudges them a comfortable income. Helping the sick is difficult work and requires extensive training. This tension between altruism and self-interest is unavoidable in medicine (6). Financial rewards to the doctor should ideally be secondary to fostering patients' well-being, not the physician's primary goal.

Any reimbursement system can offer incentives to physicians to act contrary to patients' best interests. Fee-for-service reimbursement provides incentives to increase services and to give services of little or no benefit, thereby raising the cost of health care (*see* Chapter 31). Incentives to control costs might lead physicians to withhold beneficial care. Undue influence can occur subconsciously.

The concern about financial incentives is not simply that unscrupulous physicians will deliberately subordinate the patient's interests to their own financial self-interest or the interests of hospitals or insurance plans. Financial conflicts of interest may not be more serious or more common than nonfinancial conflicts of interest. However, financial relationships are within the experience of the public, can be quantified, and are more feasible to manage than nonfinancial relationships.

HOW SHOULD CONFLICTS OF INTEREST BE ADDRESSED?

When physicians face a conflict of interest, they should take the following steps (Table 29-1), which are discussed in detail in subsequent chapters that address specific conflicts of interest.

Reaffirm that the Patient's Interests Are Paramount

Individual physicians and the medical profession need to reaffirm their fiduciary responsibility to their patients. The doctor's primary responsibility is to foster the well-being of patients.

TABLE 29-1. Managing Conflicts of Interest
Reaffirm that the patient's interests are paramount
Disclose conflicts of interest
Manage the situation to protect patients
Prohibit certain actions and situations

To check whether they are acting in the patient's best interest, doctors might ask what they would recommend if they were working under the opposite reimbursement system. Physicians paid by salary might ask whether they would recommend the intervention under fee-for-service. Similarly, fee-for-service physicians might ask what they would recommend if they or the hospital would lose money doing the procedure. The answer is simple: Physicians should recommend care that is in the patient's best interests, no more and no less. A well-designed incentive should prompt the physician to consider more carefully what he or she does with clinical uncertainties and borderline options; it should not induce him or her to forego what he or she believes is clearly in the patient's interest (7).

Disclose Conflicts of Interest

Disclosure is essential for several reasons. First, disclosing financial relationships and incentives to patients, health care institutions, or the public might prevent physicians and organizations from making unacceptable arrangements. If the physician would find it hard or awkward to justify a situation, it probably presents an unacceptable conflict of interest. Second, patients who know about a conflict of interest might make more informed decisions by placing the physician's recommendations in context and compensating for any bias. However, it is generally unrealistic to expect patients to assess whether a situation has biased the physician's judgment. Indeed, some behavioral science research suggests that disclosure may be counterproductive (5, 8). Finally, unless conflicts of interest are disclosed, society and health care institutions cannot judge whether they need to be managed or prohibited.

Manage the Situation to Protect Patients

In some circumstances, society may determine that additional steps beyond disclosure are needed to safeguard patients or the public. Physicians' actions may be regulated and their discretion limited. In clinical care, patients should be able to appeal denials of coverage and have a prompt response (*see* Chapter 32). Physician ownership of medical facilities to which they refer patients is regulated. In clinical research, review by an institutional review board is required (*see* Chapter 28).

Prohibit Certain Actions and Situations

Although disclosure and precautions are necessary steps, they might still be insufficient to protect patients. Some actions and situations present such strong and direct conflicts of interest that they should be prohibited. Because "it is difficult if not impossible to distinguish cases in which financial gain does have improper influence from those in which it does not," it might be prudent to prohibit certain actions and situations (9). For example, drug companies that sponsor accredited continuing medical education may not influence the choice of topics or speakers (*see* Chapter 33).

SUMMARY

1. Conflicts of interest might harm patients, impair physician judgment, and undermine trust in the medical profession.
2. The patients' interests should be primary, and the physician's self-interest or the interests of third parties should be secondary.

References

1. Shaw GB. *The Doctor's Dilemma*. London: Penguin Books; 1946.
2. Lo B, Field M. *Conflict of Interest in Medical Research, Education, and Practice*. 2009. Available at: http://www.nationalacademies.org/hmd/Reports/2009/Conflict-of-Interest-in-Medical-Research-Education-and-Practice.aspx. Accessed November 30, 2012.
3. Gillers S. *Regulation of Lawyers: Problems of Law and Ethics*. 10th ed. New York: Aspen Publishers; 2015.
4. Lo B, Ott C. What is the enemy in CME, conflicts of interest or bias? *JAMA* 2013;310:1019-1020.

5. Lo B, Field M. *Conflict of Interest in Medical Research, Education, and Practice*. Washington, DC: National Academies Press; 2009.

6. Jonsen AR. Watching the doctor. *N Engl J Med* 1983;308:1531-1535.

7. Morreim EH. *Balancing Act: The New Medical Ethics of Medicine's New Economics*. Boston: Kluwer Academic Publishers; 1991:124.

8. Sah S, Fugh-Berman A. Physicians under the influence: social psychology and industry marketing strategies. *Journal of Law, Medicine & Ethics* 2013;41:665-671.

9. Thompson DF. Understanding financial conflicts of interest. *N Engl J Med* 1993;329:573-576.

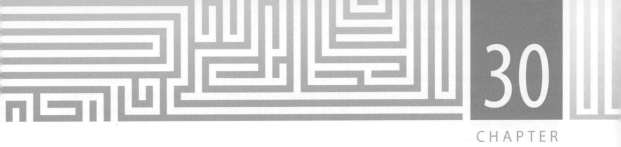

Health Outcomes, Access, and Cost in the United States

HEALTH OUTCOMES, ACCESS, AND COSTS

The United States spends far more on health care than other countries, yet has worse health outcomes and lower access to health insurance. In 2017, the United States spent over $10,000 per person for health care, almost two-and-a-half times the average of 36 advanced and emerging countries in the Organisation for Economic Co-operation and Development (OECD)(1). In 2017, the percentage of the US Gross Domestic Product spent on health care rose to 17.2%. This continued increase in health care spending in the United States is unsustainable because spending for health care cannot be spent on other important purposes, such as education, infrastructure, parental leave, preschool programs, or defense, or on reducing taxes and government expenditures and deficits, or the national debt (2).

The major drivers of higher US health expenditures are higher prices of labor and goods, including pharmaceuticals, and administrative costs (3). Moreover, physicians, who order most health expenditures, do not know the prices of interventions, do not pay the costs, and in some cases may receive higher compensation from increased expenditures (2).

Despite high expenditures for health care, health outcomes in the United States trail outcomes in other countries. Life expectancy in the United States is now almost two years below the average of the other countries, although it was above the average in 1970 (4). In the United States, social determinants of health are unequally distributed across population groups and are important drivers of health disparities (5).

Furthermore, the United States lags all but one other OECD country in access to health care (1), despite recent increases in insurance coverage in the United States. Even when insurance coverage exists, it may be inadequate. In 2016, 22% of the US population skipped medical visits, and 18% did not purchase prescribed medicines because of cost, over double the rate of skipping care in other countries (4). Poor access is particularly serious for low-income families, with 43% of low-income adults reporting unmet care needs because of the cost of care (4). In other countries, universal access to adequate health insurance is considered a fundamental societal commitment.

Thus, although health care expenditures are a formidable problem in the United States, costs must be viewed in the context of poor health outcomes and inconsistent access to health insurance (5a). Measures to reduce costs may be challenging because they should not worsen health outcomes or further reduce access to health care.

Social Determinants of Health

Because of deaths from drug overdoses, suicide, and alcoholic liver disease, total mortality is rising among US non-Hispanic whites (5b). This increase in mortality is marked among those with a high school education or less. Many other social determinants of health contribute to the mortality in the United States, including low education, racial segregation, low social support, poverty, and income inequality (6). The number of annual deaths attributable to low social support is similar to the number of deaths from lung cancer.

Neighborhoods with concentrated poverty often lack grocery stores with fresh food, adequate public transportation, adequate employment prospects, access to health care services, and good schools, and often they are situated near environmental hazards (6). Eleven percent of US households, comprising almost 40 million individuals, lack reliable access to a sufficient quantity of affordable, nutritious food (6).

Policies that reduce social disadvantage can reduce health inequalities. The emphasis in the US health system on medical treatments for acute problems has yielded benefits for some, but has not achieved higher overall levels of population health or increased longevity as in other nations (5). Overcoming US health disadvantages may require rebalancing priorities to prevent or ameliorate health-damaging social conditions and behavioral choices. The challenge is not how much money is spent on health, but rather how to spend those health dollars to provide the greatest benefit to the country as a whole (5).

GUIDING FRAMEWORK

Thus the triple challenge for US health policy is to simultaneously reduce health care spending, improve health care outcomes, and broaden health care access. The analysis of the causes of problems in the US health care system suggests a guiding framework.

Focus on Greatest Opportunities for Improvement

Although US health care has excelled at the care of serious acute illness, there are many opportunities to make gains in primary and secondary prevention and to better implement evidence-based practice guidelines that are known to improve health outcomes. Furthermore, persons with multiple chronic conditions and functional disability are at risk for poor health outcomes, hospitalizations and emergency visits, and high costs. Shifting resources from acute medical care to in-home supportive services may improve outcomes and reduce costs (7). Furthermore, some of most important drivers of poor health outcomes are social determinants of health, which can lead to opioid addiction, smoking, and obesity. Primary prevention of these conditions and preventing relapse should have a high priority.

Try to Reduce Disparities in Health

Attention to those who people who suffer the worst disparities in health outcomes not only can improve overall health outcomes, but it also improves fairness within society. Some interventions effectively address social determinants of health disparities but could be much more widely accessible, such as early childhood education and nutritional programs for infants and children, whose brains are developing.

Take a Problem-Solving Approach

Improved health outcomes will require more than improvements in better medical diagnosis, treatment, and delivery of medical care. Addressing social determinants of health will require physicians and health care systems to reach out to new partners, including community-based organizations, charitable organizations, and faith-based communities, who are working to provide social services in the community. The problems of health outcomes, quality, and costs are complicated, and many plausible approaches have proved unsuccessful. It is important that attempts to address a part of the problem be assessed with empirical evidence, to find out what interventions work, which do not, and what the unintended consequences of an intervention might be. Otherwise effort and money will be misdirected and fail to achieve their goals.

References

1. OECD. *OECD Health Statistics 2018*. Available at: http://www.oecd.org/els/health-systems/health-data.htm. Accessed July 5, 2018.
2. Emanuel EJ. The real cost of the US health care system. *JAMA* 2018;319:983-985.
3. Papanicolas I, Woskie LR, Jha AK. Health care spending in the United States and other high-income countries. *JAMA* 2018;319:1024-1039.
4. OECD. *Health at a Glance 2017: OECD Indicators*. 2017. Available at: ww.oecd.org/health/health-systems/health-at-a-glance-19991312.htm. Accessed July 7, 2018.
5. Adler NE, Glymour MM, Fielding J. Addressing social determinants of health and health inequalities. *JAMA* 2016;316:1641-1642.
5a. Blumenthal D, Abrams MK. Tailoring complex care management for high-need, high-cost patients. *Jama* 2016;316:1657-1658.
5b. Case A, Denton A. Mortality and morbidity in the 21st century. 2017. Brookings Papers on Economic Activity. Available at: https://www.google.com/search?client=firefox-b-1&ei=7qlQW5nXMsm0_AammLGICg&q=Anne+Case+Decreased+life+expectdancy+in+US&oq=Anne+Case+Decreased+life+expectdancy+in+US&gs_l=psy-ab.3...3822.6093.0.6420.7.6.1.0.0.0.144.557.4j2.6.0....0...1c.1.64.psy-ab..1.0.0....0.66y8WS_gneA. Accessed July 19, 2018.
6. Daniel H, Bornstein SS, Kane GC. Addressing social determinants to improve patient care and promote health equity: an american college of physicians position paper. *Ann Intern Med* 2018;168:577-578.
7. Roundtable on Quality Care for People with Serious Illness. *Financing and Payment Strategies to Support High-Quality Care for People with Serious Illness: Proceedings of a Workshop*. Washington, DC: National Academies Press; 2018.

31

Payments to Health Care Providers

HEALTH CARE PAYMENTS THAT DO NOT INCENTIVIZE HIGH-VALUE CARE

To reduce the unsustainably rising costs of health care, alternative models of payment that incentive high value care have been proposed. Rather than describing each model in detail, this chapter will provide conceptual framework on the ethical concerns raised by these models of payment.

Fee-for-Service Payments

Currently, fee-for-service is the most common type of health care payment in the United States. It offers incentives to increase all services, not only those that are effective or have high value. In two recent examples, physicians, many of whom believed their reimbursement was unfairly low, adjusted their practice to increase their revenue, even though patients received little or no benefit and significant harm.

Medicare reimbursed oncologists for intravenous chemotherapy drugs at much higher levels than the cost at which doctors could purchase them. Many oncologists believed that this reimbursement still did not cover office expenses for administering the drugs. Medicare reduced reimbursement for specific drugs that offered high profit margins for oncologists but did not offer patients clear clinical advantages over other, less expensive drugs. Oncologists responded by switching from drugs that experienced the largest cuts in reimbursement to other high-margin drugs (1). Moreover, some doctors switched from oral to intravenous chemotherapy despite inconvenience and higher copayments for patients.

In renal dialysis, basic payments have not kept pace with inflation. When dialysis providers were reimbursed separately for injectable erythropoietin-stimulating agents, use of these drugs soared (2), despite lack of evidence that they are effective. In fact, randomized clinical trials found no benefit with higher doses of erythropoietin-stimulating agents targeted to higher hemoglobin levels and probable harm from increased overall mortality and cardiovascular events (3). Medicare now includes injectable drugs in a bundled payment rate for dialysis patients. With this reversal of financial incentives, the use of these injectable drugs decreased (4).

Fee-for-service reimbursement schedules also encourage physicians to carry out invasive procedures rather than talk with patients about decisions or counsel them about preventive care (5). For example, Medicare reimburses a cardiologist a professional fee for inserting a temporary pacemaker, a procedure that takes about 30 minutes, that is four times greater than the reimbursement for a 1-hour family meeting to discuss goals of care.

Payers and purchasers now are modifying fee-for-service payments to incentivize quality and value, for example rewarding adherence to evidence-based practice guidelines and paying for coordination of care and health care information technology (6).

Physician Ownership of Health Care Facilities

Physicians can have an ownership stake in health care facilities in several ways. Doctors might carry out clinical laboratory testing, electrocardiograms, and chest x-rays in their own offices. Physicians might also invest in freestanding imaging centers, ambulatory surgery centers, or anatomic pathology services, to which they refer patients. Such self-referral raises ethical concerns about overuse of services and conflicts of interest.

Physicians who self-refer order significantly more imaging studies and generate higher radiology costs and total costs than other physicians (7, 8). After physicians acquire a financial interest in MRI scanners, they order significantly more scans (9). It is believed that many of these additional studies are not warranted. In general, greater use of medical services is not associated with better patient outcomes (10). The percentage of inappropriate MRI studies is greater when self-referring physicians order studies (11). Moreover, the growth in imaging services by self-referring physicians is several times greater than the growth among physicians who do not have such financial arrangements (12). Similarly, surgeons who own specialty hospitals are significantly more likely to operate on patients than non-owners, including procedures that have been shown to have no clinical benefit (13). Thus the weight of the evidence is that self-referral increases the cost of care and the utilization of inappropriate services.

Justification for Physician-Ownership of Health Facilities

One rationale for self-referral is patient convenience, including facilitating authorization and scheduling, same-day testing and care, and one-stop continuity of care (12). Proponents also argue that such physician investment increases access to state-of-the-art technology that would not be available otherwise (14). However, the evidence does not support claims of increased access. None of the physician-owned radiation therapy centers in Florida was located in rural areas or inner cities that lack centers (15). Physicians who invest in ambulatory surgical centers tend to refer insured patients to them, while referring Medicaid patients to university clinics (16).

Ethical and Legal Issues Regarding Physician-Ownership of Health Facilities

A conflict of interest occurs when physicians recommend services from which they profit financially. The American Medical Association states that self-referral might "undermine the commitment of physicians to professionalism" (14). Even the appearance that physicians are trying to increase profits might erode patient trust. Financial reward for physicians is traditionally regarded as a consequence of caring for patients, not as a goal to be pursued for its own sake.

Disclosure of physician ownership of outside facilities is ethically required, as with any conflict of interest. Disclosure, however, does not decrease referrals by physician-investors to facilities in which they have a financial interest (17). Patients who know that the physician has a financial incentive to increase referrals cannot judge whether recommendations for testing or treatment are sound. In addition, patients might be afraid of offending the physician if they do not go to the facility in question.

It is illegal for physicians to refer Medicare or Medicaid patients for services to facilities in which they or their family have a financial interest. However, there are many exceptions to this prohibition, including for in-office ancillary services, group practices, rural areas, and services personally performed or supervised by another physician in the same group practice (12).

In-Office Services

Ordering tests or treatments carried out by the physician can be distinguished from referral to outside facilities in which the physician has a financial interest (14). Procedures such as endoscopy, bronchoscopy, coronary angiography and angioplasty, and surgery are an integral part of specialist care. It would make little sense for one surgeon or cardiologist to evaluate the patient and then refer the patient to another physician for the actual procedure.

Nonfinancial Incentives to Provide More Services

Social and psychological factors reinforce the financial incentives in fee-for-service medicine to provide more services (18). In the United States, both the public and physicians regard high-technology procedures, such as MRI scans, as the epitome of excellent medical care. The prestige that hospitals and physicians gain by providing these services encourages their wider use. In addition, physicians commonly respond to the uncertainty inherent in clinical medicine by performing an additional test. The malpractice system encourages *defensive medicine*, the ordering of interventions of small marginal benefit to patients to prevent potential lawsuits. Finally, faced with an individual patient who requests an intervention of questionable appropriateness, physicians might recommend it even though they would not recommend it as a general clinical guideline (19).

Ethical Issues with Fee-for-Service Payments

Fee-for-service payments incentivize health care organizations and physicians to provide more services, even though the benefit and value to patients may be marginal or absent. Moreover, fee-for-service payments raise concerns about conflicts of interest; ordering more interventions in fee-for-service is in the self-interest of physicians, but might not be in the best interest of the patient. Patients are often in a poor position to judge the benefit and value of interventions that physicians recommend.

VALUE-BASED PAYMENTS

Many proposals have been considered or enacted to change payment mechanisms to increase the value of services provided to patients. Because there are so many proposals and variations, rather than analyzing specific proposals, this chapter will focus on the ethical issues regarding priorities, trade-offs, and unintended consequences.

The term *value-based pricing* refers to payments that are in part based on the quality and cost of care, not solely on the number of services provided.

- *Bundled payments* pay a fixed amount for an episode of care, such as for a heart attack, coronary bypass surgery, or hip replacement. Such reimbursement encourages collaboration among physicians and health care institutions, which can improve patient outcomes. The bundled payment for surgery would include, for example, not just the operation but also rehabilitation, postoperative care, and treatment of complications.
- *Global payments* for management of patients in a population with a chronic condition, such as cancer or coronary artery disease, encourage continuity of care and coordination among providers, including specialists, nurses, pharmacists, dieticians, and physical therapists. Some proposals make health care providers accountable for a population of patients, so that they have incentives to provide preventive care and to coordinate care for complex, high-cost patients.
- *Global budgets* may cover all health care or a percentage of care for a defined population.

Medicare and Medicaid policy makers are phasing in changes from fee-for-service, at first making them voluntary and offering physicians the opportunity to earn bonuses, without putting them at risk for loss of income.

Fee-for-service payment may be modified by *quality incentives* (so-called *pay for performance*). Common incentives reward adherence to evidence-based practice guidelines (such as for cancer screening hypercholesterolemia, or asthma), reduction of hospital-acquired infections, use of electronic health records, and patient satisfaction.

Payment arrangements between insurers and health care systems and hospitals may differ from how individual physicians are paid. Some large integrated health providers, such as Mayo Clinic,

Group Health, and Kaiser Permanente, pay physicians a *salary;* this reduces incentives to perform more services even if they are not high value.

COST SHARING BY PATIENTS

Patient Cost Sharing at the Point of Service

To control costs, many insurers are increasing deductibles and copayments for patients. However, the recent increases in cost sharing raises several concerns. First, such cost-sharing leads to underinsurance (that is, insured people must pay a large share of their income at the point of service to access care). In 2014, 23% of US adults were underinsured compared with 13% in 2005.

Second, cost sharing at the point of service often induces poor decision-making. In response to higher cost sharing patients reduce the use of appropriate and high-value services such as preventive care and management of chronic diseases, as well as reducing inappropriate services (20). Greater cost-sharing at the point of service is associated with higher utilization of inpatient and emergency department services among patients with chronic illness (21).

Although lowering or eliminating copayments has been suggested as a means of increasing adherence to very effective, low-cost drugs such as generic statins and beta-blockers (21), evidence shows raising copayments are much more potent than lowering copayments in changing patient behavior (22).

Patient Cost Sharing When Choosing Health Plans

Employers who provide health insurance are requiring employees to pay an increasing portion of the monthly premiums. Typically employers contribute a fixed amount, so employees who want a more expensive plan have to pay an additional amount. The least expensive plans are health maintenance organizations (HMOs), which contract with physician groups to provide comprehensive medical care in return for capitated payments, a fixed amount per patient regardless of the actual costs of care. Patients in HMOs select a primary physician or physician group and must obtain covered services through them. Employees who want a greater choice of physicians can select other types of plans, which require them to make greater monthly contributions to premiums. In preferred provider organizations (PPOs), "preferred" physicians and hospitals accept discounted fee-for-service reimbursement rates and administrative controls in exchange for a flow of patients. PPO patients can also visit nonpreferred providers, but with higher co-payments. Point of service plans allow a still greater choice of physicians or hospitals for even higher premiums and co-payments. When choosing a health care plan and paying health insurance premiums, patients usually want to control costs; however, when patients are sick and need medical care, they often want all interventions that might benefit them, even if they are expensive and the additional benefits are small.

Incentives for Health Promotion

Persons with unhealthy lifestyles, such as obesity and smoking, have higher costs for health care. Many insurers are offering employees financial incentives to exercise, stop smoking, and lose weight. Many people want to adopt these behaviors, but find it difficult to carry out their intentions. Several ethical issues need to be considered (23, 24).

First, it may be unfair to hold people responsible for behaviors they cannot change. Heavy smokers are addicted to nicotine. People may be unable to exercise because they live in an unsafe neighborhood or may not be able to lose weight because they lack access to grocery stores that sell healthy foods. People from lower socioeconomic levels (SES) levels, who are already worse off, are more likely to face such challenges. Others may not be able to exercise because of arthritis, back pain, or heart disease. It may be unfair if some people have great difficulty gaining the incentive, even if they try hard. Moreover, it may be unfair to reward people for doing what others have already done already on their own without rewards.

Second, some employment-based programs raise concerns about privacy, undue influence by employers, and employment discrimination.

Third, the design of incentives involves trade-offs between effectiveness, acceptability, and fairness. Should wellness programs incentivize results or attempts? The former will be more effective but may be less acceptable to employees. Should incentives be penalties or rewards? Again, the former will be more effective but less acceptable. Finally, should employees simply offer financial incentives, or also take steps to facilitate the desired behavioral changes. For example, companies could provide walking paths, healthier food in the cafeteria, and exercise classes on site to facilitate employees meeting targets, and thus possibly reduce days away from work because of illness.

ETHICAL ISSUES WITH HEALTH CARE PAYMENTS

Withholding Beneficial Care

Ideally, incentives to control costs would lead physicians to eliminate only expensive services that offer little or no marginal benefit to a population of patients. During the managed care era, strong incentives to control costs were believed to also restrict medically appropriate care. Incentives for quality of care, such as adherence to evidence-based practice guidelines, are intended to alleviate these concerns. More fundamentally, physicians need to appreciate that policies that are beneficial to a population of patients may be harmful to an individual patient. In some cases, an exception to clinical guidelines for an individual patient is clinically and ethically justified (25, 26).

Undermining the Physician's Fiduciary Role

The treating physician is in a unique position to identify and justify exceptions. Health care organizations and payers should allow legitimate exceptions and have in place appeals procedures that are not unduly burdensome for physicians and patients.

Incentives to physicians to reduce costs might lead patients to question whether physicians are acting in their best interests, which thereby reduces patient trust in physicians (27, 28). Furthermore, an emphasis on cost containment and efficiency may lead physicians to become entrepreneurs focused on profits instead of healers focused on patient well-being (29).

Educating Patients and Physicians About the Value of Medical Interventions

Patients need guidance from physicians as to whether interventions are worth the out-of-pocket cost (22); however, physicians may not know which interventions have low value. Many patients seek and need guidance from physicians regarding what interventions are worth the out-of-pocket cost (22). To give such advice, physicians need to be better informed about the out-of-pocket cost of the medications and services they order. The complexity and opacity of the prices of drugs and tests makes it unrealistic for physicians to remember or know such information; it would need to be incorporated into electronic health records.

Patient-centered decision aids may help patients better understand the effectiveness and risk of options regarding their care (30). Compared with usual care across a wide variety of decision contexts, patients exposed to decision aids feel more knowledgeable, better informed, and clearer about their values, and they probably have a more active role in decision-making and more accurate risk perceptions. There is growing evidence that decision aids may improve values-congruent choices. Decision aids have no adverse effects on health outcomes or satisfaction, and they also modify patient choices, resulting in fewer patients choosing major elective invasive surgery in favor of more conservative options, prostate-specific antigen screening for prostate cancer, and increased starting medications for diabetes; these choices are consistent with evidence-based clinical guidelines.

Adverse Effects on Health Disparities

Under value-based payments, physicians who care for medically or socially complex populations may be at a financial disadvantage. Adjustment for case mix and severity of illness can be administratively complex and controversial, and fail to capture important social determinants of poor health outcomes (31). For example, reimbursement may penalize hospitals that care for a disproportionate share of patients with low income, low educational levels and health literacy, unstable housing, and other social determinants of health, who are more expensive to care for than other patients. Thus, the goal of restraining health care costs may conflict with the goal of reducing health disparities. Proposals to address this dilemma include directly rewarding hospitals that disproportionately care for high-risk populations and paying for improvements in outcomes for populations that have high levels of negative social determinants of health (31).

To improve their outcomes, physicians and hospitals may respond to prospective payments by avoiding patients who are sicker, more complicated, or have social factors that adversely affect health outcomes. If this unintended consequence occurs, more complicated patients may have difficulty accessing health care, and health disparities may worsen (32, 33).

Empirical Testing of Consequences of Payment Reforms

Design of payment systems is complex. Crucial details include the size of value-based payments (6), whether payments reward improvement, achievement, or both, and whether incentives for value should be rewards, penalties, or both (33). Still another challenge is aligning payment mechanisms from health insurers or government agencies to health care institutions with payments to physicians, who are responsible for ordering interventions (6). Changes in payment may be more effective if coupled with physician education and more transparency regarding prices of interventions.

In light of many approaches to payment reform, it is essential to gather and assess evidence on the outcomes of new payments systems. After all, plausible ideas may not achieve their intended effects or may have unintended adverse consequences. At its core, health care is an enterprise that is committed to benefitting patients and avoiding harm to them; thus, practices and policies regarding payment need to be empirically tested to see whether they work or not and whether they cause more net good than harm.

The interpretation of empirical evidence will depend on values and trade-offs. For example, payment reforms may have a different balance of benefits and burdens for different groups of patients. People may have philosophical differences in how they view the impact on persons who are worse off because of social determinants of poor health. Some people will want to help patients who are least well off as a matter of compassion and fairness. Other people, however, believe that government intervention, even if well-meaning, worsens problems by fostering dependence and undermining individual responsibility (21). Such beliefs should be articulated clearly and respectfully but also be open to reassessment in light of empirical evidence.

SUMMARY

1. All payment systems create incentives that may lead physician to provide too many or too few interventions to some patients.
2. Reforms to reimbursement systems need to be assessed for outcomes, both intended and unintended.

References

3. Jacobson M, Earle CC, Price M, et al. How Medicare's payment cuts for cancer chemotherapy drugs changed patterns of treatment. *Health Aff (Millwood)* 2010;29:1391-1399.
4. Winkelmayer WC, Chertow GM. The 2011 ESRD prospective payment system: an uncontrolled experiment. *Am J Kidney Dis* 2011;57:542-546.
5. Palmer SC, Navaneethan SD, Craig JC, et al. Meta-analysis: erythropoiesis-stimulating agents in patients with chronic kidney disease. *Ann Intern Med* 2010;153:23-33.
6. Fuller DS, Bieber BA, Pisoni RL, et al. International comparisons to assess effects of payment and regulatory changes in the United States on anemia practice in patients on hemodialysis: the dialysis outcomes and practice patterns study. *J Am Soc Nephrol* 2016;27:2205-2215.
7. Hsiao WC, D.L. D, Verrilli DK. Assessing the implementation of physician payment reform. *N Engl J Med* 1993;328:928-933.

8. Nussbaum S, McClellan M, Metlay G. Principles for a framework for alternative payment models. *JAMA* 2018;319:653-654.

9. Hughes DR, Sunshine JH, Bhargavan M, et al. Physician self-referral for imaging and the cost of chronic care for Medicare beneficiaries. *Med Care* 2011;49:857-864.

10. MedPAC. *June 2009 Report to Congress*. Available at: http://www.medpac.gov/.../ancillary services_public_Feb 2011.pdf. Accessed November 19, 2011.

11. Baker LC. Acquisition of MRI equipment by doctors drives up imaging use and spending. *Health Aff (Millwood)* 2010;29:2252-2259.

12. Brownlee S, Chalkidou K, Doust J, et al. Evidence for overuse of medical services around the world. *Lancet* 2017;390:156-168.

13. Kouri BE, Parsons RG, Altert HR. Physician self-referral for diagnostic imaging: review of the empiric literature. *AJR Am J Roentgenol* 2002;179:843-850.

14. Adashi EY, Kocher RP. Physician self-referral: Regulation by exceptions. *JAMA* 2015;313:457-458.

15. Mitchell JM. Effect of physician ownership of specialty hospitals and ambulatory surgery centers on frequency of use of outpatient orthopedic surgery. *Arch Surg* 2010;145:732-738.

16. Council on Ethical and Judicial Affairs AMA. Conflicts of interest: physician ownership of medical facilities. *JAMA* 1992;267:2366-2369.

17. Mitchell JM. The prevalence of physician self-referral arrangements after Stark II: evidence from advanced diagnostic imaging. *Health Aff (Millwood)* 2007;26:w415-424.

18. Gabel JR, Fahlman C, Kang R, et al. Where do I send thee? Does physician-ownership affect referral patterns to ambulatory surgery centers? *Health Aff (Millwood)* 2008;27:w165-174.

19. *Financial Arrangements Between Physicians and Health Care Businesses*. Washington, D.C.: Office of the Inspector General, U.S. Dept. of Health and Human Services; 1989.

20. Zikmund-Fisher BJ, Kullgren JT, Fagerlin A, et al. Perceived barriers to implementing individual choosing Wisely recommendations in two national surveys of primary care providers. *J Gen Intern Med* 2017;32:210-217.

21. Redelmeier DA, Tversky A. The discrepancy between medical decisions for individuals and for groups. *N Engl J Med* 1990;322:1162-1164.

22. Chernew ME, Fendrick A. Improving benefit design to promote effective, efficient, and affordable care. *JAMA* 2016;316.

23. Saloner B, Sabik L, Sommers BD. Pinching the poor? Medicaid cost sharing under the ACA. *N Engl J Med* 2014;370:1177-1180.

24. Volpp KG, Loewenstein G, Asch DA. Choosing wisely: Low-value services, utilization, and patient cost sharing. *JAMA* 2012;308:1635-1636.

25. Volpp KG, Asch DA, Galvin R, et al. Redesigning employee health incentives—lessons from behavioral economics. *N Engl J Med* 2011;365:388-390.

26. Madison KM, Volpp KG, Halpern SD. The law, policy, and ethics of employers' use of financial incentives to improve health. *J Law Med Ethics* 2011;39:450-468.

27. Kmetik KS, O'Toole MF, Bossley H, et al. Exceptions to outpatient quality measures for coronary artery disease in electronic health records. *Ann Intern Med* 2011;154:227-234.

28. Ellrodt AG, Conner L, Riedinger M, et al. Measuring and improving physician compliance with clinical practice guidelines. *Ann Intern Mec* 1995;122:277-282.

29. Blendon RJ, Brodie M, Benson JM, et al. Understanding the managed care backlash. *Health Affairs* 1998;17:80-94.

30. Kao AC, Green DC, Zaslavsky AM, et al. The relationship between method of physician payment and patient trust. *JAMA* 1998;280:1708-1714.

31. Kassirer JP. Managing care -- should we adopt a new ethic? *N Engl J Med* 1998;339:397-398.

32. Stacey D, Legare F, Lewis K, et al. Decision aids for people facing health treatment or screening decisions. *Cochrane Database Syst Rev* 2017;4:Cd001431.

33. Chaiyachati KH, Bhatt J, Zhu JM. Time for value-based payment models to adopt a disparities-sensitive frame shift. *Ann Intern Med* 2018;168:509-510.

34. Roland M, Dudley RA. How financial and reputational incentives can be used to improve medical care. *Health Serv Res* 2015;50:2090-2115.

35. Joynt Maddox KE, Sen AP, Samson LW, et al. Elements of program design in Medicare's value-based and alternative payment models: a narrative review. *J Gen Intern Med* 2017;32:1249-1254.

Bedside Rationing of Health Care

INTRODUCTION

Physicians are ethically obligated to act in patients' best interests (*see* Chapter 4). Acting in the best interests of one patient, however, might sometimes preclude physicians from acting on behalf of another patient who is much more likely to benefit from care or from stewarding scarce resources. Dilemmas are inevitable because resources, such as critical care beds and physician time, are in limited supply and people have different priorities for limited resources.

This chapter discusses the ethical considerations that arise when one patient's interests conflict with another patient's. In addition, this chapter analyzes whether the scarcity of financial resources justifies limiting the care of an individual patient.

The terms used to discuss these issues are often used inconsistently and commonly evoke strong emotions (1). In this book *allocation* refers to decisions that set levels of funding for programs rather than determine care for individual patients. For example, funds must be allocated between Medicaid and other social programs, such as education and transportation, and, within Medicaid, between inpatient services and prenatal care. Sometimes these policy-level choices are termed *macroallocation*. In contrast, this book uses the term *rationing* to refer to decisions at the bedside or in the office to limit care for individual patients because of limited resources. The term *rationing* often connotes limiting beneficial care because it is too expensive. The term *microallocation* is also used in this context. The term *rationing* excludes clinical decisions that are a straightforward implementation of macroallocation policies, such as health plans' decisions not to cover cosmetic surgery or a societal decision on prioritization of candidates for transplantation.

Unlike other countries, such as Great Britain, the United States has not developed coherent societal allocation policies. The ethical issue is whether, in the absence of a fair societal agreement on allocation, physicians can ethically carry out rationing at the bedside (2).

RATIONING BECAUSE OF LIMITED MEDICAL RESOURCES

CASE 32.1 Limited coronary care beds

Mr. H presents to the emergency department with substernal chest pain. An electrocardiogram (ECG) shows an acute anterior myocardial infarction, multifocal ventricular premature beats, and some couplets. The cardiac care unit (CCU) and intensive care unit (ICU) are full. One of the patients in the CCU is a 73-year-old man who had an emergency operation for a ruptured aortic aneurysm. A week after the operation, he is comatose, septic, in ventilatory and renal failure, and hypotensive despite vasopressors. Another patient in the CCU experienced chest pain after an angioplasty earlier in the day but has no persistent ECG changes and has normal cardiac enzymes. The physicians consider whether to transfer one of these patients out of the CCU to free a bed for Mr. H.

In Case 32.1, the patient with multisystem failure is so sick that he is highly unlikely to survive even if CCU care is continued. The post-angioplasty patient is receiving only monitoring, not active treatment, and is highly likely to have a good outcome even if he is transferred out of critical care to a monitored bed on a step-down unit. In contrast, Mr. H might benefit greatly from timely revascularization and antiarrhythmic therapy, which can be administered only in intensive care. If CCU beds were allocated on a strictly first-come, first-served basis, Mr. H would be denied substantial benefits.

Arguments Against Bedside Rationing

Traditionally, bedside rationing by physicians has been considered unethical because doctors should act as fiduciaries and patient advocates, helping patients receive all the beneficial care that the system allows (3, 4). One eminent physician wrote, "Physicians are required to do everything that they believe may benefit each patient without regard to costs or other societal considerations. In caring for an individual patient, the doctor must act solely as the patient's advocate, against the apparent interests of society as a whole" (5). This fiduciary role maintains patient trust. Moreover, in the absence of priorities and rules that are socially agreed on, rationing decisions might be arbitrary and based on ethically irrelevant considerations such as ethnicity, gender, and gender orientation (6). In other roles as citizens and professional leaders, physicians should help determine how resources should be allocated.

Arguments in Favor of Bedside Rationing

In recent years, as the rise in medical care costs continues to exceed inflation, it has become clear that physicians cannot avoid choices among interventions that vary in value. An absolute prohibition against bedside rationing, therefore, is ethically problematic.

Beneficence Is Not an Absolute Duty

An absolutist view of patient advocacy would not serve patients well in the long run because health care would become unaffordable to all but the most wealthy. Although the physician's primary goal is the well-being of patients, foregoing a small clinical benefit for an individual patient may promote the well-being of the population as a whole or permit larger clinical benefits to other patients (7).

The physician's ethical obligation to act in an individual patient's best interests is not absolute. In several circumstances physicians are ethically or legally required to act against an individual patient's best interests to benefit third parties. For example, although maintaining confidentiality of medical information is in a patient's best interest, it is overridden when infectious diseases or threats of physical violence might harm third parties (*see* Chapter 5).

The guideline of beneficence has been specified in ways that allow physicians not to do literally everything that might benefit a particular patient. The American Medical Association declares that "physicians must advocate for any care they believe will materially benefit their patients" (8). Other advocates of the fiduciary role enjoin physicians to practice "parsimonious" or "efficient" medicine, without specifying those terms (3, 4). The Charter on Medical Professionalism requires physicians to promote a "just distribution of societal resources" (9). All these views allow some forms of rationing, without calling it such. It would be more honest to acknowledge that such limits occur and to consider the circumstances when rationing is justified.

Microallocation Without Physicians Harms Patients

If treating physicians were not involved in microallocation, these clinical decisions would be made according to utilization review guidelines or by health care administrators. Such a process would fail to take into account meaningful differences in individual patient circumstances that are too complex to be captured in simple guidelines or rules (10, 11). Physicians can often bring to bear pertinent clinical information that justifies an exception to a general rule limiting interventions (12).

Other Patients Might Be Seriously Harmed

Providing care to one patient might deny care to another patient who would receive much greater medical benefit from limited resources, including physician time. In these situations informal rationing is standard medical practice that has strong ethical justification.

Triage Because of Limited Physician Time

CASE 32.2   Limited physician time

Mr. M, a 48-year-old man, comes to the physician's office after 40 minutes of crushing substernal chest pain and shortness of breath. At the same time, a 21-year-old woman with asthma comes to the office with worsening shortness of breath for the past day, despite increasing use of inhaled bronchodilators. These patients do not have appointments, and the physician's schedule is already full.

Because their time is limited, physicians must decide which patients deserve higher priority. In a life-threatening emergency such as a probable myocardial infarction in Case 32.2, a delay of care might cause grave harm and takes priority over other cases. Mr. M needs to be stabilized and transported to the emergency department. Regularly scheduled patients presumably would agree to wait because they would want similar priority if they should find themselves in a serious emergency. However, how is an emergency defined? If care is promptly instituted for the woman with an asthma exacerbation, her symptoms will be relieved more rapidly and hospitalization might be avoided. However, it is a value judgment as to how much benefit or potential harm to the asthma patient justifies asking regularly scheduled patients to wait. Referring the asthma patient to the emergency department only pushes the dilemma back a step, since patients presenting for care there are routinely triaged.

Patients and society expect physicians to allocate their time. It is difficult to imagine that anyone other than a physician or nurse would decide who should wait. General rules can be set—for example, patients with serious emergencies should take priority over scheduled patients with minor or self-limited illnesses. Physicians, however, need to interpret those general rules in a particular case—for example, deciding whether a patient's asthma attack warrants asking other patients to wait.

In Case 32.1 essential medical resources—CCU beds—are in short supply. In clinical practice, physicians frequently transfer patients to allow others to receive intensive care. When the CCU or ICU is full, physicians identify patients who are too sick to benefit from continued intensive care and set more restrictive standards for admission to the unit. Increasing the supply of critical care beds will not resolve the problem of rationing but only postpone the dilemma of the last bed. Transferring patients to other hospitals with open CCU beds would be problematic for patients who need immediate treatment and are already patients at a hospital site.

RATIONING BECAUSE OF FUTURE SCARCE MEDICAL RESOURCES

In Case 32.1 a specific patient would be seriously harmed if care were not rationed. In the following case an unidentified future patient will predictably be harmed unless care is rationed.

CASE 32.3   Shortage of blood products

A 36-year-old man with alcoholic cirrhosis is admitted for severe variceal bleeding and encephalopathy. He is not a candidate for liver transplantation because of active alcohol and amphetamine use and nonadherence with physician visits and prescribed medications. The surgeons do not believe he will survive a portacaval shunt operation. After 3 days he has consumed 42 units of blood and continues to bleed briskly despite endoscopic sclerotherapy, administration of octreotide, and a percutaneous placement of a transjugular intrahepatic portal-systemic shunt. The regional blood bank has only three more units of his type despite appeals for donations. It is New Year's Eve, when many automobile accident victims will need transfusions.

In Case 32.3 there is no identified individual who will be harmed if blood products are not rationed, but the existence of such an individual is virtually certain. Many persons with trauma can recover completely with vigorous emergency care. Thus, a future patient is likely to be seriously harmed if all available blood were given to the patient in Case 32.3, who has not improved despite maximal care.

Physicians might be reluctant to ration interventions to patients who are already receiving care because of loyalty or fidelity—that is, doctors might believe that they have implicitly promised to provide ongoing care and not to curtail it to benefit other patients. The emotional appeal of this position is clear, and keeping promises is an important ethical guideline. However, maintaining fidelity should refer to appropriate ongoing care, not to unlimited care regardless of the benefits to the patient or the harms to others.

Although limitations on transfusions are justified in Case 32.3, there are challenges in implementing such limits in a fair manner. Various physicians might set different limits in practice. Some physicians might stop after 40 units, others after 60 units. More specific practice standards and institutional policies and procedures, including an interdisciplinary committee with public members, would make such decisions more consistently and, therefore, more fairly.

Policies and Procedures to Address Drug Shortages

Recently hospitals have experienced nationwide shortages of key medications, including cancer chemotherapy and drugs commonly used in emergency departments, such as intravenous saline solution and injectable potassium, opioids, and epinephrine.

If individual physicians address these shortages on a case-by-case basis, decisions are likely to be inconsistent in similar cases. More ethically troubling, some patients may be denied effective medications for clinically irrelevant characteristics such as ethnicity, gender, age, or skin color (6).

Institutional policies and procedures have much stronger ethical justification. All clinically similar patients should be treated as similarly deserving of consideration and limited medications should be distributed according to clinical need and predicted effectiveness (7, 13). Ability to pay, ethnicity, citizenship, and social worth should not be considered (13). Patients should have the right to appeal decisions. The process should be led by an interdisciplinary institutional committee that includes patient representatives, and the policy and process should be publicly transparent. An additional advantage of an institutional approach is that measures can be taken to increase availability of available supplies, for example, through repackaging into smaller dose units to avoid wasted medications.

RATIONING ON THE BASIS OF COST

In a recent national survey, 53.1% of physicians reported having personally refrained within the past 6 months from using specific clinical services that would have provided the best patient care because of health system cost (14). The most frequently limited interventions were medications and MRI scans.

In the previous cases, compelling ethical arguments exist for limiting care to one patient to provide much more beneficial clinical services to other patients. When rationing is done primarily to save money rather than to benefit other patients directly, however, the reasons are generally weaker. The following case illustrates these issues.

CASE 32.4   **Expensive care for a patient with poor prognosis and quality of life**

Mrs. D is a 76-year-old nursing home resident with severe dementia. She recognizes her family only occasionally and does not respond to health care workers' questions or requests. She develops chronic renal failure and symptoms of uremia. While competent, she had never expressed her preferences about renal dialysis. Although her primary physician and nephrologist recommend that renal dialysis not be performed, her family insists on it. They believe that as long as she recognizes them and smiles, her life should be prolonged. They understand that dialysis likely causes a sharp decline in her functioning and that most patients like her do not survive a year after initiating dialysis (15).

At the time, the public hospital is considering closing obstetrical and substance abuse services because of budget deficits. The physicians feel they are accomplices to an unjust health care system if they use resources on this patient when more pressing health needs are unmet. A vascular surgery consultant writes in the medical record, "In the current climate of out-of-control medical costs, it is unconscionable to provide expensive care for this patient."

As discussed in Chapter 14, it would be appropriate to provide renal dialysis to Mrs. D because it would achieve the family's goal of prolonging her life at a quality they consider acceptable. The physicians, however, believe that Mrs. D's quality of life is so poor that the cost of dialysis is not justified.

Objections to Bedside Rationing on the Basis of Cost

Physicians should support more enlightened policies regarding allocation, but in most circumstances attempts by physicians to ration care on the basis of costs at the level of the individual patient, although well intentioned, are not justified.

No Public Policy Authorizes Physicians to Ration

Although the physicians caring for Mrs. D felt partly responsible for the soaring cost of health care, no public policy authorizes physicians to limit the care of patients on renal dialysis to save resources for other patients. On the contrary, US public policy pays for dialysis to all patients with end-stage renal failure. In the 1960s, selecting patients for a limited number of renal dialysis machines on the basis of prognosis or quality of life proved so controversial that Congress singled out end-stage renal disease for universal coverage under the Medicare program.

Bedside Rationing Based on Costs Would Be Unfair

It would be inconsistent and, therefore, unfair if one physician or hospital withheld dialysis from Mrs. D, but another might provide it. Indeed, the public nursing home in the area provided chronic dialysis to numerous patients with severe Alzheimer disease. It violates the ethical guideline of justice to treat similar patients unequally. Whether or not Mrs. D receives dialysis should not be based on the choice of physician or hospital.

Bedside rationing might also be unfair if only certain patients or interventions are singled out for review. It makes little sense to limit one health care intervention as not cost-effective without looking at the cost-effectiveness of other interventions as well. Many people would object to limiting dialysis for Mrs. D if other interventions, such as intensive care for patients with extremely poor prognoses, were not similarly scrutinized.

Money Saved by Rationing Cannot Be Reallocated

Physicians in the United States who save money on the care of an individual patient generally cannot redirect those resources to patients or projects with higher priority (16). If physicians withheld dialysis from Mrs. D, they could not redirect funds to more pressing medical or social needs, such as prenatal care or childhood immunizations. Furthermore, in managed care organizations savings from limiting care to patients might be directed toward higher salaries for administrators or greater profits for investors rather than to more cost-effective interventions. In the absence of broader health care reform, attempts to limit health care costs at the bedside are likely to be ineffective gestures.

Limiting care for one patient to make resources available to other patients is more strongly justified if several conditions are met (17). First, saved resources would be reallocated to interventions that provide greater benefits for the population of patients receiving care. Second, the physicians would not benefit directly from saving resources. Third, the limitations in care are applied to all similar patients with no exceptions based on privileged social status.

Opponents of bedside rationing would argue that physicians in Case 32.4 fulfilled their ethical obligations to use limited resources prudently by discussing with Mrs. D's family her limited life expectancy on dialysis and making a strong recommendation against it.

RECOMMENDATIONS FOR PHYSICIANS

Physicians who are considering rationing life-sustaining interventions at the bedside should take several actions (Table 32-1). Hospitals should have policies and procedures incorporating these recommendations.

TABLE 32-1. Suggestions for Physicians Considering Bedside Rationing
Try to get more resources for the patient within the system
Make decisions openly
Get a second opinion
Notify patients or surrogates when care is rationed

Try to Get More Resources Within the System

Physicians should try to obtain more resources within the system. For example, in Case 32.1, beds in the postoperative recovery room might be used as temporary ICU beds. Such efforts, however, might lead to other problems, such as disrupting operating room schedules.

Make Decisions Openly

Discussing rationing dilemmas explicitly can identify unquestioned assumptions and hidden value judgments. When people must make their arguments and values explicit, others can present rebuttals or disagreements or suggest ways to resolve the problem.

Get a Second Opinion

Eliciting a second opinion from an interdisciplinary institutional committee can improve decision-making. For example, such a review might suggest other options or point out unwarranted value judgments.

Notify Patients or Surrogates When Care Is Rationed

Patients or their surrogates should be notified when beneficial care will be rationed. It is disrespectful to transfer patients out of intensive care or stop transfusions without explaining to them or their families what is happening. If possible, it is preferable to make such explanations before an actual clinical crisis occurs.

SUMMARY

1. Bedside rationing may be ethically appropriate if restricting services that provide only limited benefit to one patient would allow another patient to receive much greater medical benefits.
2. Decisions to ration to save money are ethically problematic if funds cannot be redirected to patients or projects with clearly higher priority.
3. Physicians facing bedside rationing decisions should take steps to help ensure that these decisions are consistent and fair. Hospitals should have institutional policies and procedures to help ensure consistency and fairness.

References

1. Walker RJ, Egede LE. Rationing of Care: Conceptual Ambiguity and Transparency in Data Collection and Synthesis. *J Gen Intern Med* 2016;31:1415-1416.
2. Scheunemann LP, White DB. The physician as rationer: uncertainty about the physician's role obligations. *Semin Respir Crit Care Med* 2012;33:421-6.
3. Pellegrino ED, Thomasma DG. *For the Patient's Good: The Restoration of Beneficence in Health Care.* New York: Oxford University Press; 1988.
4. Kassirer JP. Managing care—should we adopt a new ethic? *N Engl J Med* 1998;339:397-398.
5. Levinsky NG. The doctor's master. *N Engl J Med* 1984;311:1573-1575.
6. Rosoff PM. Who Should Ration? *AMA J Ethics* 2017;19:164-173.
7. Jagsi R, Spence R, Rathmell WK, Bradbury A, Peppercorn J, Grubbs S, et al. Ethical considerations for the clinical oncologist in an era of oncology drug shortages. *Oncologist* 2014;19:186-92.

8. Council on Ethical and Judicial Affairs. *Code of Medical Ethics: Current Opinions with Annotations*. Chicago: American Medical Association; 1998. 143.

9. Medical professionalism in the new millennium: a physician charter. *Ann Intern Med* 2002;136:243-6.

10. Hall MA, Berenson RA. Ethical practice in managed care: a dose of realism. *Ann Intern Med* 1998; 128:395-402.

11. Hillman AL. Managing the physician: rules versus incentives. *Health Aff (Millwood)* 1991;10:138-146.

12. Ellrodt AG, Conner L, Riedinger M, Weingarten S. Measuring and improving physician compliance with clinical practice guidelines. *Ann Intern Mec* 1995;122:277-282.

13. Rosoff PM, Patel KR, Scates A, et al. Coping with critical drug shortages: an ethical approach for allocating scarce resources in hospitals. *Arch Intern Med* 2012;172:1494-1499.

14. Sheeler RD, Mundell T, Hurst SA, et al. Self-reported rationing behavior among US physicians: a national survey. *J Gen Intern Med* 2016;31:1444-1451.

15. Kurella Tamura M, Covinsky KE, Chertow GM, et al. Functional status of elderly adults before and after initiation of dialysis. *N Engl J Med* 2009;361:1539-1547.

16. Daniels N. Why saying no to patients in the United States is so hard. *N Engl J Med* 1986;314:1380-1383.

17. Pearson SD. Caring and cost: the challenge for physician advocacy. *Ann Intern Med* 2000;133:148-153.

ANNOTATED BIBLIOGRAPHY

1. Daniels N. Why saying no to patients in the United States is so hard. *N Engl J Med* 1986;314:1380-1383. Points out that in the US system there is no way to direct money saved on one patient to more cost-effective purposes.

2. Scheunemann LP, White DB. The physician as rationer: uncertainty about the physician's role obligations. *Semin Respir Crit Care Med* 2012;33:421-426. Analyzes the appropriate role of physicians in rationing.

3. Pearson SD. Caring and cost: the challenge for physician advocacy. *Ann Intern Med* 2000;133:148-153. Suggests criteria for ethically appropriate bedside rationing.

4. Rosoff PM. Who Should Ration? *AMA J Ethics* 2017;19:164-173. Analyzes rationing in the context of drug shortages and describes policies and procedures at one hospital system.

Gifts from Drug Companies

INTRODUCTION

Gifts from drug companies to physicians formerly were ubiquitous. A 2001 study found that 97% of residents were carrying at least one item, such as reference books (90%), pens (79%), or information cards (70%) that had pharmaceutical insignia (1). Small gifts bearing the company or product name included pens and message pads, as well as more expensive items such as umbrellas, flashlights, and clocks. However, drug companies no longer provide such branded gifts because of concerns about conflicts of interest. This chapter presents arguments for and against accepting gifts from drug companies or medical device manufacturers and suggests guidelines for such gifts (2).

TYPES OF GIFTS

In 2012, pharmaceutical manufacturers spent more than $15 billion for drug detailing to US physicians and almost $6 billion for drug samples—around $26,000 per physician. The total amount spent for promotional activities was almost double the amount spent for research and development.

Continuing Medical Education

Drug companies spend over $2 billion dollars a year on educational and promotional meetings. More than 60% of funding for accredited continuing medical education (CME) now comes from commercial sources, including drug company support, advertising, and exhibitor fees (3). Accredited CME programs must comply with requirements for disclosure of drug company payments to the course and to speakers and review speakers' presentations for bias. Drug companies commonly work with publishing and education companies to develop CME programs. Compared with CME programs sponsored by academic institutions, CME programs from these companies present fewer sessions on such topics as prevention, lifestyle changes, and doctor–patient communication (4).

Drug companies provide presentations and slides for talks, as well as speaker training, to physicians on their speakers bureaus. The companies then pay honoraria and expenses when members of the speakers bureau give talks.

Companies also host nonaccredited talks for physicians, accompanied by dinners at desirable restaurants. Formerly physicians attending those talks were commonly given "consultants' fees" for suggesting ways to market the product.

Meals and Hospitality

Drug companies provide lunch or refreshments at hospital conferences or CME courses. Conference organizers often solicit these subsidies to increase attendance. Drug detailing staff can also pay for lunches for physicians and office staff.

Drug Detailing

Drug representatives provide individualized information and gifts to physicians, together with free drug samples for patients. Many physicians depend on drug representatives as convenient sources of information about new drugs. Studies suggest that physician exposure to information from drug companies is associated with more prescriptions, higher drug costs, and lower quality of prescribing (5, 6). Drug representatives have a prescribing profile for each physician, which is obtained from prescription records purchased from pharmacies. These profiles enable drug representatives to tailor their message to the individual doctor and to assess its impact (7, 8). Drug representatives are trained to assess physicians' personality styles and to establish a personal connection with them (9, 10).

REASONS FOR DRUG COMPANIES TO OFFER GIFTS

There is evidence that gifts from drug companies strengthen physicians' recognition of products (11). One study found that doctors who attended a drug company–sponsored CME or who accepted funds for travel or lodging for educational symposia were more likely to prescribe the sponsor's medications. This occurred even if physicians forgot the sponsors' names or believed that they could not be influenced. Doctors who met with pharmaceutical representatives or accepted industry-paid meals were more likely to request formulary additions or to prescribe in nonrational ways. Physicians who received gifts from pharmaceutical manufacturers, even practice-related gifts, were more likely to believe that gifts did not affect prescribing behavior. Physicians who accepted free drug samples were more likely to prescribe newer (and more expensive) medications for hypertension than older medications that are recommended by practice guidelines as initial therapy (12).

REASONS FOR ACCEPTING DRUG-COMPANY GIFTS

Gifts from drug companies subsidize continuing education courses and, thereby, might enhance medical education and professional society meetings. Providing lunches, travel expenses, and honoraria for hospital conferences might improve educational programs by increasing attendance and enabling smaller hospitals to invite nationally prominent experts. Thus, some argue that drug-company gifts and subsidies have, overall, more benefit than harm. If physicians refused all gifts and subsidies from drug companies, then patients would pay the same amount for drugs but their physicians would receive less education. Some physicians believe that drug samples provide medications to indigent and uninsured patients; however, a lower percentage of indigent or uninsured patients report receiving drug samples than do wealthy or insured patients (13).

OBJECTIONS TO ACCEPTING DRUG-COMPANY GIFTS

Table 33-1 summarizes objections to accepting gifts from drug companies.

TABLE 33-1. Objections to Accepting Gifts from Drug Companies
Gifts impair objectivity
Gifts undermine patient and public trust
Gifts demean the medical profession
Gifts create the expectation of reciprocity
Gifts increase the cost of health care

Gifts Impair Objectivity

Objectivity of presentations might be compromised if a drug company selects speakers and topics, writes or edits talks, provides slides, and trains the presenters (14). A speaker might selectively present or emphasize data favorable to a sponsor's drug or class of drugs rather than draw from the overall body of available data. Drug company representatives informed US physicians of harms of drugs in only 39% of interactions and rarely mentioned serious adverse events, even for drugs that had a "black box" warning from the Food and Drug Administration (15).

Gifts Undermine Patient and Public Trust

Even if gifts from pharmaceutical companies do not actually influence a physician's therapeutic decisions, they might undermine public trust. After all, physicians are not choosing medications for their own use and paying the costs themselves; they are prescribing for their patients. According to an older survey, patients are more likely than physicians to believe that gifts are not appropriate and that they influence physician behavior (16). About 30% of patients believe that even small gifts such as a mug, pen, or lunch would influence a physician's behavior, compared with about 10% of physicians (16). More recent studies have found that patients who know or believe their physician has accepted payments from drug companies rated their physicians lower on honesty, fidelity, or trust (17, 18).

Outside of medicine, society has enacted strict rules regarding conflicts of interest that might undermine trust in public officials. Judges are expected to refuse gifts from persons or companies who have a financial stake in their professional decisions. Government officials may not accept gifts of more than nominal value from persons or organizations who would be affected by or gain financially from their decisions. By analogy, it might be inappropriate for physicians to accept drug-company gifts that create even the appearance of a conflict of interest.

Gifts Demean the Medical Profession

Dependence on drug-company subsidies to support CME programs demeans physicians (19). If the public believed that physicians attend conferences only if lunch is provided or the registration fee is subsidized, then they might infer that physicians place little value on keeping up-to-date with medical advances.

Gifts Create the Expectation of Reciprocity

Gifts create relationships and obligations in the recipient, such as grateful conduct, goodwill, and reciprocation (9, 20). The problem is not that physicians immediately change prescribing practices after receiving a free lunch. Drug company representatives are trained to use small gifts, such as meals, to develop relationships with physicians and their staff and to persuade physicians to prescribe a target drug (10, 21).

Gifts Increase the Cost of Health Care

Ultimately, patients and their insurers pay for drug-company gifts to physicians. Given the sharply rising cost of drugs, it might be unseemly for physicians to receive even small gifts from drug companies. One physician criticized, "Am I supposed to believe that the members of a clinical department are so impoverished that they cannot buy their own pens or pizza and beer?" (19). There is evidence suggesting that accepting gifts from drug companies is associated with prescribing brand name drugs rather that equally effective generic drugs of same pharmaceutical class (22).

RECOMMENDATIONS

Disclose Gifts to the Public

Speakers at CME programs must disclose any honoraria or consulting fees from commercial entities in the course syllabus and at the beginning of their presentations. Under the Physician Payment Sunshine Act, drug, device, and biotechnology companies must report all payments to physicians by name that total more than US$100 a year to a publicly available database (2). Thus, members of the public can to determine how much money a physician received from drug companies.

Physicians might find it difficult to determine what gifts are acceptable and what are not. A helpful rule of thumb is, "What would your patients or the public think if they knew you had accepted these gifts?" (23). In borderline cases, it would be judicious to err on the side of declining gifts.

Allow Certain Other Practices

Some types of gifts or support are widely considered acceptable, with disclosure and appropriate management. At professional society meetings, drug companies often underwrite the printing of abstract books; such support is publicly acknowledged. For accredited CME courses, educational grants from commercial sponsors are permitted, provided that the sponsors may not influence the selection of speakers or the choice of topics. The CME course director is responsible for reviewing presentations from speakers who have financial relationships with drug or device manufacturers to ensure there is no bias. Bias in CME presentations could be more rigorously and comprehensively identified, for example by asking whether presentations compare options for managing the condition, use a critical literature review or meta-analysis to summarize the totality of the evidence, discuss the limitations of data for new therapies, and consider what important pertinent topics are missing (3, 24).

In promotional talks sponsored by drug companies, which do not offer CME credit and are often held at restaurants, there are no requirements for lack of bias (21). Defenders of promotional meals argue that there is no definitive evidence that that they harm patients. However, this absence of evidence does not establish a lack of harm. Moreover, no empirical studies suggest that meals from drug manufacturers improve patient outcomes (21).

Forbid Certain Practices

Certain types of gifts and support from drug companies are so likely to raise questions about bias and impropriety that they should be banned (2). For example, the American College of Physicians, the American Medical Association, the Accreditation Council for Continuing Medical Education, and the Pharmaceutical Manufacturers Association agree that it is unethical for physicians to accept direct payments to attend activities that have no educational value. The pharmaceutical industry has declared that occasional meals provided in conjunction with informational presentations must be modest (25). Drug company representatives may no longer provide items for the personal benefit of health care professionals, such as tickets to a recreational event, or mugs, pens, and similar items (25).

Several prominent medical centers have taken strong, comprehensive policies regarding interactions with pharmaceutical companies (2). Physicians may not accept any industry gifts, including drug samples, on campus or at clinical sites. This includes meals with conferences. Furthermore, industry representatives are not permitted in patient care areas except for in-service training on devices and are permitted in nonclinical areas only by appointment. Policies restricting detailing by drug representatives were associated with modest but significant decreases in prescribing in detailed drugs across multiple drug categories in most institutions (26).

SUMMARY

1. Gifts from drug companies might impair objectivity, undermine public trust, and increase the cost of health care.
2. The primary concern of physicians should be their patients' best interests, not their own personal convenience or well-being.

References

1. Sigworth SK, Nettleman MD, Cohen GM. Pharmaceutical branding of resident physicians. *JAMA* 2001; 286:1024-1025.
2. Lo B, Field M. *Conflict of Interest in Medical Research, Education, and Practice.* 2009. Available at: http://www.iom.edu/Reports/2009/Conflict-of-Interest-in-Medical-Research-Education-and-Practice.aspx. Accessed November 30, 2012.

3. Barnes B. Financial conflicts of interest in continuing medical education: implications and accountability. *JAMA* 2017;317:1741-1742.

4. Katz HP, Goldfinger SE, Fletcher SW. Academia-industry collaboration in continuing medical education: description of two approaches. *J Contin Educ Health Prof* 2002;22:43-54.

5. Spurling GK, Mansfield PR, Montgomery BD, et al. Information from pharmaceutical companies and the quality, quantity, and cost of physicians' prescribing: a systematic review. *PLoS Med* 2010;7:e1000352.

6. Fickweiler F, Fickweiler W, Urbach E. Interactions between physicians and the pharmaceutical industry generally and sales representatives specifically and their association with physicians' attitudes and prescribing habits: a systematic review. *BMJ Open* 2017;7.

7. Manz C, Ross JS, Grande D. Marketing to physicians in a digital world. *N Engl J Med* 2014;371:1857-1859.

8. Grande D. Prescriber profiling: time to call it quits. *Ann Intern Med* 2007;146:751-752.

9. Sah S, Fugh-Berman A. Physicians under the influence: social psychology and industry marketing strategies. *Journal of Law, Medicine & Ethics* 2013;41:665-671.

10. Fugh-Berman A, Ahari S. Following the script: how drug reps make friends and influence doctors. *PLoS Med* 2007;4:e150.

11. Wazana A. Physicians and the pharmaceutical industry: is a gift ever just a gift? *JAMA* 2000;283:373-380.

12. Ubel PA, Jepson C, Asch DA. Misperceptions about beta-blockers and diuretics: a national survey of primary care physicians. *J Gen Intern Med* 2003;18:977-983.

13. Cutrona SL, Woolhandler S, Lasser KE, et al. Characteristics of recipients of free prescription drug samples: a nationally representative analysis. *Am J Public Health* 2008;98:284-289.

14. Avorn J. Rethinking the use of physicians as hired expert lecturers. *Ann Intern Med* 2014;161:363-364.

15. Mintzes B, Lexchin J, Wilkes MS, et al. Pharmaceutical sales representatives and patient safety. *J Gen Intern Med* 2013;28:1395.

16. Gibbons RV, Landry FJ, Blouch DL, et al. A comparison of physicians' and patients' attitudes towards pharmaceutical industry gifts. *J Gen Intern Med* 1998;13.

17. Grande D, Shea JA, Armstrong K. Pharmaceutical industry gifts to physicians: patient beliefs and trust in physicians and the health care system. *J Gen Intern Med* 2012;27:274-279.

18. Hwong AR, Sah S, Lehmann LS. The effects of public disclosure of industry payments to physicians on patient trust: a randomized experiment. *J Gen Intern Med* 2017;32:1186-1192.

19. Waud DR. Pharmaceutical promotions: a free lunch? *N Engl J Med* 1992;327:351-353.

20. Dana J. How psychological research can inform policies for dealing with conflicts of interest in medicine. In: Lo B, Field M, eds. *Conflict of Interest in Medical Research, Education, and Practice*. Washington, DC: National Academies Press; 2009. 358-374.

21. Lo B, Grady D. Payments to Physicians: Does the Amount of Money Make a Difference? *JAMA* 2017;317:1719-1720.

22. DeJong C, Aguilar T, Tseng CW, et al. Pharmaceutical industry-sponsored meals and physician prescribing patterns for Medicare beneficiaries. *JAMA Intern Med* 2016;176:1114-1122.

23. Coyle SL. Physician-industry relations. Part 1: individual physicians. *Ann Intern Med* 2002;136:396-402.

24. Lo B, Ott C. What is the enemy in CME, conflicts of interest or bias? *JAMA* 2013;310:1019-1020.

25. PhRMA. *Code on Interactions with Health Care Professionals*. 2008. Available at: http://www.phrma.org/about/principles-guidelines/code-interactions-healthcare-professionals. Accessed May 5, 2018.

26. Larkin I, Ang D, Steinhart J, et al. Association between academic medical center pharmaceutical detailing policies and physician prescribing. *JAMA* 2017;317:1785-1795.

ANNOTATED BIBLIOGRAPHY

1. Lo B, Field M. *Conflict of Interest in Medical Research, Education, and Practice*. 2009. http://www.iom.edu/Reports/2009/Conflict-of-Interest-in-Medical-Research-Education-and-Practice.aspx. Accessed November 16, 2011.
Consensus report from the Institute of Medicine on conflicts of interest in medicine, including gift from drug companies. Summarizes empirical data on the topic and makes policy recommendations.

2. Lo B, Ott C. What is the enemy in CME, conflicts of interest or bias? *JAMA* 2013;310:1019-1020.
Identifying and eliminating bias directly can address many concerns about conflicts of interest.

3. Larkin I, Ang D, Steinhart J, et al. Association between academic medical center pharmaceutical detailing policies and physician prescribing. *JAMA* 2017;317:1785-1795.
   Empirical study of impact of drug detailing policies on prescribing by physicians.
4. Sah S, Fugh-Berman A. Physicians under the influence: social psychology and industry marketing strategies. *Journal of Law, Medicine & Ethics* 2013;41:665-671
   Describes social psychology mechanisms by which marketing by drug companies influence physician prescribing.

CHAPTER

Disclosing Errors

INTRODUCTION

An estimated 40,000 Americans die every year because of medical errors (1). In a 2002 survey, 42% of the public and 35% of physicians reported that an error had occurred in their own care or a family member's care (2). In only 30% of cases was the patient or family told that an error had occurred (2). Many physicians find it difficult to disclose errors to patients and colleagues because of possible recriminations from patients, setbacks to their professional reputation or livelihood, and malpractice suits. Patients want more disclosure of errors than physicians say they typically provide (3).

This chapter discusses the reasons for and against disclosing errors and suggests how physicians can respond to errors. An *error* is a failure of a plan to be completed as intended or the use of a wrong plan to achieve an aim. Errors can be either acts or omissions. Errors might—or might not—result in harm to patients; when no harm is done, the incident is called a *near miss* or a *close call*. Errors might or might not be avoidable. Adverse events are defined as undesired patient outcomes that result from medical care rather than from the underlying disease; they include situations in which the treatment plan was appropriate and carried out correctly, such as side effects of drugs.

The following case illustrates dilemmas posed by physicians' errors.

CASE 34.1 | **Overdose of insulin**

A 54-year-old man with diabetes is hospitalized for congestive heart failure. The resident prescribes 100 units of insulin rather than the patient's usual dose of 10 units, and the patient receives the higher dose. He develops hypoglycemia, seizures, and coma. Upon recovery, the patient and his family ask physicians why the seizures occurred. The health care team is reluctant to tell them that an error occurred, fearing that he would get angry and perhaps sue them.

Traditionally, such errors were blamed on individuals who were deficient in knowledge, effort, or conscientiousness. The modern view is that most errors are due to inherent limitations in human cognition and attention and to system failures. In this view, blaming the physician is problematic (1, 4, 5). First, errors like the one in Case 34.1 usually are due to a momentary loss of concentration or attention, which is beyond the doctor's voluntary control. A "slip of the pen" or a lapse in concentration could happen to the most expert and careful physician. Second, errors generally have multiple system causes. The pharmacist who dispensed the medication and the nurse who administered it failed to detect the incorrect dosage. The attending physician might have provided closer supervision. These system problems are "accidents waiting to happen." More training for individual health care workers will be less effective overall in preventing such errors than redesigning the health care delivery system (6), including computerized ordering of medications, checklists, bar coding, and improved teamwork among physicians, pharmacists, and nurses. Focusing on improving the system of health care, rather than blaming individuals, is likely to result in higher quality of care for the population of patients as a whole.

SHOULD ERRORS BE DISCLOSED TO PATIENTS?

Since the 2001 report *To Err Is Human* from the Institute of Medicine, disclosure of errors to patients has become the standard of care (7). The Joint Commission, which accredits health care institutions, requires hospitals to tell patients when unanticipated outcomes of care occur. Finally, several states have enacted laws that require the disclosure of unanticipated outcomes of care.

Reasons Not to Disclose Errors to Patients or Surrogates

Physician Is not Really Responsible for the Error

Physicians understandably do not want to take the blame for errors if they are not morally responsible. Only a few errors result from negligent or intentional violations of a clear standard of care or performance (4). Most are caused by systems flaws and limits in human cognition, which are beyond the physician's control.

Disclosure Would Harm Health Care Professionals

Physicians might fear that patients or families might respond to disclosure of errors by becoming angry, changing providers, or filing a lawsuit. Indeed, many patients report that they would change physicians if their physician committed a life-threatening error (3). The reluctance of physicians to acknowledge errors, however, creates a vicious circle: If physicians are not forthright about errors, patients become more upset and likely to sue. Students and residents might worry that their careers will be damaged if they disclose a serious error to a supervising physician and that colleagues and supervisors might respond punitively rather than supportively (8).

Reasons to Disclose Errors to Patients or Surrogates

Disclosure Respects the Patient

Almost all patients would want even minor errors disclosed to them (9). Patients want to know what happened, why it happened, how adverse consequences will be mitigated, and how recurrences will be prevented (9-11). In addition, patients seek an apology (9).

Unless the patient in Case 34.1 is told about the insulin overdose, he cannot understand this incident. He might well fear that seizures and coma will recur or that he has a grave problem, such as a brain tumor. Fearing a recurrence, he might change jobs or cut back on activities, such as driving or travel. Under the doctrine of informed consent, physicians have an affirmative duty to provide the patient or surrogate with pertinent information about his condition and the options for care. This duty to disclose goes beyond responding honestly to questions from patients. In thinking about disclosure, physicians might imagine how they would feel if a relative was harmed by an error and the health care team was not forthright about what happened.

Disclosure Benefits the Patient

Disclosure enables patients or surrogates to mitigate the harms that the error caused, for example, through additional tests, treatment, or follow-up care. Patients or families are more likely to cooperate with such measures if they understand the reasons for them. Disclosure might also allow patients to be compensated for harms resulting from errors. In Case 34.1, the patient required intensive care, a prolonged hospitalization, and a computed tomography (CT) scan following the error. It is unfair to ask the patient or an insurer to pay for this additional care. Moreover, most patients want charges for such care to be waived (12). Furthermore, it seems reasonable and fair to compensate patients for lost income or serious disability resulting directly from errors. Patients cannot seek such compensation unless they or their surrogates are aware that an error occurred.

Disclosure Benefits the Physician

Disclosure might also mitigate adverse impacts on the physician's livelihood. Health care institutions can institute programs that disclose adverse outcomes, offer an apology, set up a quality-improvement process to prevent similar errors in the future, and offer compensation for medical errors (13). Such programs do not increase malpractice claims. Although disclosing an error does not shield a physician from legal liability, nondisclosure might increase the legal risk (14).

WHAT TO SAY TO PATIENTS ABOUT ERRORS?

In Case 34.1, the physician clearly made an error, the patient suffered serious harm, and the error caused a poor outcome. Under these circumstances, the physician's responsibility to the patient should prevail over any self-interest in concealing the error. The physician should take the initiative in disclosing relevant information. First, physicians should explicitly acknowledge that an error occurred and offer an apology (15, 16). When a person harms another, apologizing is the expected social response and a prerequisite to making amends and being forgiven (17). Many states do not allow expressions of sympathy made after an unanticipated outcome to be used as evidence in lawsuits. These laws, however, have major limitations: They protect institutions, not individual physicians, and do not shield explanations of the cause of errors or admissions of fault. Thus, these laws may not address physician's concerns about liability for giving patients the comprehensive disclosure and apologies that they seek (18). Second, the physician needs to explain the error and its consequences. Third, the physician should explain what can and will be done to mitigate the resulting harms to the patient and to prevent the error from recurring (10).

Some physicians might make only limited disclosure of errors—for example, telling the patient and family in Case 34.1 only that the patient's blood sugar got too low because he received more insulin than he needed, without saying that an error occurred (15). Other physicians might say, "I am sorry about what happened," but not take responsibility for the error. Patients and families, however, might regard a partial apology as evasive and mean-spirited. Ethically, an appropriate response to concerns about a lawsuit in Case 34.1 would be for the risk manager to offer a fair out-of-court settlement. Current best practice is to disclose the error, offer an apology, explain how the institution will institute a quality-improvement process to prevent similar errors in the future, and also to proactively offer compensation for medical injuries (13). The process of root cause analysis and quality improvement helps develop a culture that prizes patient safety.

RESPONSIBILITY FOR ERRORS

The vast majority of errors are caused by systems defects or limitations in human attention and cognition, which are beyond the control of the individual physician. Few errors are caused by deficiencies in knowledge, skill, or due care. A strong argument can be made that people should not be held responsible for actions and conditions beyond their control.

The current systems approach to errors has led to calls for a "blame-free" culture because overall patients benefit more from putting in place systems to prevent errors, catch them before harm occurs, or reduce harms that do occur (6). However, health care workers should be held accountable for deliberate, egregious errors, for example, habitual and willful errors (19). Individual physicians are still held responsible for errors in several ways, including malpractice suits. Moreover, settlements are reported to the National Practitioner Data Bank when applying for staff privileges, even if the error was beyond the physician's control. Movements are underway to have state licensing boards close cases of errors that have gone through a process of disclosure, root cause analysis, quality improvement, and offer of fair compensation, without reporting them to the National Practitioner Data Bank (20).

SITUATIONS IN WHICH DISCLOSURE IS CONTROVERSIAL

In many cases, it might be unclear whether the physician should disclose an error to the patient or take responsibility for it.

The Error Caused No Harm

Errors that cause no harm to patients are called *near misses*.

CASE 34.2 | **Incorrect prescription**

A physician prescribed a sulfonamide antibiotic to a patient with a history of allergy to those medications. A nurse discovered the error, and the prescription was changed after two doses. No adverse effects occurred.

Such near misses need to be reported to quality-improvement programs to prevent similar errors that could harm patients. Should they also be disclosed to the patient? In Case 34.2, some physicians might argue that if the prognosis or future care of the patient is not altered, there is no point in telling the patient of the error. Such physicians might hesitate to burden patients with all the uncertainties and adjustments made in the course of care. In addition, patients might lose confidence in physicians and hospitals.

Even in this case, however, there are strong reasons to disclose the error to patients. Disclosure is likely to strengthen the doctor–patient relationship because patients respect physicians for being honest. Disclosure might also promote patient well-being by allowing reconsideration of the diagnosis of drug allergy. Furthermore, patients might call attention to errors—for example, after noticing that the medication has changed. If this occurs, physicians might find it awkward to explain the change if the patient had not been told immediately. Finally, there is little risk to physicians in disclosing "near misses" because patients who suffer no harm are unlikely to get angry and cannot sue.

Outcome Would Have Been Poor Even Without the Error

In other cases, the physician makes an error and the patient suffers a poor outcome, but the poor outcome would very likely have occurred even if there had been no error. For example, the adverse outcome might be due to the underlying disease.

CASE 34.3 | **Failure to administer appropriate treatment**

A 72-year-old man developed headache, dizziness and vomiting, and ataxia and became comatose. MRI showed a large bilateral pontine hemorrhage and hydrocephalus. Previously he had said that he feared having a stroke and living with severe difficulties, as happened with his father, with alertness, thinking, and caring for himself. On the basis of his wishes, his family declined intensive care or neurosurgery and agreed to palliative care to allow the patient to die in the emergency department. Just before this death, radiology reported that his chest x-ray showed a small infiltrate.

In this case, the physicians did not check the results of the x-ray, and an apparent pneumonia was not treated with antibiotics. However, antibiotics would not have altered the grave prognosis of the brainstem hemorrhage or the family's decision for palliative care. The error did not contribute to the patient's death.

In this case, the physician's focus should be on reassuring the family that the patient did not suffer because he was comatose and to support them in their grief. It would be appropriate not to discuss the pneumonia, unless the patient required oxygen for comfort and the family asked what caused the lack of oxygen. Physicians must recognize, however, that determining whether an error caused an adverse outcome is difficult (6) and that their belief that the error caused no harm might be biased or self-serving. Consultation with an experienced colleague might help physicians evaluate their judgment and actions accurately.

As an opportunity for quality improvement, however, the hospital should follow up on how x-rays are read and reported in the emergency department, to assure that films on critically ill patients are read promptly and results reported to the treating physician.

Adverse Outcome Could Not Have Been Avoided

Some procedure-related adverse events are due to a mishap, such as poor technique or a slip of the instrument. System factors, such as inadequate training or supervision, might be contributing factors. In other cases, however, the procedure was carried out skillfully and yet an adverse event occurs.

CASE 34.4	Foreseeable complication of an invasive procedure

A 43-year-old man with interstitial lung disease undergoes a bronchoscopy and transbronchial biopsy. The procedure is performed following standard procedures. He suffers a pneumothorax that requires insertion of a chest tube for 2 days. The patient was informed of this risk prior to the procedure.

In this case, the patient suffered a known complication of an invasive procedure that was appropriately and skillfully performed. The bronchoscopy service needs to review the case to be certain that the standard of care was followed. The patient agreed to the procedure and accepted the risks. Although the physician must explain the unintended adverse outcome and should express regret over it, the doctor is not to blame for this complication.

DISCLOSING ERRORS BY TRAINEES TO AN ATTENDING PHYSICIAN

In teaching hospitals, errors by trainees might not be reported to attending physicians (21, 22).

Disclosure of Serious Errors by Trainees to Supervising Physicians

Students, house officers, and fellows might be reluctant to tell supervisors about errors lest they jeopardize their grades, recommendations, or future positions. Supervisors might respond judgmentally rather than supportively.

Attending physicians are ethically and legally responsible for patient care. They cannot perform this role properly if significant information about the patient is withheld. Furthermore, attending physicians might learn of such errors even if trainees do not disclose them. Most supervising physicians believe that failure to disclose errors is worse than making them in the first place (22, 23). Although trainees are expected to make some errors, covering them up raises doubts about reliability, trustworthiness, and character. Disclosing appropriate errors is considered a requirement of professionalism (16).

Responses to Errors by Trainees

Supervising physicians need to respond to trainee errors on several levels.

Elicit and Acknowledge the Trainee's Emotional Distress

Appropriate emotional support needs to be provided (21, 24). The supervisor can put the trainee's feelings in context: Although it causes distress to admit an error, it is a sign of responsibility and caring. Understanding this link between emotional distress and learning might offer the resident some solace.

Review the Medical Issues and Decisions

The supervisor can help the trainee learn from the error and make constructive changes to prevent similar errors in the future, for example, seeking advice in difficult cases, reading more about the medical problem, and confirming key clinical data personally rather than relying on someone else's report (22). Discussing errors explicitly also helps other trainees avoid similar errors and contributes to a culture of safety.

Discuss How to Disclose the Error to the Patient or Surrogate

If disclosure is appropriate, then the attending physician should inform the patient together with the trainee. Such joint discussions offer trainees emotional support and role modeling.

ERRORS BY OTHER HEALTH CARE WORKERS

A physician might become aware of an error by another health care worker that harmed a patient. For example, in Case 34.1 another clinical service or a different hospital might have made the overdose of insulin. Even if the current physician did not make the error, the patient still needs to understand what happened and try to mitigate the resulting harms. Thus, the current physician might consider whether to disclose the error to the patient.

Ethical Issues Regarding Errors by Other Health Care Workers

Patients need disclosure of errors regardless of who committed them. Physicians, however, often find it more difficult to deal with errors by other health care workers. The facts of the case might be unclear, even if the physician reviews the medical record. In addition, disclosure might conflict with the current physician's self-interest (25). The other physician or institution might become irate or stop referring patients. Physicians in training who notice a serious error by a senior physician might fear retaliation (*see* Chapter 36). In addition, the patient or family might vent their anger on the current physician, who bears no responsibility for the error. On the other hand, if the current physicians do not discuss the earlier error, the patient and family may feel that there is a cover-up.

Responses to Errors by Other Health Care Workers

Faced with a clear and serious error by another health care worker, the current physician might take several steps (25).

Waiting for the patient to ask is ethically problematic because physicians have an affirmative obligation to disclose relevant information to patients.

Usually it is helpful for the current physician to consult colleagues with relevant expertise to ensure that they agree that an error occurred, rather than a difference of opinion about care. The current physician should then contact the other physician to discuss the case. It is important to gather all the relevant facts before making a judgment or taking action.

In some cases, there will be disagreement over whether an error occurred or how to respond. If this is the case, institutional processes for quality improvement should be activated, for example a case conference or peer review committee, with a view toward informing the patient if it is determined that an error occurred (25).

If the patient is still receiving care at the institution in which the error occurred, then a joint conference might be held with the current physician, the previous physician, and relevant specialists (25), with a view toward informing the patient if it is determined that an error occurred.

SUMMARY

1. The decision to acknowledge an error ideally should be based on ethical guidelines, not on expedience.
2. Disclosure of errors is difficult, but failure to disclose errors undermines physicians' credibility and compromises their integrity.
3. When disclosure of errors is accompanied by a root cause analysis and implementation of a quality-improvement plan, similar errors can be prevented in the future.

References

1. Kohn LT, Corrigan JM, Donaldson M. *To Err Is Human: Building a Safer Health System. 2000.* Available at: https://www.nap.edu/catalog/9728/to-err-is-human-building-a-safer-health-system. Accessed June 15, 2018.
2. Blendon RJ, DesRoches CM, Brodie M, et al. Views of practicing physicians and the public on medical errors. *N Engl J Med* 2002;347:1933-1940.
3. Gallagher TH, Levinson W. Disclosing harmful medical errors to patients: a time for professional action. *Arch Intern Med* 2005;165:1819-1824.

4. Runciman WB, Merry AF, Tito F. Error, blame, and the law in health care—an antipodean perspective. *Ann Intern Med* 2003;138:974-979.

5. Reason J. Human error: models and management. *BMJ* 2000;320:768-770.

6. Wachter RM, Pronovost PJ. Balancing "no blame" with accountability in patient safety. *N Engl J Med* 2009;361:1401-1406.

7. Gallagher TH, Studdert D, Levinson W. Disclosing harmful medical errors to patients. *N Engl J Med* 2007;356:2713-2719.

8. Wu AW, Folkman S, McPhee SJ, et al. Do house officers learn from their mistakes? *JAMA* 1991;265: 2089-2094.

9. Gallagher TH, Waterman AD, Ebers AG, et al. Patients' and physicians' perspective regarding the disclosure of medical errors. *JAMA* 2003;289:1001-1007.

10. Mazor KM, Greene SM, Roblin D, et al. More than words: Patients' views on apology and disclosure when things go wrong in cancer care. *Patient Educ Couns* 2013;90:341-346.

11. O'Connor E, Coates HM, Yardley IE, et al. Disclosure of patient safety incidents: a comprehensive review. *Int J Qual Health Care* 2010;22:371-379.

12. Mazor KM, Simon SR, Yood RA, et al. Health plan members' views about disclosure of medical errors. *Ann Intern Med* 2004;140:409-418.

13. Moore J, Bismark M, Mello MM. Patients' Experiences with communication-and-resolution programs after medical injury. *JAMA Intern Med* 2017;177:1595-1603.

14. Mazor KM, Reed GW, Yood RA, et al. Disclosure of medical errors: what factors influence how patients respond? *J Gen Intern Med* 2006;21:704-710.

15. Gallagher TH, Garbutt JM, Waterman AD, et al. Choosing your words carefully: how physicians would disclose harmful medical errors to patients. *Arch Intern Med* 2006;166:1585-1593.

16. Levinson W, Yeung J, Ginsburg S. Disclosure of medical error. *JAMA* 2016;316:764-765.

17. Lazare A. Apology in medical practice: an emerging clinical skill. *JAMA* 2006;296:1401-1404.

18. Mastroianni AC, Mello MM, Sommer S, et al. The flaws in state 'apology' and 'disclosure' laws dilute their intended impact on malpractice suits. *Health Aff (Millwood)* 2010;29:1611-1619.

19. Shojania KG, Dixon-Woods M. 'Bad apples': time to redefine as a type of systems problem? *BMJ Qual Saf* 2013;22:528-531.

20. Gallagher TH, Farrell ML, Karson H, et al. Collaboration with regulators to support quality and account-ability following medical errors: the communication and resolution program certification pilot. *Health Serv Res* 2016;51:2569-2582.

21. Fischer MA, Mazor KM, Baril J, et al. Learning from mistakes. Factors that influence how students and residents learn from medical errors. *J Gen Intern Med* 2006;21:419-423.

22. Wu AW, Cavanaugh TA, McPhee SJ, et al. To tell the truth: ethical and practical issues in disclosing medical mistakes to patients. *J Gen Intern Med* 1997;17:770-775.

23. Bosk CL. *Forgive and Remember: Managing Medical Failure.* Chicago: University of Chicago Press; 1979.

24. Wu AW. Medical error: the second victim. The doctor who makes the mistake needs help too. *BMJ* 2000;320:726-727.

25. Gallagher TH, Mello MM, Levinson W, et al. Talking with patients about other clinicians' errors. *N Engl J Med* 2013;369:1752-1757.

ANNOTATED BIBLIOGRAPHY

1. Kohn LT, Corrigan JM, Donaldson M. *To Err Is Human: Building a Safer Health System. 2000.* Available at: https://www.nap.edu/catalog/9728/to-err-is-human-building-a-safer-health-system.
   Landmark consensus report concluding that most errors are due to system problems and limits of human cognition and attention. Recommends a confidential system of reporting errors to prevent future errors.

2. Wu AW, Folkman S, McPhee SJ, et al. Do house officers learn from their mistakes? *JAMA* 1991;265: 2089-2094.
   House officers who accepted responsibility for serious mistakes were more likely to make constructive changes in practice, but were also more likely to experience emotional distress. Attending physicians were told of serious mistakes only 54% of the time, and patients or families were told of the mistake in only 24% of cases.

3. Gallagher TH, Studdert D, Levinson W. Disclosing harmful medical errors to patients. *N Engl J Med* 2007;356:2713-2719.

   Describes growing incentives and pressures to disclose errors to patients and presents evidence suggesting that malpractice costs may decrease with greater disclosure.

4. Gallagher TH, Mello MM, Levinson W, et al. Talking with patients about other clinicians' errors. *N Engl J Med* 2013;369:1752-1757.

   Thoughtful analysis of how to respond to errors by other physicians.

Impaired Colleagues

INTRODUCTION

Physicians who are impaired or incompetent might harm patients. Society relies on the medical profession to regulate itself, yet colleagues of impaired physicians are often reluctant to intervene, even in egregious cases. Ethically, there needs to be an appropriate balance between protecting patients from impaired physicians and rehabilitating impaired physicians so they can return to practice, help future patients, and earn their livelihood. The following case illustrates common dilemmas regarding impaired colleagues.

CASE 35.1	Drinking alcohol while on call

Dr. New, a young internist who has recently joined a group practice, is at a party. She overhears a senior colleague, Dr. Elder, answer a page. Dr. Elder has been drinking and has slurred speech. Over the phone he prescribes 2.50 mg of digoxin, an unusually large dose. From what she hears of the conversation, Dr. New suspects that she has covered this patient, an elderly man with mild renal insufficiency, a recent hip fracture repair, and postoperative pneumonia.

Although Dr. New suspects that the patient is at risk of a drug overdose, she cannot be sure. Should she intervene to protect the patient from this suspected mistake? If so, should she confront Dr. Elder or talk to the house officer or nursing supervisor covering the service? What about other patients Dr. Elder might harm? Dr. New wants to prevent harm to patients, but she is reluctant to jeopardize a colleague's career or her own.

This chapter discusses intervening with impaired colleagues, reasons to take action, concerns about doing so, and practical suggestions. Chapter 34, which discusses errors, contains related materials. Errors by impaired or incompetent colleagues are more serious than other errors because they are more likely to be repeated. Although many medical errors are due to system problems, those discussed in this chapter are due primarily to shortcomings of an individual physician.

Common causes of impairment include alcoholism, substance abuse, and psychiatric and medical illness, such as depression and Alzheimer disease. The prevalence of these conditions is at least as high in physicians as in the general population. Alcohol abuse or dependence in physicians is more common than in the general public and is associated with recent major medical errors (1).

Many impaired physicians can be treated effectively in programs whose approach is confidential rehabilitation rather than punishment. Physicians might also be incompetent because of inadequate knowledge and skills or careless behavior—for example, failing to round on patients.

REASONS FOR INTERVENING WITH IMPAIRED COLLEAGUES

Physicians have an ethical obligation to be competent, based on the ethical guidelines of refraining from causing harm and acting in their patients' best interests. There are also compelling ethical

TABLE 35-1. Reasons for Intervening with Impaired Colleagues
To prevent harm to patients
To carry out professional self-regulation
To help the impaired colleague

reasons for physicians to intervene with seriously impaired colleagues, even though the patients who might be harmed are not their own (Table 35-1).

Prevent Harm to Patients

People have a duty to prevent serious harm to others when it can be done at minimal risk or inconvenience to themselves (2). Modern professional codes of ethics also require physicians to protect patients from impaired colleagues (3, 4). An impaired physician's colleagues might be in a unique position to prevent harm to patients because they have both the expertise to evaluate the quality of care and also the opportunity to do so.

In other occupations, workers whose impairment might endanger the public are aggressively identified. For example, airline pilots and train engineers are required to submit to drug testing before hiring, after accidents, and on a random basis (5). A commercial pilot who is suspected of drinking while on duty may be removed from the cockpit. Critics charge that in comparison, the treatment of impaired physicians is too lax.

Carry Out Professional Self-Regulation

Society grants the medical profession considerable autonomy to regulate itself through selecting applicants for medical school and residency, defining standards of practice, certifying physicians, and disciplining members. The rationale for such professional autonomy is that laypeople do not have the expertise to determine whether physicians are impaired or incompetent. In return, society expects the profession to screen out practitioners who might endanger patients. If people believe that physicians are covering up for impaired or incompetent colleagues, they will lose trust in the medical profession and society might regulate physicians more directly.

Help the Impaired Colleague

Impaired physicians might harm themselves and their families, as well as their patients, through automobile accidents, violent episodes, or lapses in judgment. Furthermore, impaired physicians might destroy their livelihood and their families' economic security. Intervening with impaired colleagues might avert such destructive outcomes.

REASONS NOT TO INTERVENE WITH IMPAIRED COLLEAGUES

State licensing boards provide strong evidence that physicians are reluctant to intervene with impaired colleagues. Compared with the estimated prevalence of impairment, state boards receive few reports about impaired physicians. There might be several reasons for such reluctance.

Uncertainty Whether Patients Are at Serious Risk

Physicians might be uncertain whether colleagues suspected of impairment are actually placing patients at risk, as in Case 35.1. Dr. New does not know the complete story. Perhaps the patient needed a high dose because he had uncontrolled atrial fibrillation or intestinal malabsorption.

Reluctance to Criticize Colleagues

Physicians rely on their colleagues' skills, knowledge, and judgment. Thus, doctors might hesitate to admit that a colleague is impaired because it calls such trust into question. Physicians are understandably reluctant to criticize someone who is respected. Dr. New may also feel a debt of gratitude to Dr. Elder if he has helped her establish her practice and referred patients to her. Physicians might also hesitate to probe matters that are often considered private, such as alcohol consumption. Dr. New, for example, might be reluctant to act on the basis of a personal telephone conversation that she accidentally overheard. Furthermore, doctors are understandably reluctant to undermine a colleague's reputation and livelihood. Subconsciously, physicians might identify with impaired colleagues. If they question a colleague's competence, might other physicians in turn criticize them harshly after a minor error?

Retaliation Against Whistle-Blowers

Whistle-blowers often face personal retaliation. If Dr. New confronts Dr. Elder, then he might get angry or tell her to mind her own business. If she tells other people, colleagues might label her a snitch or a tattletale. Dr. Elder might accuse her of trying to ruin his reputation or trying to build up her own practice. He might even retaliate by criticizing her work and discouraging other physicians from referring patients to her. Dr. Elder could potentially even sue her for defamation of character or lost income. Even the threat of a lawsuit might deter Dr. New from pursuing the matter. Dr. New's natural concern about her own career might conflict with her desire to prevent harm to vulnerable patients.

LEGAL ISSUES REGARDING IMPAIRED COLLEAGUES

Reporting Laws

Many states have adopted laws concerning reporting of impaired or incompetent colleagues. The specific provisions of reporting laws vary from state to state. In Massachusetts, physicians must report to the state licensing board colleagues whom they suspect are practicing medicine while impaired. Other states permit such reporting but do not require it. Most states grant legal immunity from civil suits to physicians who report colleagues in good faith.

The Health Care Quality Improvement Act

In 1986, Congress passed legislation regarding reporting of incompetent physicians. This law requires hospitals and state licensing agencies to report to the National Practitioner Data Bank most disciplinary actions related to professional incompetence or misconduct (6). In addition, insurance companies must report malpractice payments above US$10,000. To prevent incompetent or impaired physicians from simply resigning from one hospital staff, relocating, and continuing to practice elsewhere, hospitals are required to obtain information from the National Practitioner Data Bank when physicians apply for hospital privileges and periodically thereafter.

The law also confers legal immunity on persons and hospitals who report impaired colleagues in good faith. Specifically, immunity is given to persons who provide "information to a professional review body regarding the competence or professional conduct of a physician" (7). In addition, peer review bodies and persons who work with or assist them are granted legal immunity. Note, however, that in Case 35.1, these provisions would not protect Dr. New if she dealt with Dr. Elder outside the formal peer-review process.

Physician Health Programs

Most states have set up physician health programs to treat and rehabilitate impaired physicians (8, 9). Often these are run by the state medical society rather than the medical licensing bureau. These programs have a high success rate in returning physicians to practice. The Joint Commission requires all hospitals to have a physician wellness committee that is coordinated with the state physician wellness program. The goal is to rehabilitate impaired physicians in a confidential manner while protecting patients. The physician may have to suspend practice or may be permitted to continue to practice in a monitored situation, depending on the circumstances (9). On the one hand, some physician advocates physician health programs have been criticized for conflicts of interest and lack of due process (8). In many states, state licensing boards suspend the licenses of physicians who voluntarily seek treatment or revoke licenses if physicians do not cooperate with evaluation and treatment (8). These critics charge that such provisions deter physicians from voluntarily seeking help. On the other hand, patient advocates criticize these confidential programs for favoring the interests of physicians rather than the patient safety, asserting that patients should know whether a physician has undergone treatment for impairment so that they can make informed decisions about their choice of physician.

Institutional Responsibilities in Physician Impairment

Hospitals and clinics have responsibilities for staff credentialing and patient safety and should have programs for responding to concerns about impaired physicians. Health care institutions are setting up programs to identify physician impairment before incidents raise concerns about patient safety. As physicians become older, they are at risk for declines in cognition, dexterity, and sensorimotor agility (10), which can impair patient care. Some institutions have implemented mandatory cognitive evaluation and anonymous peer observation of actual patient care at a certain age (11). Other professionals whose work involves the safety of third parties, such as airline pilots, are subject to age-related screening and restrictions on practice.

DEALING WITH IMPAIRED COLLEAGUES

Physicians can deal with impaired colleagues in several ways (Table 35-2).

Protect Patients from Immediate Harm

If Dr. New believes that Dr. Elder's order might seriously harm the patient, then she should take immediate action. She might consider saying, "I'm sorry to intrude, but I thought I heard you say 2.50 mg of digoxin. I'm afraid the nurses might have heard the wrong dose as well." If the matter is not resolved satisfactorily, then Dr. New could call the hospital and ask the nursing supervisor at the hospital to look into the case. Dr. New should also intervene if Dr. Elder is apparently drunk on call, even if she had no direct evidence that he had made a questionable medical decision. If Dr. Elder does not agree to have a colleague take calls for him, then it would be prudent to notify another senior physician or the chief of the department and arrange for someone else to take calls, at least until Dr. Elder regains sobriety.

Determine Whether Further Action Is Needed

After preventing immediate harm to patients, Dr. New needs to assess whether additional action is needed. Gathering more information about the impaired colleague can usually be done discreetly.

Because whistle-blowing is emotionally difficult and personally risky, physicians might take smaller steps to prevent harm to patients. Many physicians would stop referring patients to such a colleague, but would otherwise let the matter drop. Other physicians cover up for impaired colleagues rather than confront them. For example, a physician might review a colleague's work and correct that doctor's errors. Although well-intentioned, such actions are ineffective in the long run. Monitoring a colleague's clinical activities is impractical and also counterproductive because it allows the physician to deny the impairment.

TABLE 35-2. Dealing with Impaired Colleagues
Protect patients from immediate harm
Determine whether further action is needed
Talk with the colleague directly
Report the problem to responsible officials

Talk with the Colleague Directly

A physician will often want to talk with an impaired colleague directly, particularly if the colleague is a friend. Although such conversations are uncomfortable, they can be effective. The matter can be resolved if the impaired colleague agrees to seek help—for example, by enrolling in a rehabilitation program. Alternatively, physicians impaired by physical illness might decide to retire or to restrict the scope of their practice.

Report the Problem to Responsible Officials

Dr. New does not need to solve the problem of the impaired colleague by herself. She needs only to decide whether there is sufficient suspicion of impairment to warrant further investigation. In Case 35.1, Dr. New directly observed potential harm to a patient. She can discharge her ethical obligations by reporting impaired colleagues to officials who can investigate and take appropriate action. Such officials include the chief of service, the chief of staff of the hospital, or, if a trainee is involved, the director of a training program or student clerkships. These persons are responsible for ensuring the quality of patient care and the competence of medical staff. Alternatively, Dr. New might refer her colleague to the hospital's employee assistance programs or to the state medical society's physician health program. In cases of egregious impairment or incompetence, notifying the state licensing board directly might also be advisable.

Physicians often are reluctant to confront impaired colleagues or refer them to appropriate resources. In a recent survey, about one third of physicians reported that they were not prepared to deal with incompetent colleagues [12]. About 17% had direct personal knowledge of such a colleague in the past 3 years; however, only one third of them had reported them to the hospital, clinical, or relevant authority [12]. The most common reasons were that they thought someone else would do so, that nothing would happen after the report, and fear of retribution.

In an earlier survey of physicians, although 96% of house officers agreed that they should report impaired or incompetent colleagues, 45% of respondents who had encountered such physicians had not reported them [13]. The case's specific circumstances influence how physicians prefer to respond to an impaired or incompetent colleague. Most house officers said they were willing to confront a fellow house officer who was impaired by alcohol but preferred to tell the chief resident or the chief of medicine about an impaired attending physician. House officers, however, were less comfortable confronting a fellow house officer who was incompetent rather than impaired and preferred to refer such matters to a more senior physician [13].

SUMMARY

1. There are understandable practical reasons why physicians hesitate to intervene with impaired colleagues.
2. There are cogent ethical reasons for physicians to take action to prevent impaired colleagues from harming patients.
3. Physician wellness programs offer a way to rehabilitate physicians in a confidential manner, while protecting patients from harm.

References

1. Oreskovich MR, Kaups KL, Balch CM, et al. Prevalence of alcohol use disorders among American surgeons. *Arch Surg* 2012;147:168-174.
2. Beauchamp TL, Childress JF. *Principles of Biomedical Ethics*. 7th ed. New York: Oxford University Press; 2012.
3. Taub S, Morin K, Goldrich MS, et al. Physician health and wellness. *Occup Med (Lond)* 2006;56:77-82.
4. Snyder L. American College of Physicians Ethics Manual: sixth edition. *Ann Intern Med* 2012;156:73-104.
5. Pham JC, Pronovost P, Skipper G. Identification of physician impairment. *JAMA* 2013;209:2101-2102.

6. U.S. Department of Health & Human Services. *National Practitioner Data Bank*. Available at: https://www .npdb.hrsa.gov/index.jsp. Accessed November 11, 2018.
7. Health Care Quality Improvement Act. 42 U.S.C.A. §§11101-11151 (1990).
8. Lenzer J. Physician health programs under fire. *BMJ* 2016;353:i3568.
9. Candilis PJ. Physician health programs and the social contract. *AMA J Ethics* 2016;18:77-81.
10. Kaups KL. Competence not age determines ability to practice: ethical considerations about sensorimotor agility, dexterity, and cognitive capacity. *AMA J Ethics* 2016;18:1017-1024.
11. Dellinger EP, Pellegrini CA, Gallagher TH. The aging physician and the medical profession: a review. *JAMA Surg* 2017;152:967-971.
12. DesRoches CM, Rao SR, et al. Physicians' perceptions, preparedness for reporting, and experiences related to impaired and incompetent colleagues. *JAMA* 2010;304:187-193.
13. Reuben DB, Noble S. House officer responses to impaired physicians. *JAMA* 1990;263:958-960.

ANNOTATED BIBLIOGRAPHY

1. Taub S, Morin K, Goldrich MS, et al. Physician health and wellness. *Occup Med (Lond)* 2006;56:77-82. Policy paper by the American Medical Association on the clinical, ethical, and practical issues regarding impaired physicians.
2. Dellinger EP, Pellegrini CA, Gallagher TH. The aging physician and the medical profession: a review. *JAMA Surg* 2017;152:967-971. Thoughtful analysis of growing problem of aging physicians, arguing that physicians' ability to do their clinical responsibilities be evaluated at a certain age.

36

Ethical Dilemmas Students and House Staff Face

INTRODUCTION

Students and residents face particular ethical dilemmas either because they are not able to provide expert care or because they depend on supervising physicians for grades or recommendations. Both trainees and patients benefit when these issues are addressed openly. Ideally, patient welfare should be paramount. In addition to trainees, other health care workers and the institution itself also have responsibilities to address these dilemmas appropriately.

LEARNING ON PATIENTS

Introducing Trainees to Patients

CASE 36.1 Introducing students as physicians

The attending physician introduces a medical student on a third-year clerkship to the patient as "Doctor." When the student expresses concerns outside the patient's room, the attending physician shouts that students have to get over their "hang-ups" about taking responsibility, grow up, and be a good team player. "If you don't want to be doctor, give up your place to someone who does."

The attending physician adds, "Patients who come here know that students will be taking care of them. If they didn't agree, they would go somewhere else."

Several reasons are offered for introducing students as physicians, for example, that patients might not trust trainees or worry needlessly about their care. There are compelling reasons, however, to introduce students truthfully. Patient trust cannot be built on misrepresentation. Patients who are misled about a health care provider's role might feel betrayed if (or more realistically when) they discover the trainee's actual status. As a practical matter, it is likely that patients will learn that the student is not yet a physician. For example, a nurse or consultant might correct the patient's misunderstanding. Informed consent requires physicians to disclose pertinent information to patients (*see* Chapter 3). The claim that patients who seek care at teaching hospitals have given implied consent to be "teaching material" is untenable. The concept of "implied consent" applies only to emergency situations in which delaying treatment would seriously harm a patient who is unable to give consent. State laws and accreditation requirements may also require trainees to disclose their educational status to patients (1).

The medical school and hospital should set clear standards for introduction of trainees and abusive behavior. Attending physicians should introduce themselves and the other members of the team, explaining roles, supervision, and how they contribute to care. Trainees have time to research literature and talk with patients. There is no strong and consistent evidence that the quality of care overall is substantially better or worse in teaching hospitals compared with nonteaching hospitals (2, 3). Most patients agree that trainees enhance the quality of their care and want to contribute to education (4, 5).

To give patients more transparency about their physicians, some hospitals now provide each hospitalized patient a list of all members of the medical team, with a brief explanation of their roles. Some hospitals also give trainees cards with their picture, name, and level of training, similar to cards of baseball players, to help patients identify the many physicians providing them care. In Case 36.1, the student and resident might later talk privately with the patient to clarify the roles of team members and invite questions. Generally patients appreciate such honesty.

Learning Basic Clinical Skills

To learn to take a history, perform a physical examination, draw blood, and start intravenous lines, medical students need to practice on patients. Although patients are not subjected to any serious medical risks, they might be inconvenienced, lose privacy, or experience some discomfort. Out of respect for patients, the attending physician or resident should ask permission first. When asked, almost all patients agree to have students listen to a heart murmur or perform a history and physical examination. But although it is reasonable to ask many patients to spend up to an hour with a student, it is inappropriate to ask them to spend several hours with a student learning to do a history and physical examination, to miss their meals, or to lose sleep.

Learning Intimate Examinations

Although patient consent to participation by trainees in their care is always important, it is particularly important for intimate examinations, such as pelvic, rectal, breast, and testicular examinations (6). Most medical schools have students learn such examinations with people who are paid to do this and are trained to provide feedback to students on their performance (6). This process benefits students by decreasing their anxiety and enhancing their skills. When students carry out intimate exams with real patients, as a matter of respect for patients, they should obtain explicit permission (7). When asked in advance without feeling pressured, the great majority of patients allow such examinations (6).

Pelvic examinations done under anesthesia offer opportunities for students to master a difficult skill. Because a woman's muscles are relaxed under anesthesia, a more thorough examination is possible. Senior physicians sometimes ask students to perform pelvic examinations on an anesthetized patient in the operating room without her consent. Consent for surgery, however, does not include consent for examination by students so that explicit consent for student examinations is required. In several states, laws prohibit trainees from performing a pelvic examination on an anesthetized or unconscious patient without informed consent, unless the examination is within the scope of their care for the patient (7).

Learning Invasive Procedures

CASE 36.2	Performing an invasive procedure

Obviously tired after a 9-hour wait in the emergency room, a woman with an asthma exacerbation is finally admitted to her hospital room. "Oh no, not another needlestick!" she groans, as a medical student approaches to draw arterial blood gases. The medical student gulps because his previous few attempts have been unsuccessful despite multiple punctures.

Every clinician has attempted a procedure knowing that someone else could do it more skillfully. The trainee's self-interest in learning and long-term goal of benefiting future patients might conflict with the short-term goal of providing the best care to current patients. Learning invasive procedures might present inconvenience, discomfort, or even physical risk to patients.

Trainees might not discuss their participation in invasive procedures with patients, fearing that patients will request more experienced physicians. Such requests are understandable; many physicians might not be willing to have a trainee perform the procedure on themselves or a close relative.

In their training, medical students might worry that they are taking unfair advantage of patients but hesitate to discuss their concerns with supervisors (8). They fear that their reputation or career might suffer or that they will be viewed as reluctant to take responsibility. However, students who do not address their concerns may suffer moral distress.

Both trainees and patients benefit when learning procedural skills is addressed openly. Learning invasive procedures requires an institutional solution, as well as individual student commitments not to perform a procedure that they are not comfortable performing or that the patient has not agreed to let them do. The best practice for learning procedures is graduated training in procedural competency. First, trainees learn and demonstrate proficiency in simulated settings, using simulators or manikins (9). Second, trainees learn to carry out procedures on real patients only under direct supervision and with patient consent. Many teaching hospitals now have "proceduralist" services where residents spend a rotation carrying out procedures with an attending physician, assuring a sufficient number of supervised cases to gain proficiency. The senior physician should take over the procedure, if needed.

When informed and given a choice, most patients allow trainees to do procedures. Almost all patients are willing to have students perform simple procedures, such as suturing or starting an IV (10). For more invasive procedures, 27% of emergency department patients would not allow a resident to perform a lumbar puncture and 52% would not allow a resident to perform intubation (10). The vast majority patients agree to have interns and residents participate in their surgery (11). However, with more information, patients are less willing to agree to involvement of less experienced trainees in surgery (11). Patients may be more willing to accept resident participation when they have an opportunity to voice their concerns and to have explained how residents are prepared, supervised, and contribute overall to their care. Patient requests to have a more experienced physician perform the procedure should be honored, if possible.

Trainees should carry out procedures only under adequate supervision. Without it, the patient might be placed at unnecessary risk and the trainee will not learn from the experience. The hospital has a responsibility to provide such supervision, and the trainee has a corresponding responsibility to ensure it is in place before starting the procedure.

Learning on Dead Patients

Trainees face further dilemmas if they are asked to learn on a newly deceased patient without explicit consent to do so. After a patient dies, the resident might instruct interns and students to practice intubation and insertion of a central venous catheter. "The patient is dead. You can't hurt her, but you might hurt a live patient later if you don't practice now." Such practice increases skill and thereby benefits future patients (12). Some argue that dead bodies cannot be harmed. Invasive procedures, however, might be regarded as disfiguring, offensive, or a violation of the corpse's dignity (12, 13). Dead patients are not "teaching material." They should be treated with respect.

Some physicians suggest that practicing invasive procedures should be permitted unless relatives specifically object. Unless family members, however, are informed of this practice, they might not know to raise objections. A better policy would be to obtain consent from survivors for practicing invasive procedures on newly dead patients (12-16). Empirical studies show that it is feasible to seek and obtain consent from relatives, even in this stressful situation (17). When consent is sought candidly and compassionately, generally family members give permission (14, 18). In a predominantly non-Caucasian sample, however, fewer than one half of respondents would agree to placement of an endotracheal tube and almost one half of respondents would be angry if asked to allow trainees to learn invasive procedures on a newly deceased relative (19). Permission from survivors also helps trainees to resolve their own ambivalence over learning on patients and to appreciate that their training depends on patient altruism.

Taking Too Much Clinical Responsibility

Trainees sometimes assume too much decision-making responsibility without adequate supervision, putting patients at risk (20). For instance, a resident on a busy service might give a subintern a signed but blank physicians' order sheet, saying "You're a good student, and you can page me if you have a real question." It is unrealistic to expect a student to distinguish routine orders from serious management decisions. Errors in judgment or dosage can occur even with "routine" orders. Furthermore, the resident is giving the student a mixed message: "Call me for serious problems, but if you're a good student you won't bother me." Discouraging trainees' questions also reduces opportunities for learning. Students who request adequate supervision implicitly criticize the resident and might experience retaliation in grades and evaluations. They might be labeled as "insecure," "reluctant to assume responsibility," or "not a team player."

Both the teaching institution and the trainee should be accountable. The institution should clarify expectations for supervising trainees, establish a culture of asking for help, and set up procedures to respond when a team has too many patients relative to staffing. Trainees should not take too much responsibility or place patients at inappropriate risk. Trainees should know their own limitations and not exceed them.

ABUSE OF TRAINEES

The attending physician's yelling, insults, and disrespect in Case 36.1 to the student are disrespectful, abusive, and unprofessional (21). Other examples of abusive, disruptive behavior include disrespect, yelling, insults, and refusal to complete tasks (22). Such behavior is not uncommon. In a survey of 2017 graduates of US medical schools, around 39% reported that they had been subjected to unwanted sexual advances, been subjected to remarks or names that were offensive sexually, racially, or ethnically, or received lower evaluations or grades solely because of gender, race, or ethnicity rather than performance (23). The Joint Commission, which accredits health care organizations, considers such behavior a sentinel event alert because it fosters environment in which medical errors become more likely and patient safety threatened (22).

Risks to Whistle-Blowers

Fear of retaliation is a serious and realistic concern for trainees who consider reporting such abusive behavior (23). Reporting carries a risk of retaliation, even if it is done confidentially, because the attending physician in Case 36.2 can infer who made the complaint. The power hierarchy in academia is steep; trainees depend on attending physicians for grades and recommendations. If the clerkship is in the specialty the student plans to enter, a positive recommendation from this attending physician is essential. Even if the student receives a good grade, a comment such as not being a "team player" can be damning. As in other occupations, whistle-blowers might suffer harm even if their accusations prove valid. Individual trainees need to decide how much personal risk as a whistle-blower they are willing to accept relative to the harm they might prevent.

Responding to Abusive Behavior

Case 36.1 illustrates how other persons and the health care institution need to take responsibility for responding to abusive behavior, as well as the person who is subjected to the abuse.

At the time of the incident, people who are the brunt of such behavior or who witness it should not ignore or trivialize it. People can defuse the situation by distracting the perpetrator or directly addressing the problem, while supporting the person subjected to abuse. People are exhorted to be brave, step up, and say something (24). "I feel" statements can be effective, such as "This behavior makes me feel uncomfortable" or "I feel disrespected by such remarks."

Shortly after the incident, after rounds, other people on the team can support the student. This group behavior reinforces the norm that such behavior is unacceptable.

Later, the institution's procedures for reporting such abuse should be activated. Depending on the institution, the clerkship director, dean of education, chief resident, chief of service, or ombudsman should be notified. Health care organizations must have a process to investigate incidents, discipline perpetrators, and prevent future abusive and disruptive behavior.

UNETHICAL PATIENT CARE BY OTHER PHYSICIANS

Trainees might be involved in cases in which senior physicians apparently violate ethical guidelines (25, 26).

CASE 36.3 | **Failure to obtain informed consent for sterilization**

An attending obstetrician performs a tubal ligation on a 32-year-old Latina on Medicaid who has just delivered her sixth child by cesarean section. According to the chart, the patient refused sterilization at her last prenatal visit. The resident who delivered the baby and served as the translator for the patient is outraged. The delivery room nurse confirms that no informed consent was obtained but cautions, "Don't ruin your career over this."

Some disagreements reflect reasonable differences of clinical judgment or misunderstanding by the trainee. In Case 36.3, however, the attending physician is violating the ethical guideline of respecting patient autonomy, as well as legal requirements on informed consent. The resident felt outraged at the event, frustrated at being powerless, guilty that she did not intervene, and ashamed that she had become an accomplice in an unethical deed. She believed that the attending physician's action was sexist and racist. The resident is experiencing moral distress because her desire to do what is morally correct—protect the patient from an unwanted surgery that ends her reproductive capacity—is thwarted by her role as a trainee and her dependence on senior physicians for career advancement.

Trainees might also observe grossly substandard care by senior physicians in other situations, as when they fail to round on patients, write progress notes, or answer pages (25, 26). In cases of clearly inadequate care, the trainee has an ethical obligation to try to protect patients and to not mislead them. In addition, there is an ethical obligation to try to prevent harm to future patients if a pattern of impairment exists (*see* Chapter 35).

Suggestions for Trainees

Involve More Senior Physicians

Trainees often feel that they have to resolve these troubling situations by themselves. However, they should discuss the situation with trusted colleagues and senior physicians. These discussions allow trainees to verify that they have observed unethical misconduct or markedly substandard care, rather than a reasonable difference of judgment. Such reality testing is often crucial for their peace of mind and sense of integrity. In addition, these leaders might provide emotional support, give advice, and intervene constructively. The chief resident, clerkship or residency director, and chief of service have an obligation to address issues of unethical or incompetent behavior. Furthermore, every hospital should have procedures, such as quality-assurance programs or a patient ombudsperson, for investigating such cases.

Decide What to Tell the Patient

In addition to informing appropriate senior physicians, the trainee needs to consider what to tell the patient, if anything. There are strong reasons why patients should have truthful information about events that will affect their future medical care and life plans. The sterilized woman in Case 36.3 cannot make informed decisions about reproduction unless she knows that a tubal ligation was performed.

Trainees do not need to inform the patient personally if they inform some responsible senior physician, such as the chief of service. Trainees, however, do need to answer truthfully if the patient asks the trainee directly what happened.

Protecting Whistle Blowers from Retaliation

Hospitals and clinics have a responsibility to establish a process for health care workers to report cases of unethical care. Because of the power that more senior physicians have over trainees, however, trainees who voice ethical concerns need to be protected from retaliation to the greatest extent possible. However, perpetrators may be able to infer who made the accusation. Whistle blowers should have input into the timing of investigations. If there is no imminent preventable harm to patients, a trainee may want the allegations investigation only after the clerkship or rotation evaluations have been filed.

Protect Your Own Interests

Trainees who fulfill their obligations to patients should minimize risks to themselves (26). Some measures, such as writing an angry note in the chart or directly accusing the attending physician of being unethical, are likely to inflame the situation. Involving more senior physicians can reduce the risk of reprisals. Trainees who are unwilling to be identified as accusers can still discuss episodes confidentially with an ombudsman or chief of staff. In this way, if other people are willing to come forward and be named, there will be corroborating evidence. In addition, trainees should keep records to document how they raised their concerns and how more senior physicians at the institution responded. Moreover, the trainee would be prudent to send copies of this information to trusted others to document what they did at the time.

RELATIONSHIPS WITH COLLEAGUES

CASE 36.4	Lying or equivocating on rounds

A 54-year-old man is admitted with severe pancreatitis. Overnight he required large volumes of fluid to maintain his blood pressure. While the intern is presenting the patient on rounds, the attending physician asks, "So what happened to his calcium?" The intern remembers that calcium is a prognostic factor that should be followed in pancreatitis. Although he checked the patient's laboratory tests, the intern cannot remember whether he specifically reviewed the calcium. He thinks he would have noticed if the calcium had not been normal.

In Case 36.4, the intern feels a tension between making a good impression on the attending physician and acting for the patient's benefit. If the intern says that the calcium was normal when it was not, then the subsequent plan of care might be inappropriate. Hence, the ethical analysis is clear: The intern should say what he did and offer to verify the value at the nearest computer terminal.

The culture of the hospital and team is important. An attending physician who tends to sharply criticize trainees deters them from telling the truth and learning. A teaching style that stresses or shames interns is counterproductive. Slips in which a person forgets something are an unavoidable aspect of human nature (27). Usually they are due to the limits of human cognition, not negligence. Exhorting interns to be more careful or shaming them cannot remedy slips. It is more constructive for the resident and attending physician to reinforce the value of truth-telling by stopping rounds to look up the value, by discussing why the calcium level is important in pancreatitis, and suggesting how to develop a routine or a checklist to ensure that essential labs are carried out.

LIMITS ON DUTY HOURS

Residency accreditation bodies limit house staff duty hours to no more than 80 hours a week to prevent fatigue and burnout and to reduce medical errors. Strictly observing such limits raises ethical dilemmas.

CASE 36.5	House staff duty hours

During an on-call night, an intern has admitted only two patients. After rounds, he has finished his tour-of-duty and is already checking out when he gets paged. A 78-year-old woman that he admitted with pyelonephritis now has a temperature of 39° C, a blood pressure of 100/60, a pulse of 110, and seems confused. The cross-covering resident appears stressed; she exclaims, "Look, I've already had three holdover admissions. How can you dump a patient like this?"

In Case 36.5, the harried cross-cover intern accuses her colleague of "dumping" a patient. This term highlights the way in which stressed physicians might focus their attention on their own needs, rather than the patient's. Ironically, restrictions on house staff work hours were intended to reduce stress on physicians. The intern signing out might feel that he should help his colleague by staying longer. In this case, the intern is not tired. He might be overwhelmed another day and need similar help. Moreover, a patient in early septic shock needs timely attention. It is commendable to help colleagues during unexpected urgent situations.

Many House Staff Exceed Duty Hours

In surgery, 78% of interns voluntarily exceed duty hours (28). The main reason given was to prevent adverse patient outcomes. However, about one quarter said the program or the attending physician expected it, and 7% to 9% said they were coerced to do so (28). In medicine, 87% of interns report staying past shift limits and regard it as professional to do so (29). House staff also report that they continue to work from home, doing such tasks as checking labs, dictating notes, and communicating with other health care workers. In medicine, moreover, house officers say that they routinely make trade-offs between leaving on time and lying about their hours.

Why House Staff Exceed Duty Hours

In some cases, a resident can provide a highly important and irreplaceable benefit to a patient or family by working longer than the scheduled hours. For example, a house officer might be in the middle of a discussion about withdrawing life-sustaining interventions or comforting a family member over a patient's death. It would be desirable for him to finish the conversation before signing out to the covering physician. In such situations, the rapport that the physician has developed with the patient or family is not readily handed off to another doctor. Under such circumstances, strict adherence to the time clock would undermine the ideals of acting for the benefit of patients and with compassion. Such situations, however, should remain exceptions and should not create an expectation that trainees should routinely exceed work hour limits.

Addressing Dilemmas Posed by Duty Hours Restrictions

Both institutional and individual perspectives are needed. Other professions, such as law enforcement and nursing, put much more emphasis on transition of responsibility and handoffs at the beginning and end of shifts (29). In medicine on-call systems should anticipate that on-call interns and residents might be overwhelmed and have back up readily available. In the long run, asking already busy interns on an in-patient rotation to stay additional hours to help others only leads to more stress, fatigue, and greater risk for patients. Many hospitals have a dedicated rapid response team to respond urgently to sepsis and impending hypotension. Under this system neither intern need carry out initial management of sepsis. However, the intern who admitted the patient should communicate crucial information, such as the patient's previous adverse reactions to antibiotics or risk for renal insufficiency.

Misrepresenting duty hours by house staff should not be regarded solely or primarily as a matter of individual ethics. To be sure, as Chapter 6 discusses, avoiding deception and misrepresentation are important ethical guidelines for physicians. However, institutions and the medical profession should not put trainees in the position of having to misrepresent their working hours to fulfill professional obligations to patients. Resources for adequate staffing should be found so that house staff can realistically complete their responsibilities in the allotted time. Most important, there should be no expectation or coercion that house officers routinely should violate professional and institutional rules to provide good patient care.

PROFESSIONALISM

Training programs evaluate medical students and residents for professionalism, which has been defined in terms of core values such as altruism, respect for patients and colleagues, humanism, accountability, and a lifelong commitment to learning and high-quality care (30, 31). These professional values are similar to what philosophers term virtues: characteristics and attitudes that are essential to being a good physician. Professional values are both aspirations and expectations for behavior. They often are transmitted through a hidden curriculum, using stories and cases rather than formal teaching and by residents rather than faculty members. Evaluations regarding professionalism are challenging because expectations may not be explicit or specific and because different observers may reach different subjective judgments. Moreover, as discussed in Chapter 1, there is no single definition of professionalism or its essential components that is universally accepted (30).

Training in Professionalism

Professionalism training and evaluation focuses on observable behaviors in specific scenarios (30, 32). Teaching on professionalism can bridge the gap between general professional values and specific actions that can be learned and practiced. Teaching can discuss the advantages and disadvantages of various options for action in specific situations, including suggesting to whom trainees can turn for help (30). This focus on specific clinical scenarios, actions, and decisions offers practical suggestions to trainees.

Greater emphasis on professionalism with trainees might reduce future physician misconduct. Discipline by a medical board was strongly associated with previous unprofessional behavior in the medical school (33). The strongest predictor was irresponsibility, such as unreliable attendance at clinic and not following up on patient care activities. Another factor was diminished capacity for self-improvement, including failure to accept criticism, argumentativeness, and poor attitude. The rationale for addressing such problematic behaviors during training is to change patterns of behavior that might harm patients.

Evaluations of Professionalism

Evaluations of trainees for professionalism can be problematic. Different raters can give inconsistent evaluations (34), which may overestimate the impact of the trainee's characteristics and underestimate how the situation shapes behavior (35). Furthermore, focusing on trainee's behaviors overlooks the reasoning behind the behavior (35). Finally, the expectation that trainees will speak up when lapses of professionalism occur fails to acknowledge that this is "onerously difficult," particularly in institutional environments that do not support speaking up (36). Also, trainees might complain that professional evaluations may inappropriately reward deference to senior physicians and the academic hierarchy (26). Students allege that sometimes they are termed unprofessional when they are pointing out unprofessional behavior by senior physicians. For these reasons, evaluations of professionalism might be criticized as inconsistent, arbitrary, and therefore unfair.

Differences Between Clinical Ethics and Professionalism

Although professionalism and clinical ethics overlap, there are several important differences. First, clinical ethics focuses on dilemmas in which important values are in conflict and the physician may therefore be uncertain over the appropriate course of action. In contrast, the base cases in professionalism are clear-cut shortcomings in behavior, such as disrespect to patients and colleagues. Clinical ethics also addresses situations where health care workers disagree with each other for good reasons or disagree with the patient or family. For example, in care near the end of life, well-intentioned people may disagree over what the patient would have wanted in the clinical situation at hand or what is best for a patient who can no longer make decisions for him- or herself (*see* Chapters 11 to 14).

The cases in this chapter could be framed as violations of professionalism. There is little question that abusing students, subjecting a patient to distress to learn a procedure, sterilizing a woman without her consent, and lying to an attending physician about a patient's laboratory results are ethically wrong. The challenge is to determine how to respond in the situation that does not cause serious damage to the trainee's legitimate concerns about his or her education and career.

Second, clinical ethics focuses on reasons as well as actions, which are the focus of professionalism. Ethics discusses in detail the reasons physicians should consider and processes they should use when deciding which behavior is the most appropriate in a clinical situation. Professional values are usually expressed in general terms and may not provide specific, practical guidance. It often is not clear how they should apply in a specific case.

Clinical ethics analyzes whether the reasons offered for a decision or action are convincing or not. Such analysis helps the physician clarify his or her position. Furthermore, it offers suggestions for discussing the case with other health care workers and with the patient and family. Indeed, often through such discussions, it becomes clear what the best plan for care is. It is helpful to be able to anticipate the concerns that other persons might have about the options, to understand why certain reasons are generally considered unconvincing, and to consider which communication approaches might be helpful to achieve a mutually acceptable decision and course of action.

In addition to understanding how to resolve dilemmas in the case at hand, clinical ethics helps the physician understand how to address similar cases in the future. How might the decision change if the clinical situation were changed? What characteristics of a new situation would justify a different course of action?

Examining the reasons for a decision or action has pitfalls. Reasons given after an action may be constructed to justify what has already been done (37). This book addresses reasons offered before an action is carried out. At that time, reasons can be explained to others and subjected to scrutiny, leaving open the possibility that people can change their minds about the action.

A scholar of professionalism has called for greater attention to intention and motive in professionalism activities (35). Intentions can be important in ethics (*see* the discussion of deception and misrepresentation in Chapter 6). However, intentions are complicated because they may be multiple or mixed and must be inferred from actions as well as words (*see* the discussion of double effect in Chapter 15). In a case where the physician says he or she is carrying out palliative sedation, his or her statement that he or she was intending to relieve pain, not end the patient's life, cannot be accepted without also examining whether his or her actions are consistent with that intention; that is, was the starting dose reasonable and were increases in doses carried out in response to a determination that the patient was still suffering (*see* Chapter 15). Motive is ulterior to intention; it is the reason that the person carried out the intended action. Motive is even harder to infer than intention. In the case of palliative sedation, the physician will generally say that his or her motive is to alleviate suffering but not to end the patient's life. But another motive may be that he or she did not want to have to return to the bedside regularly to evaluate whether the patient still has unrelieved distress; in turn the motive for this reluctance to monitor the patient closely may be a desire to leave the hospital to attend a wedding or a sporting event. People often judge the same action differently depending on the motive ascribed to the person carrying out the action.

SUMMARY

1. Trainees' interests in learning clinical medicine and invasive procedures might conflict with current patients' interests. The ethical guideline of preventing harm to patients might conflict with trainees' career advancement and need to learn.

2. The ethical ideal is for all trainees to act in patients' best interests, even at some personal risk or disadvantage.
3. Both the training institution and the trainee have responsibilities to address ethical dilemmas facing trainees.

References

1. Marracino RK, Orr RD. Entitling the student doctor: defining the student's role in patient care. *J Gen Intern Med* 1998;13:266-270.
2. Au AG, Padwal RS, Majumdar SR, McAlister FA. Patient outcomes in teaching versus nonteaching general internal medicine services: a systematic review and meta-analysis. *Acad Med* 2014;89:517-23.
3. Papanikolaou PN, Christidi GD, Ioannidis JP. Patient outcomes with teaching versus nonteaching healthcare: a systematic review. *PLoS Med* 2006;3:e341.
4. Kim N, Lo B, Gates EA. Disclosing the role of residents and medical students in hysterectomy: what do patients want? *Acad Med* 1998;73:339-341.
5. Magrane D, Jannon J, Miller CT. Obstetric patients who select and those who refuse medical students' participation in their care. *Acad Med* 1994;69:1004-1006.
6. Wolfberg AJ. The patient as ally—learning the pelvic examination. *N Engl J Med* 2007;356:889-890.
7. Barnes SS. Practicing pelvic examinations by medical students on women under anesthesia: why not ask first? *Obstet Gynecol* 2012;120:941-943.
8. Christakis DA, Feudtner C. Ethics in a short white coat: the ethical dilemmas that medical students confront. *Acad Med* 1993;68:249-254.
9. Sacks CA, Alba GA, Miloslavsky EM. The evolution of procedural competency in internal medicine training. *JAMA Intern Med* 2017;177:1713-1714.
10. Santen SA, Hemphill RR, Spanier CM, et al. "Sorry, it's my first time!" Will patients consent to medical students learning procedures? *Med Educ* 2005;39:365-369.
11. Porta CR, Sebesta JA, Brown TA, et al. Training surgeons and the informed consent process: routine disclosure of trainee participation and its effect on patient willingness and consent rates. *Arch Surg* 2011;147:57-62.
12. Jones JW, McCullough LB. Ethics of re-hearsing procedures on a corpse. *J Vasc Surg* 2011;54:879-880.
13. Berger JT, Rosner F, Cassell EJ. Ethics of practicing medical procedures on newly dead and nearly dead patients. *J Gen Intern Med* 2002;17:774-778.
14. Schmidt TA, Abbott JT, Geiderman JM, et al. Ethics seminars: the ethical debate on practicing procedures on the newly dead. *Acad Emerg Med* 2004;11:962-966.
15. Council on Ethical and Judicial Affairs of the American Medical Association. Performing procedures on the newly deceased. *Acad Med* 2002;77:1212-1216.
16. Goldblatt AD. Don't ask, don't tell: practicing minimally invasive resuscitation techniques on the newly dead. *Ann Emerg Med* 1995;25:86-90.
17. Makowski AL. The ethics of using the recently deceased to instruct residents in cricothyrotomy. *Ann Emerg Med* 2015;66:403-408.
18. McNamara RM, Monti S, Kelly JJ. Requesting consent for an invasive procedure in newly deceased adults. *JAMA* 1995;273:310-312.
19. Morag RM, DeSouza S, Steen PA, et al. Performing procedures on the newly deceased for teaching purposes: what if we were to ask? *Arch Intern Med* 2005;165:92-96.
20. Rosenbaum JR, Bradley EH, Holmboe ES, et al. Sources of ethical conflict in medical housestaff training: a qualitative study. *Am J Med* 2004;116:402-407.
21. Lucey C, Levinson W, Ginsburg S. Medical student mistreatment. *Jama* 2016;316:2263-2264.
22. Van Norman GA. Abusive and disruptive behavior in the surgical team. *AMA J Ethics* 2015;17:215-220.
23. American Association of Medial Colleges. *Medical School Graduation Questionnaire.* 2017. Available at: https://www.aamc.org/download/481784/data/2017gqallschoolssummaryreport.pdf. Accessed June 14, 2018.
24. Freischlag JA, Faria P. It is time for women (and men) to be brave: a consequence of the #metoo movement. *JAMA* 2018.
25. Caldicott CV, Faber-Langendoen K. Deception, discrimination, and fear of reprisal: lessons in ethics from third-year medical students. *Acad Med* 2005;80:866-873.
26. Brainard AH, Brislen HC. Viewpoint: Learning professionalism: a view from the trenches. *Acad Med* 2007;82:1010-1014.

27. Kahneman D. *Thinking, Fast and Slow*. New York: Farrar, Straus and Giroux; 2011.

28. Bilimoria KY, Quinn CM, Dahlke AR, et al. Use and underlying reasons for duty hour flexibility in the flexibility in duty hour requirements for surgical trainees (FIRST) trial. *J Am Coll Surg* 2017;224:118-125.

29. Arora VM, Farnan JM, Humphrey HJ. Professionalism in the era of duty hours: time for a shift change? *JAMA* 2012;308:2195-2196.

30. Livingston EH, Ginsburg S, Levinson W. Introducing JAMA Professionalism. *JAMA* 2016;316:720-721.

31. Medical professionalism in the new millennium: a physician charter. *Ann Intern Med* 2002;136:243-246.

32. Levinson W, Ginsburg S, Hafferty FW, et al. A practical approach to "professionalism." In: Levinson W, Ginsburg S, Hafferty FW, et al, eds. *Understanding Medical Professionalism*. Columbus, OH: McGraw-Hill Education; 2014.

33. Papadakis MA, Teherani A, Banach MA, et al. Disciplinary action by medical boards and prior behavior in medical school. *N Engl J Med* 2005;353:2673-2682.

34. Ginsburg S, Regehr G, Lingard L. Basing the evaluation of professionalism on observable behaviors: a cautionary tale. *Acad Med* 2004;79:S1-S4.

35. Ginsburg S. Duty hours as viewed through a professionalism lens. *BMC Med Educ* 2014;14:S15.

36. Wong BM, Ginsburg S. Speaking up against unsafe unprofessional behaviours: the difficulty in knowing when and how. *BMJ Qual Saf* 2017;26:859-862.

37. Haidt J. *The Righteous Mind: Why Good People Are Divided by Politics and Religion*. Vintage Books; 2013.

ANNOTATED BIBLIOGRAPHY

1. Barnes SS. Practicing pelvic examinations by medical students on women under anesthesia: why not ask first? *Obstet Gynecol* 2012;120:941-943.
   Thoughtful discussion of ethical issues in learning intimate examinations, emphasizing the need for patient consent.

2. Jones JW, McCullough LB. Ethics of re-hearsing procedures on a corpse. *J Vasc Surg* 2011;54:879-880.
   Analysis of the ethical issues regarding learning procedures on the newly dead. Recommends that informed consent from next of kin be obtained.

3. Porta CR, Sebesta JA, Brown TA, et al. Training surgeons and the informed consent process: routine disclosure of trainee participation and its effect on patient willingness and consent rates. *Arch Surg* 2011: 2011;147:57-62.
   Patients want to be informed how residents are involved in surgery, but such disclosure may make them less willing to have residents participate.

4. Lucey C, Levinson W, Ginsburg S. Medical student mistreatment. *JAMA* 2016;316:2263-2264.
   Suggests how students and residents should respond to mistreatment by attending physicians.

5. Arora VM, Farnan JM, Humphrey HJ. Professionalism in the era of duty hours: time for a shift change? *JAMA* 2012;308:2195-2196.
   Residents who stay after work hour limits face unrealistic faculty expectations about professionalism and training.

6. Levinson W, Ginsburg S, Hafferty FW, et al. Understanding medical professionalism. *Understanding Medical Professionalism*. Columbus, OH: McGraw-Hill Education; 2014.
   Comprehensive textbook for medical students on professionalism.

VI

Ethical Issues in Clinical Specialties

37

Ethical Issues in Pediatrics

INTRODUCTION

Children are immature, cannot make informed decisions, and depend on their parents or guardians emotionally and financially. They must be protected from the consequences of unwise decisions that they or others make. It is tragic if a child dies or suffers serious harm because a simple, effective medical treatment was not provided.

HOW ARE ETHICAL ISSUES IN PEDIATRICS DIFFERENT?

Children Are Not Autonomous

Young children cannot weigh risks and benefits, compare alternatives, or appreciate the long-term consequences of choices and therefore are incapable of making informed decisions. Hence, autonomy is less important in pediatrics than in adult medicine. Children's objections to beneficial medical interventions do not have the same ethical force as adults' informed refusals by competent adults. Because children are immature and vulnerable, they need an adult to make decisions for them and to look after their best interests.

Physicians Should Be Advocates for Children

Doctors have a unique opportunity to identify when a child's health and well-being are seriously jeopardized by their parents' decisions or actions. Physicians therefore have special responsibilities in these situations to prevent children from suffering serious, long-lasting harm.

Respect the Child's Potential to Become Autonomous

Children's potential to become autonomous adults deserves respect. Parents mold children, and parental values deserve great deference. However, when children reach maturity they might choose different values from their parents'. Physicians need to help ensure that parental decisions do not close off a child's open future as a unique person. As children grow, they become capable of making informed decisions, and their involvement in care should increase. Physicians should provide children with information about their conditions and opportunities to participate in decisions about their care, in developmentally appropriate ways (1).

WHO SHOULD DECIDE FOR CHILDREN?

The Presumption of Parental Decision-Making

Parents are presumed to be the appropriate decision makers for their children (1). Generally, love motivates them to do what is best for their children. In addition, parents have long-term relationships with and obligations to their children. Furthermore, children mature and develop in the context of a family. In most cases, parents concur with physicians' recommendations—for example, agreeing to antibiotics for strep throat, bronchodilators for asthma, and surgery for appendicitis.

American culture prizes parental responsibility, family integrity, and strong parent–child relationships. Parents or guardians have considerable latitude, but not unlimited discretion, in raising children according to their values. Within limits set by society, parents may inculcate their values in children and make choices for rearing their children. For example, children must attend school, but parents may choose the type of school.

Physicians speak of *parental permission* rather than consent to distinguish what people may decide for themselves from what they may decide for their children. Although informed adults have a right to refuse any medical intervention, parents do not have absolute power to refuse care for their children (1). As noted, parental permission should be supplemented with the child's assent when developmentally appropriate.

Parents commonly ask physicians what they would do if it were their child. Physicians need to clarify what the parents are asking (2). They might be asking what care would optimize their child's outcome, requesting the physician's medical judgment and reasoning, seeking guidance, looking for a human connection, or asking whether they are making the right choice (2, 3). The physician's response needs to be supportive and compassionate. If the parents want to know what the physician personally would do, it is helpful for physicians to describe the process of decision-making they would use, including talking with relatives and friends, as well as what factors they would consider. If parents still want to know what the physician would do, then it is appropriate to offer a recommendation on the basis of the parents' values and goals, keeping in mind that they may differ from the physician's own preferences.

Who Are Parents?

Many children now are raised by single parents or by gay, lesbian, or transgender parents. Gamete donors, custody arrangements after divorce, and remarriage also lead to families that differ from historical nuclear families. Some health care workers may have personal objections to these new types of families or believe that only traditional families can provide nurturing parenting. Health care professionals should distinguish their personal preference or religious beliefs from conclusions based on trustworthy empirical evidence and focus on the individual child in specific family context rather than broad generalization. Moreover, professionals should respect the values of caring parents.

Exceptions to Parental Decision-Making

Some parents are estranged from their children or unwilling to be involved in their care. Other parents lack the capacity to make informed decisions, for example, because of substance abuse or developmental disability. Still other parents severely harm their child through neglect, abuse, or incest. Physicians have a special responsibility to identify and try to prevent such grave harm to children.

Strictly speaking, parents should make decisions for children unless a court has appointed someone else as guardian. Informal arrangements, however, are often made for another relative, such as an aunt, uncle, or grandparent, to make decisions when parents are absent, incapable of making decisions, for fail to provide a minimally acceptable level of care.

Emergencies

In an emergency, when a parent or guardian is not available and a delay in treatment would jeopardize the child's life or health, the physician should act in the child's best interests and immediately provide appropriate treatment without waiting for parental permission (4).

Adolescent Patients

As children mature, they develop the capacity to make informed decisions about their health care. Most states allow 18-year-olds to give informed consent or refusal to medical care without parental involvement. Other state laws allow younger minors make their own decisions about health care because of their status or the condition for which treatment is sought (5). State laws regarding the medical care of adolescents balance several countervailing policy goals: fostering access to treatment for important public health problems, respecting adolescents who are functionally adults, and encouraging parental involvement in their children's care. Because statutes vary according to state and medical condition, physicians need to know the laws in their jurisdiction.

Status of the Minor

Mature minors are capable of giving informed consent. Ethically, mature minors should be allowed to consent to or refuse medical treatment. Generally, adolescents above 14 or 15 years of age have such decision-making capacity, but younger children commonly have difficulty entertaining alternatives, appreciating the consequences of decisions, and appraising their future realistically. In most states, a court must declare an adolescent a matured minor.

Emancipated minors are recognized as *de facto* adults because of marriage, service in the armed forces, or living apart from parents and managing their own finances. Many states require a judicial hearing and declaration of emancipation by the courts (6).

Treatment of Specified Conditions

Most states allow minors to obtain treatment without parental permission for sensitive conditions, such as sexually transmitted diseases (STDs), contraception, pregnancy, sexual assault, substance abuse, and psychiatric illness (6). The rationale is not that adolescents who seek treatment for such conditions are making informed decisions—indeed, these conditions might impair judgment or result from unwise choices. Instead, the justification is that requiring parental permission would deter many adolescents from obtaining effective treatment for important, treatable public health problems.

Parental Involvement in Care of Adolescents

Even when adolescents are allowed to consent to treatment for sensitive conditions, parents' involvement in their subsequent care will generally be beneficial. State laws on informing parents of the adolescent's care vary according to the condition and by state (6). For some sensitive conditions, physicians are required to notify parents or are permitted (but not required) to do so. In other conditions, physicians are prohibited from informing parents without the minor's consent. In still other conditions, doctors may use their judgment about disclosing to parents.

Generally, physicians should encourage adolescents to discuss medical decisions with their parents, who usually provide useful support and advice (7). Often it is impossible to keep the parents from learning about the child's condition because of the condition's nature, the practicalities of obtaining treatment, or the need to pay for care. Doctors can offer to help adolescents disclose information to their parents. In some situations, disclosure might be counterproductive or dangerous, as in cases of domestic violence. In such situations, it would be desirable for the adolescent to confide in a trusted adult relative.

Parental Requests for Treatment

Parents might request that the physician test an adolescent for illicit drug use or pregnancy without telling the child (8). Although parents are naturally concerned, surreptitious testing is unacceptable because it violates the adolescent's emerging autonomy, creates mistrust and suspicion in the family, and undermines the physician–child relationship.

WHAT STANDARDS TO USE IN DECIDING FOR CHILDREN?

Because children cannot make informed decisions, beneficence—acting in the child's best interest—is the primary ethical guideline in pediatrics.

The Child's Best Interests

Generally parents have the authority to decide what they consider best for their children. The concept of "best interests," however, emphasizes that children are persons separate from their parents, with their own interests and rights. Generally parents' decisions and ongoing involvement in a child's care promote the child's best interests, so there is a strong presumption against intervening in a parent's decisions. In some cases, however, parental decisions may forego substantial clinical benefits or place the child at serious risk. In such cases, another adult, such as the physician, needs to advocate on behalf of the child. Assessments of a child's best interests, however, may be contested, with reasonable people disagreeing over which outcomes are desirable, what risks are acceptable, and how to weigh the benefits and burdens of interventions.

A child's best interests include both the duration and quality of life. Although quality-of-life judgments seem unavoidable, they might also be ethically problematic. It is difficult to predict a child's future quality of life. Healthy people tend to underestimate the quality of life of persons with chronic illness. Although some people believe that Down syndrome is a fate worse than death, many children with this condition experience happiness and are prized by their parents. Chapter 4 discusses best interests in detail.

The Child's Preferences

To the extent that children have or are developing the capacity to make informed decisions about their medical care, their choices should be respected. Chapter 10 discusses how to determine whether a patient has the capacity to make medical decisions.

Even when children are not capable of giving informed consent, their *assent* to interventions is still ethically important if it is developmentally appropriate. It is disturbing to force interventions on a child who cannot understand what will be done and is actively resisting it. A child's objections to care authorized by the parents, however, are not necessarily decisive. For instance, a toddler who objects to shots authorized by the parents should still receive childhood immunizations. Forced therapy, however, becomes problematic if children are older, the effectiveness of the intervention is uncertain, or the side effects are more probable, more serious, or longer lasting. The physician should listen to and respond in an age-appropriate manner to the child's reasons for dissenting from treatment. If interventions are carried out despite the child's objections, it is appropriate for the doctor to apologize to the child.

Parents' and Other Family Members' Interests

Although the child's best interests are of primary concern, parents and other family members have interests that should also be taken into account (9). Promoting some of the child's interests might set back interests of other family members or the family as a unit (9). Moreover, living in a flourishing family is desirable for the child. Parents cannot be expected to devote all their energy and resources to one child, no matter how the interest of other family members or the family as a whole are adversely impacted. For example, parents might choose not to buy a house in the best school district, but instead to live closer to their jobs or to save for their retirement. However, parents are expected to make some sacrifices for the sake of their children, and most do so gladly.

PHYSICIAN–CHILD–PARENT RELATIONSHIP

Disclosing of information to children, protecting confidentiality, and truth-telling show respect for children, lead to beneficial consequences, and foster trust in the medical profession.

Disclosure of Information to Children

Physicians should provide children pertinent information about their care in terms they can understand. Children who cannot understand medical details might still want to know what will be done to them. Doctors should also obtain the child's assent if this is developmentally appropriate.

Some parents do not want their children to know about serious diagnoses, such as advanced cancer or HIV infection. Physicians should elicit the parents' and child's concerns and fears. Most children and adolescents with cancer already have some understanding of what is happening and have distressing symptoms (10). Parents might believe that the child will not be able to handle bad news. Physicians can explain how talking honestly about prognosis can help both them and the child cope better. One study of children who died of cancer found that no parent regretted talking with their child about death, but about one quarter of parents who did not later regretted it (11).

Physicians can repeat conversations about prognosis over time by asking parents what their hopes and fears are, as well as hopes and fears of the child and what he or she knows about the disease (10).

Physicians should give forthright but compassionate answers when children ask directly about their diagnosis. Deceiving the child would compromise the physician's integrity and patients' trust in the medical system.

Confidentiality

Exceptions to Confidentiality

Although confidentiality is a fundamental aspect of the doctor–patient relationship (*see* Chapter 5), in some situations physicians must override confidentiality to protect vulnerable children from a high likelihood of serious harm. Physicians and other health care workers must report cases of suspected child abuse or neglect to child protective services agencies. To be justified in reporting a case, physicians do not need definitive proof of abuse and neglect, but only sufficient information to warrant a fuller investigation. In evaluating possible cases of child abuse, physicians should treat parents with respect, keeping in mind that most parents are trying their best to deal with a difficult situation. Intervention might enable parents to obtain enough assistance and support to prevent further abuse. In extreme cases, protective service agencies may remove the child from parental custody.

Disclosure to Schools

Physicians might need to disclose health information to schools so that they can respond appropriately to the child's medical needs. Whenever information is disclosed, physicians should disclose only information that is truly needed. For example, a school does not need to know the diagnosis, but only that the child's absence was medically indicated. Doctors might also need to arrange for the child to receive medications at school. It is useful for physicians to discuss how parents, the child, and school personnel might respond to inquiries about the child's health in ways that maintain confidentiality to the greatest extent possible.

Confidentiality with Adolescents

Adolescents commonly wish to keep certain information confidential from their parents—for instance, that they are receiving care for mental health, STDs, pregnancy, or substance abuse (7). Assurances of confidentiality make adolescents more willing to seek needed health care, particularly for such sensitive conditions, and to disclose information candidly to physicians. Because concerns about confidentiality deter adolescents from seeking needed care, physicians should routinely discuss confidentiality with adolescents and offer them an opportunity to talk privately, apart from parents. However, physicians should not provide absolute assurances of confidentiality, but explain that exceptions to confidentiality are made in specific situations (12). Moreover, it cannot be guaranteed that parents will not learn of the adolescent's medical situation, for example, through bills or insurance records.

REFUSAL OF MEDICAL INTERVENTIONS

Disagreements Between Parents and Physicians

Parents sometimes refuse care that physicians believe is in the child's best interests or provide suboptimal care for the child at home. Doctors need to try to persuade parents to accept effective interventions that have few side effects (*see* Chapter 4). In addition, physicians, together with social workers and nurses, can mobilize emotional support and social resources to help the parents provide better care. If disagreements persist, then the physician's response to parents' refusal of treatment will depend on the clinical circumstances, the benefits and burdens of treatment, and, in some situations, the child's wishes.

Interventions of Limited Effectiveness or Great Burdens

Physicians should respect parents' informed refusals of interventions that have limited effectiveness, impose significant side effects, require chronic treatment, and are controversial. Such interventions are clearly not in the child's best interest.

Effective Interventions with Few Side Effects

Parents sometimes refuse treatments that are highly effective in restoring a child with life-threatening illness to health, are short term, and have few side effects. For example, Jehovah's Witnesses commonly refuse blood transfusions for children who suffer major trauma. Christian Scientist parents often refuse antibiotics for life-threatening bacterial infections. Physicians who are unable to persuade parents to accept such interventions in these situations should seek a court order to administer the treatment (13). A court order is important because it signifies that society regards the parent's refusal as unacceptable. As one court declared, although "parents may be free to become martyrs themselves," they are not free to "make martyrs of their children" (14). Courts have also reasoned that saving the child's life in such situations allows him or her to survive to an age where he or she can make autonomous decisions about his or her own religious beliefs. Children who receive court-ordered treatments over parental objections are generally accepted back into the family and community.

Overriding parents through the courts may be unrealistic in chronic conditions. Even if a child with asthma or diabetes is not receiving medications regularly, disrupting the parent–child bond causes emotional distress for the child. Foster placement or institutionalization might be worse for the child than care from well-meaning parents who are trying to cope with difficult circumstances.

For parental refusal of vaccinations, see Chapter 44.

Effective but Burdensome Therapy

Parents sometimes refuse interventions that cure a fatal disease in the vast majority of cases but are highly burdensome, such as bone marrow transplantation in acute lymphocytic leukemia or combination chemotherapy in testicular carcinoma. If parents continue to refuse such therapy after repeated attempts at persuasion, some physicians seek court orders to compel treatment (15). In doing so, physicians need to take into account the need for long-term parental cooperation with the child's care. Physicians should listen to the parents' objections and show respect for their opinions and ongoing responsibility for the child. In situations where treatment is less successful, the physician's obligation to advocate for it is correspondingly weaker.

Adolescents' Refusal of Interventions

In some cases, adolescents themselves refuse effective treatments. The physician's response should depend on the seriousness of the clinical situation, the effectiveness and side effects of treatment, the reasons for refusal, the parents' preferences on treatment, and the burdens of insisting on treatment. It is difficult to force adolescents to take ongoing therapies, such as insulin shots for diabetes or inhalers for asthma. The most constructive approach is to try to understand the reasons for refusal, to address them, and to provide psychosocial support. In several cases, adolescents have run away from home rather than accept potentially curative cancer chemotherapy that has significant side effects (16). Because it is physically difficult, as well as morally troubling, to force such treatment on resisting adolescents, these refusals have been accepted, particularly when the parents have supported the child's refusal.

INTERVENTIONS WITH QUESTIONABLE MEDICAL INDICATIONS

Parents sometimes request medications to modify their child's behavior or enhance their school performance. Stimulant medications improve distractibility, inattention, and impulsivity in children who do not meet criteria for attention-deficit/hyperactivity disorder (ADHD). If such use of stimulant medications is widespread, parents may feel pressured to use them so that their children are not at a disadvantage.

Critics contend that a better alternative to such use of medications is instruction and practice to strengthen the will of a restless and unruly child (17). In their view, proper moral education requires shaping of character. These critics contend that unlike other parental steps to help their children, such as tutoring, medications rupture the bond between effort and accomplishment and undermine the child's responsibility, self-control, and sense of right and wrong.

In rebuttal, other writers point out that these critics create a false dichotomy between medication and effort. In fact, students using stimulant medications, like those drinking coffee, still must study hard to learn. It is also an oversimplification to suggest that poor school performance results primarily from a lack of individual will and effort. In a child with significant behavioral and learning problems who does not meet criteria for ADHD, if behavioral and counseling approaches prove ineffective, it is reasonable for informed parents to carry out a trial of medications.

CARE OF EXTREMELY PREMATURE NEONATES

With technological advances in neonatal intensive care, outcomes for severely preterm infants have improved over time for infants born at 23 weeks of gestation or greater in US research-oriented neonatal centers (18). However, outcomes for infants born after only 22 weeks gestation or less have not improved, prognosis remains poor, and active treatment is not commonly carried out at many institutions. For infants born at 22 weeks gestation who receive active treatment, 23% were alive at 18 to 22 months after birth, 15% without severe impairment. In contrast, most infants born after 26 weeks of gestation do well; 76% survived without severe impairment at 18 to 22 months after birth. Outcomes for infants receiving care outside of such neonatal centers are unlikely to be as favorable. There is a self-fulfilling prophecy regarding poor outcomes (19); babies who do not receive active treatment have worse outcomes.

Current professional standards urge physicians to help parents make individualized decisions regarding the level of care for infants with extreme prematurity and life-threatening or serious congenital abnormalities. The physician's role is to provide balanced, unbiased information, individualized prognostic estimates using all available information, offer ongoing support and realistic hope to parents undergoing a very emotionally difficult experience (20, 21), help parents understand the information presented, identify and clarify their values and preferences, offer recommendations, and respect their informed decisions. Misconceptions about the experience of raising an extremely premature child are ubiquitous (21).

The 1985 federal "Baby Doe Regulations" set limits on decisions to withhold medical treatment from disabled infants less than 1 year old. They are intended to ensure interventions such as surgery for tracheal–esophageal fistula in infants with Down syndrome. Under these regulations, treatment other than "appropriate nutrition, hydration, or medication" need not be provided if (a) the infant is irreversibly comatose, (b) treatment would merely prolong dying, (c) treatment would not be effective in ameliorating or correcting all life-threatening conditions, (d) treatment would be futile in terms of survival, or (e) treatment would be virtually futile and inhumane. Decisions to withhold medically indicated treatment may not be based on "subjective opinions" about the child's future quality of life. Subsequently, the Born-Alive Infants Protection Act of 2002 was intended to reject the idea that a child's care should vary according to "whether that child's mother or others want him or her" (22).

The Baby Doe Regulations have been sharply criticized for excluding parents from decision-making (22, 23). A further criticism is that maximal medical interventions must be provided unless they are futile or the child is irreversibly comatose or dying. In other clinical settings, the mere possibility of survival does not require the physicians and families to employ all available medical technology (24).

SUMMARY

1. Parents are generally given great discretion to make decisions for their children, on the assumption that they will act in the child's best interests. Generally, parents and physicians should make shared decisions about the child's care.
2. A parent may not forego interventions that almost always save the child's life and restore the child to full health and have very few serious medical adverse effects.
3. Parents may refuse interventions that have a very low likelihood of success and great adverse effects.
4. As children gain maturity, they should play an increasing role in decision-making, as appropriate for their developmental stage.

References

1. Committee on Bioethics American Academy of Pediatrics. Informed consent, parental permission, and assent in pediatric practice. *Pediatrics* 1995;95:314-317.
2. Kon AA. Answering the question: "Doctor, if this were your child, what would you do?" *Pediatrics* 2006; 118:393-397.
3. Korones DN. What would you do if it were your kid? *N Engl J Med* 2013;369:1291-1293.
4. Consent for emergency medical services for children and adolescents. *Pediatrics* 2011;128:427-433.
5. English A, Ford CA, Santelli JS. Clinical preventive services for adolescents: position paper of the Society for Adolescent Medicine. *Am J Law Med* 2009;35:351-364.
6. *Consent in adolescent health care.* 2018. Accessed June 1, 2018, from http://www.uptodate.com/contents/consent-in-adolescent-health-care
7. English A, Ford CA. More evidence supports the need to protect confidentiality in adolescent health care. *J Adolesc Health* 2007;40:199-200.
8. Knight JR, Mears CJ. Testing for drugs of abuse in children and adolescents: addendum—testing in schools and at home. *Pediatrics* 2007;119:627-630.
9. Brudney D, Lantos JD. Whose interests count? Pediatrics 2014;134 Suppl 2:S78-80.
10. Rosenberg AR, Wolfe J, Wiener L, et al. Ethics, emotions, and the skills of talking about progressing disease with terminally ill adolescents: a review. *JAMA Pediatrics* 2016;170:1216-1223.
11. Kreicbergs U, Valdimarsdottir U, Onelov E, et al. Talking about death with children who have severe malignant disease. *N Engl J Med* 2004;351:1175-1186.
12. Ford C, English A, Sigman G. Confidential health care for adolescents: position paper for the society for adolescent medicine. *J Adolesc Health* 2004;35:160-167.
13. American Academy of Pediatrics Committee on Bioethics. Conflicts between religious or spiritual beliefs and pediatric care: informed refusal, exemptions, and public funding. *Pediatrics* 2013;132:962-965.
14. Prince v. Massachusetts. 321 U.S. 158 (1944).
15. Hord JD, Rehman W, Hannon P, et al. Do parents have the right to refuse standard treatment for their child with favorable-prognosis cancer? Ethical and legal concerns. *J Clin Oncol* 2006;24:5454-5456.
16. Traugott I, Alpers A. In their own hands: adolescents' refusals of medical treatment. Arch *Pediatr Adolesc Med* 1997;151:922-7.
17. Beyond Therapy: *Biotechnology and the Pursuit of Happiness.* 2003. Accessed September 12, 2012, from http://bioethics.georgetown.edu/pcbe/reports/beyondtherapy/
18. Younge N, Goldstein RF, Bann CM, et al. Survival and neurodevelopmental outcomes among periviable infants. *N Engl J Med* 2017;376:617-628.
19. Marlow N. The elephant in the delivery room. *N Engl J Med* 2015;372:1856-1857.
20. Ecker JL, Kaimal A, Mercer BM, et al. Periviable birth: interim update. *Am J Obstet Gynecol* 2016;215: B2-B12.e1.

21. Brunkhorst J, Weiner J, Lantos J. Infants of borderline viability: the ethics of delivery room care. *Semin Fetal Neonatal Med* 2014;19:290-295.

22. Sayeed SA. The marginally viable newborn: legal challenges, conceptual inadequacies, and reasonableness. *J Law Med Ethics* 2006;34:600-610.

23. Bell EF. Noninitiation or withdrawal of intensive care for high-risk newborns. *Pediatrics* 2007;119:401-403.

24. Kopelman LM. Are the 21-year-old Baby Doe rules misunderstood or mistaken? *Pediatrics* 2005;115:797-802.

ANNOTATED BIBLIOGRAPHY

1. Committee on Bioethics, American Academy of Pediatrics. Informed consent, parental permission, and assent in pediatric practice. *Pediatrics* 1995;95:314-317.
Lucid discussion of distinctions between assent by children, permission from parents for care, and informed consent by adults.

2. Brudney D, Lantos JD. Whose interests count? *Pediatrics* 2014;134:S78-S80.
Thoughtful analysis of the interests of children, parents, other family members, and the family itself.

3. Olson KA, Middleman AB. *Consent in adolescent health care*. 2018. Available at: http://www.uptodate.com/contents/consent-in-adolescent-health-care
Comprehensive and current review of legal and ethical issues regarding confidentiality in caring for adolescents.

4. American Academy of Pediatrics Committee on Bioethics. Conflicts between religious or spiritual beliefs and pediatric care: informed refusal, exemptions, and public funding. *Pediatrics* 2013;132:962-965.
Analysis of physician's ethical obligations when parental refusal of medical care based on religious or spiritual beliefs will lead to preventable death or serious disability.

Ethical Issues in Surgery

INTRODUCTION

Surgery differs from other specialties in clinically significant ways. First, surgeons intentionally cause short-term injury to patients to achieve long-term therapeutic goals. Although all medical interventions involve risk, many surgical adverse effects are certain, rather than possible, and occur before any benefit can be realized. Patients undergo operative risks, experience pain, and emerge with scars. Second, patients turn over control of their bodies to the surgical team in the operating room (1). Third, operations are not standardized in the sense that drug therapies have standard dosages. The surgeon's technical skill, judgment, experience, and confidence are crucial. Individual surgeons vary in their choice of incision, use of electrocautery and stapling, and selection of suture material or implanted devices. This chapter discusses how these distinctive clinical characteristics of surgery have important ethical implications.

HOW ARE ETHICAL ISSUES IN SURGERY DIFFERENT?

Several ethical guidelines are particularly salient in surgery.

1. Acting in the patient's best interests takes on added importance because patients are completely dependent on the surgical team during operations. Neither patients nor their surrogates can look out for their interests during surgery.
2. Informed consent is especially important because surgery is a major bodily invasion. Some operations, such as mastectomy, colostomy, or amputation, dramatically alter the patient's body image, sense of self, and daily functioning. Patients differ in what surgical risks they are willing to accept for what prospect of benefit.
3. Learning procedural skills differs from learning cognitive skills. More senior physicians can supervise decision making by trainees so that the risk of mistakes is greatly reduced. With procedural skills, however, the trainee has manual control of the procedure and can make a mistake before the supervising surgeon can intervene. Furthermore, there is a learning curve for surgical procedures. After surgeons complete residency or fellowship, they continue to learn new techniques, such as robotic procedures.
4. Individual surgeons are held responsible for the outcomes of surgery. Perioperative deaths raise the question of whether the surgeon erred in judgment or technique. Postoperative deaths need to be reported to the coroner. In surgical morbidity and mortality conferences, surgeons must justify why they operated and how the case was managed (2). Increasingly, hospital- and surgeon-specific clinical outcomes are tracked and made available to the public or insurers. Moreover, surgeons usually feel personally responsible for outcomes because of their "hands-on" involvement in care (1).

INFORMED CONSENT IN SURGERY

Patients need information that is pertinent to their decision to have an operation. As part of the informed consent process, surgeons need to discuss information about the operation, the benefits and risks, the likely consequences, and the alternatives. The consent process is crucial for building a trusting relationship and allaying the patient's concerns about surgery.

Disclosure of Alternative Approaches

Evidence-based medicine has demonstrated that for some conditions, several options have similar outcomes. In benign prostatic hypertrophy, transurethral resection of the prostate, medical treatment, and watchful waiting are all acceptable approaches. For localized breast cancer, lumpectomy followed by radiation offers survival rates similar to more extensive surgery, but less disfigurement. A number of states legally require that women with breast cancer be informed of breast-conserving treatments. The importance that the patient places on side effects of different approaches will be decisive. Hence, the surgeon should discuss all standard options with the patient even if the doctor believes that one is superior. However, surgeons do not need to discuss alternative or unconventional therapies whose effectiveness has not been demonstrated or that no respected subset of physicians has adopted.

Concurrent Surgery

In concurrent surgery, after completing critical portions of the operation in one patient, the attending surgeon moves to a second operating room to begin a critical portion of an operation on a second patient. The rationale for concurrent surgery is to allow timely access to specialized or sought-after surgeons who otherwise may have unacceptable waiting times (3). Concurrent surgery must be distinguished from overlapping surgery, where an attending surgeon is responsible for critical portions of operations in two different patients simultaneously. Overlapping surgery is considered unethical, similar to "ghost surgery," because the attending surgeon who obtained consent is not carrying out critical portions of the operation (3). Concurrent surgery raises a number of concerns that need to be addressed (3, 4).

Definition of Critical Parts of the Operation

There is no standard definition of what the critical parts of an operation are. Opening and closing the surgical field are not considered critical, but beyond that the attending surgeon decides what the critical aspects of the operation are. Standardization of what parts of common operations are critical would improve accountability and public acceptance of the practice.

Judgment of the Attending Surgeon

The clinical judgment of the attending surgeon is crucial for minimizing risks of concurrent surgery. The surgeon should identify patients who are not appropriate for concurrent surgery, for example, because the operation is too complex or risky (5). Furthermore, the attending physician needs to be familiar with the skills of the assisting surgeons (often trainees) to be confident that they are capable of carrying out the noncritical portions of the concurrent surgery (3). Moreover, the attending surgeon needs to ensure that there is attending coverage for noncritical portions of the operation if an unexpected complication occurs.

Informed Consent for Concurrent Surgery

Only a small minority of the public is aware of the practice of concurrent surgery, and only a minority support it (6). Almost all people believe that the attending surgeon should inform patients in advance and define what the critical portions of the surgery will be (6). Surveys suggest that patients and families are most uncomfortable with overlap of critical portions of operations (7). Explanations of concurrent surgery should be carried out when the patient first expresses interest in surgery, before they make a decision to have an operation with a particular surgeon (5). Discussions between attending surgeons and patients regarding concurrent surgeries must be explicit, not vague or misleading (3). Explaining the noncritical portions of the operation and the steps taken to minimize the risks of concurrent surgery will bolster patient trust (5).

Oversight of Concurrent Surgery

A few studies of the outcomes of concurrent surgery suggest that it is not associated with increased risk of patient harm, but the generalizability of these findings is unclear (5). To increase patient trust in concurrent surgery, health care institutions and professional organizations should define the critical parts of common operations, document the attending surgeon's presence and absence from the operating room, and have adverse events reported and reviewed (5).

Disclosure of Surgical Innovation

Surgical progress depends on innovations, which usually require stepwise refinements and generally are not evaluated in randomized clinical trials. Minor variations of established procedures, such as changing the incision, are common, low-risk, and can be done at the discretion of the surgeon (1). Some innovations, however, are major differences from accepted practice, pose more than minor risks to patients, and have not previously been described in textbooks and articles (8). Such innovations should be reviewed by peers, and patients should consent to the innovative nature of the procedure (8).

Disclosure of Outcomes

Surgical mortality and complication rates vary across institutions and surgeons. For some operations, low-volume hospitals and surgeons have markedly higher surgical mortality rates, despite overall improvements in outcomes (9). Outcomes reporting for operations raises a number of concerns, including inadequate risk adjustment, random variation in relatively small samples, and the unintended consequence of hospitals avoiding high-risk cases. Dissemination of hospital- or surgeon-specific outcomes can spur quality improvement in poor-performing hospitals, provided that the data are risk-adjusted and reliable (10, 11). For example, hospitals with higher mortality in pancreatectomy have higher blood loss, less invasive monitoring, and less use of epidural anesthesia (12). In New York and other states, public release of outcomes for coronary bypass surgery motivated quality-improvement efforts in institutions with very poor outcomes (13, 14). Some insurers have also used outcomes data to direct patients to centers of excellence and to increase reimbursement for better outcomes or for participation in quality-improvement programs or outcomes registries (14). However, such outcomes data have not led patients to seek care at hospitals with better outcomes. Recently a number of hospital rating systems have become publicly available, but their ratings are discordant, and it is uncertain whether they predict clinical outcomes that matter to patients or will change where patients seek care (15).

Trainee Participation in Surgery

When trainees participate in surgical procedures, there is lower mortality and comparable morbidity (12, 16). Operative time and resource utilization are higher with residents, but rescue is also higher in complex operations.

The vast majority of patients want to be informed of the role of trainees during surgery and agree to have interns and residents participate in their surgery (17). However, with more information, patients were less willing to agree to greater trainee participation or to involvement of less experienced trainees in surgery (17). Thus, patients should be informed of the trainees' role during surgery and how they will be supervised (3). Many surgical residents experience moral distress that patients are not really aware of their roles and not openly informed how teaching hospitals strive for continuous quality improvement and provide structured, competency-based curricula for residents (18).

Disclosure of Experience

Some physicians urge that surgeons should discuss with patients their experience and outcomes when outcomes for the proposed operation vary in statistically and clinically significant ways (19, 20). Such disclosure can be based on both respecting patient autonomy and acting in the patient's best interests. In a recent survey, 63% of patients said that they could not decide whether to have an operation without being told the surgeon's experience and outcomes (21).

Disclosure is also an issue when experienced surgeons learn new techniques, such as laparoscopic or robotic surgery. Initially, complication rates are higher with laparoscopic procedures than with open techniques, and operating times are longer. When surgeons get more experience, complication rates become comparable to those of open procedures. Patients consider it extremely important to know a surgeon's experience with a new technique (3, 21). Surgeons, however, might be concerned that patients who learn that they are inexperienced with a technique will not trust them to do the operation, making it more difficult for them to master new skills.

Changes in the Operation due to Unanticipated Findings

A surgeon might encounter unexpected findings during an operation that require a substantially different procedure than was discussed during the informed consent process. For example, suppose that during a cholecystectomy the surgeon finds a gastric mass that is suspicious for carcinoma. Should the surgeon biopsy the mass, and, if so, should the surgeon resect the tumor if the biopsy shows carcinoma? The surgeon might believe that an opportunity to cure gastric carcinoma might be missed if biopsy and resection are not done. Furthermore, a second operation would subject the patient to additional risk. On the other hand, the patient might be upset to find that the surgeon performed a more extensive operation than discussed, even if the surgeon did so to benefit him.

How can surgeons resolve this dilemma between acting for the patient's good and respecting the patient's autonomy? Some surgeons request blanket consent to change the operation if unexpected findings occur. An alternative is to contact the next of kin in the waiting area or by phone to discuss the proposed change in care. If the family agrees with the surgeon's recommendations, both the patient's best interests and autonomy are served. It would also be acceptable to biopsy the mass if the family cannot be immediately located and to resect the mass only if a family member's consent can be obtained.

In some situations, however, deferring resection of a mass found unexpectedly at surgery might present significant risk to the patient because surgical exposure might be substantially compromised at reoperation or because of serious comorbidities.

Such cases of incidental findings need to be distinguished from cases in which the operation needs to be changed because of an anatomical variation or a major surgical complication. For instance, a surgeon might nick the spleen and a splenectomy might be required to control bleeding. In this instance, the surgeon should proceed with the splenectomy and explain to the patient after the operation that a splenectomy was done because of the intraoperative complication.

MAY A SURGEON DECLINE TO OPERATE?

In some cases, a surgeon might judge that an operation is not indicated because the risks of surgery greatly outweigh the possible benefits (22). What should the surgeon do if the patient or referring physician insists on surgery? Different reasons for not operating need to be distinguished. Some reasons are patient centered. The surgeon might believe that an operation will not benefit the patient. For instance, a patient with chronic abdominal pain might believe that the pain is caused by gallbladder disease and seek a cholecystectomy (22). If there is no objective evidence of gallstones, however, the surgeon might conclude that a cholecystectomy would be futile in a strict sense and decline to operate (see Chapter 9).

In other situations, the surgeon might judge that although the operation is not futile, the risks are prohibitive, as the following case illustrates.

CASE 38.1	Decision to not operate in a very high-risk patient

Mr. G is a 64-year-old man admitted for a myocardial infarction. He continues to have chest pain, ischemic changes on his cardiogram, and congestive heart failure. He is found to have multiple diffuse coronary lesions that cannot be revascularized. He also develops a urinary tract infection from a Foley catheter. Despite antibiotics, Mr. G subsequently develops pyelonephritis, intrarenal abscesses, and septic shock. He becomes confused and unable to participate in decisions. Percutaneous drainage guided by computed tomography is not feasible. The family appreciates that the surgery is very risky, but they believe it offers the patient the only chance of survival. The surgeon, however, believes that Mr. G's coronary disease is so unstable that he is unlikely to survive even a laparoscopic procedure.

Surgeons are traditionally permitted great discretion not to operate when they determine that surgery would not be in the patient's best interests. Surgeons often justify a refusal to operate by the shorthand declaration, "This patient is not a surgical candidate." Such surgical decisions are rarely challenged and discussed, but internists' unilateral decisions to withhold medical interventions are often extensively debated.

Is there an acceptable ethical basis for this distinction between surgeons and internists? Surgeons are held more responsible for the harmful consequences of operations than internists are for the harmful effects of drugs they prescribe. Making a surgical incision causes much more certain and direct harm to the patient than writing a prescription does. Furthermore, because surgery requires manual manipulations, it is undesirable to require surgeons to perform operations they consider inadvisable. An unwilling surgeon might place the patient at additional risk because of lapses of concentration or lack of confidence.

Surgeons need to appreciate that the patient may have a different threshold for risk than they do. Some patients might accept severe short-term harms and unfavorable odds of success, for example, if the patient will very likely die without an operation that has high mortality (23). In this situation, an institutional dispute resolution process could be more desirable than a unilateral decision by a surgeon. At a minimum, another surgeon should be asked if he or she would be willing to operate. Surgeons should decline to operate only if the risks are substantially greater than the likely benefits, as opposed to only slightly increased. Surgeons must guard against misrepresenting information to patients because of their own bias. For example, they should never overstate an operation's risks because they recommend against it. Furthermore, they must be careful to base decisions on medical outcomes, not their personal judgments that the patient's quality of life is unacceptably poor.

Other reasons for not operating might be surgeon centered. In some cases, surgeons question whether the risk of contracting HIV infection or hepatitis C during an operation is acceptable in view of very limited benefits to the patient (*see* Chapter 24). In other cases, a surgeon might be reluctant to take on complex, high-risk cases that might worsen their complication rates or length of hospital stays or make it more difficult to secure contracts from managed care organizations. Yet another factor might be unreimbursed care. Surgeons might believe that they have accepted more than their fair share of charity cases. In these situations, the surgeon's self-interest must be acknowledged as a natural and legitimate concern. However, they should be addressed directly. Ultimately, the ethical ideal is for physicians to make patients' best interests paramount if they can do so without a grave setback to their own self-interest.

REQUESTS TO OPERATE IN WAYS THAT INCREASE RISK

Patients might consent to an operation but refuse specific interventions or techniques. Such restrictions might make their operation riskier and more complicated. These decisions need to be distinguished from patient refusals of the operation itself.

CASE 38.2 **Emergency surgery on a Jehovah's Witness**

Mr. D, a 64-year-old Jehovah's Witness, is admitted after a motor vehicle accident with a ruptured spleen, a hemoglobin of 6%, hypotension, chest pain, and ischemic changes on electrocardiogram. He refuses blood transfusions but agrees to surgery, understanding that he might die without transfusions. The surgeon declares, "I accept his right to refuse transfusions, but he can't make me operate with one hand tied behind my back."

In case 38.2 Mr. D has a clear indication for splenectomy. In his religion, surviving the accident is less important than avoiding the taint of transfusions, which would result in everlasting damnation (*see* Chapter 11). The risk of death, myocardial infarction, and renal failure may be increased in severe anemia.

Some surgeons might be angry because of the need for additional time and effort and the reduced margin of error. Many surgeons intuitively make a distinction between respecting the patient's refusal of transfusions and following the patient's request to have the surgery under restrictive conditions. Philosophers distinguish negative and positive rights. Negative rights are claims to be left alone; they protect patients from unwanted interventions on their bodies. Positive rights require others to act in certain ways. Negative rights are generally considered stronger than positive rights. Thus, patients have a strong right to refuse unwanted interventions, but less authority to specify how surgeons carry out their work.

Faced with requests to carry out operations with specific restrictions, surgeons generally have a legal right to decline to operate and to transfer care to another surgeon. In many cases, a more fruitful approach is to consider how to minimize additional risks due to foregoing transfusions. Severe blood conservation, including blood salvage interventions, administration of acceptable alternative blood fraction, and use of epoetin alpha may reduce operative risk. Jehovah's Witnesses have undergone cardiac surgery with no increase in complications or mortality (24). Moreover, surgeons should keep in mind the ethical ideal of putting the patient's best interests paramount. A skilled and experienced surgical team offers the patient the best chance at a favorable outcome.

In the following case, the patient objects to certain aspects of the proposed operation after the physician brings up the nature of the operation.

CASE 38.3 **Patient refusal of emergency colostomy**

Mr. N, a 74-year-old man, is admitted to the hospital with an acute abdomen. He is found to have free air under the diaphragm. The surgeon believes that the patient has perforated a peptic ulcer or a carcinoma of the colon. The surgeon explains that if the perforation is in the colon, she will perform a colostomy, which might not need to be permanent. Mr. N adamantly refuses a colostomy. "A friend got one and had one complication after another. He was so ashamed of that bag. I'd rather be dead than go through that humiliation." There is no time for the patient to talk to people who have adapted well to a colostomy. Technically, an end-to-end anastomosis is possible, but it has a much higher risk of complications.

A colleague suggests, "In an emergency I never discuss the details of the surgery. All that the patient needs to know is that he needs an operation to save his life and that the risks of surgery are small compared with the alternatives. Too much information can be dangerous because there is no time to correct misunderstandings. I would never do an end-to-end anastomosis. How would you justify it at a morbidity and mortality conference if he got a complication?"

In Case 38.3, the ethical dilemma is that the patient might be making an irreversible decision under time pressure that he would greatly regret later when more fully informed. The surgeon believes that the patient's refusal is based on an unrealistic appraisal of a colostomy. Most patients who are initially dismayed at the prospect of a colectomy later adjust well to living with it (25). In elective situations, most patients can be persuaded to accept a colostomy, but in an emergency there is no time for extended discussions. A surgeon dedicated to acting in the patient's best interests would want to do the less risky operation, knowing that most patients adapt to a colostomy. From this perspective, it would be terrible if the patient refused life-saving surgery because of an outcome that might not happen or might be only temporary. The colleague's concern about the morbidity and mortality conference is not just a desire to avoid personal criticism; the professional standard of care is based on what a reasonable surgeon would do under the circumstances.

In contrast, a surgeon dedicated to patient autonomy will respect the patient's refusal of colostomy even if that decision might not be fully informed. From this viewpoint, even if the operation was skillfully performed and successfully treated the perforation, it would be tragic if the patient had to live with a mutilation of his body to which he did not consent. Although the vast majority of surgical patients hold survival as their highest priority, some give higher priority to quality of life (26). Some patients might even consider a colostomy so unacceptable that they would rather die than have the operation.

The surgeon in Case 38.3 has several options. One option is to refuse to operate unless the patient agrees to a colostomy if needed. This option, however, might leave the patient worse off than having an end-to-end anastomosis. Also, if the on-call surgeon declines to operate, it might be difficult to find a colleague to take over the case without unacceptable delay.

CASE 38.3 | *Continued*

The surgeon should try to persuade the patient to accept the colostomy, even with severe time constraints. The surgeon can ask the patient to talk over the phone with his family, primary care physician, or the chaplain, and the surgeon could explain to them why a colostomy is preferable. In addition, the surgeon might paradoxically persuade the patient by giving him control. "If you decide that you won't accept the colostomy after talking to your family and your primary care doctor, I'll do the surgery in the other, riskier way. I won't force you to have an operation you don't want. But before you decide, I'd like to understand better what about the colostomy troubles you. I'd also like you to understand why I think the colostomy is the best operation for you." The surgeon might acknowledge, "Everyone finds it hard to think about a colostomy" and might say, "I wish I had a way of doing the surgery so you didn't have a colostomy and didn't have an increased risk of complications." If persuasion fails, it is ethically appropriate for the surgeon to plan an end-to-end anastomosis, based on the patient's informed choice.

To reduce the risk of complications, some surgeons might be tempted to misrepresent what they will do in the operating room. For example, they might say they will try to do an end-to-end anastomosis if possible, even though they actually intend to do a colostomy. As Chapter 6 discusses, such misrepresentation is unethical because it undermines patient trust and physician integrity.

SUMMARY

1. The unique clinical circumstances of surgery impose special ethical obligations on surgeons regarding informed consent, decisions not to operate, and patient requests to carry out the operation in certain ways.
2. Concurrent surgery requires particular attention to the informed consent process, professional and institutional responsibilities to define the critical portions of an operation, and the attending surgeon's responsibility to minimize risks.

References

1. Angelos P. Surgical ethics and the future of surgical practice. *Surgery* 2018;163:1-5.
2. Bosk CL. *Forgive and Remember: Managing Medical Failure.* Chicago: University of Chicago Press; 1979.
3. Langerman A. Concurrent Surgery and Informed Consent. *JAMA Surg* 2016;151:601-602.
4. Mello MM, Livingston EH. The Evolving Story of Overlapping Surgery. *JAMA* 2017;315:1563-1564.

5. Mello MM, Livingston EH. Managing the risks of concurrent surgeries. *JAMA* 2016;315:1563-1564.
6. Kent M, Whyte R, Fleishman A, et al. Public perceptions of overlapping surgery. *J Am Coll Surg* 2017;224:771-778.e4.
7. Edgington JP, Petravick ME, Idowu OA, et al. Preferably not my surgery: a survey of patient and family member comfort with concurrent and overlapping surgeries. *J Bone Joint Surg Am* 2017;99:1883-1887.
8. Biffl WL, Spain DA, Reitsma AM, et al. Responsible development and application of surgical innovations: a position statement of the Society of University Surgeons. *J Am Coll Surg* 2008;206:1204-1209.
9. Reames BN, Ghaferi AA, Birkmeyer JD, et al. Hospital volume and operative mortality in the modern era. *Ann Surg* 2014;260:244-251.
10. Chassin MR, Loeb JM, Schmaltz SP, et al. Accountability measures--using measurement to promote quality improvement. *N Engl J Med* 2010;363:683-688.
11. Schwarze ML. The process of informed consent: neither the time nor the place for disclosure of surgeon-specific outcomes. *Ann Surg* 2007;245:514-515.
12. Saliba AN, Taher AT, Tamim H, et al. Impact of resident involvement in surgery (IRIS-NSQIP): looking at the bigger picture based on the american college of surgeons-NSQIP database. *J Am Coll Surg* 2016;222:30-40.
13. Steinbrook R. Public report cards—cardiac surgery and beyond. *N Engl J Med* 2006;355:1847-1849.
14. Birkmeyer NJ, Birkmeyer JD. Strategies for improving surgical quality—should payers reward excellence or effort? *N Engl J Med* 2006;354:864-870.
15. Bilimoria KY, Barnard C. The new CMS hospital quality star ratings: the stars are not aligned. *JAMA* 2016;316:1761-1762.
16. Ferraris VA, Harris JW, Martin JT, et al. Impact of residents on surgical outcomes in high-complexity procedures. *J Am Coll Surg.* 2016;222:545-555.
17. Porta CR, Sebesta JA, Brown TA, et al. Training surgeons and the informed consent process: routine disclosure of trainee participation and its effect on patient willingness and consent rates. *Arch Surg* 2012;147:57-62.
18. McAlister C. Breaking the silence of the switch—increasing transparency about trainee participation in surgery. *N Engl J Med* 2015;372:2477-2479.
19. Krumholz HM. Informed consent to promote patient-centered care. *JAMA* 2010;303:1190-1191.
20. Gates EA. New surgical procedures: can our patients benefit while we learn? *Am J Obstet Gynecol* 1997;176:1293-1298.
21. Lee Char SJ, Hills NK, Lo B, et al. Informed consent for innovative surgery: a survey of patients and surgeons. *Surgery* 2013;153:473-480.
22. Sugarman J, Harland R. Acute yet non-emergent patients. In: McCullough LB, Jones JW, Brody BA, eds. *Surgical Ethics.* New York: Oxford University Press; 1998:116-132.
23. Wicclair MR, White DB. Surgeons, intensivists, and discretion to refuse requested treatments. *Hastings Cent Rep* 2014;44:33-42.
24. Ferraris VA, Davenport DL, Saha SP, et al. Surgical outcomes and transfusion of minimal amounts of blood in the operating room. *Arch Surg* 2012;147:49-55.
25. Halpern J, Arnold RM. Affective forecasting: an unrecognized challenge in making serious health decisions. *J Gen Intern Med* 2008;23:1708-1712.
26. List MA, Stracks J, Colangelo L, et al. How do head and neck cancer patients prioritize treatment outcomes before initiating treatment? *J Clin Oncol* 2000;18:877-884.

ANNOTATED BIBLIOGRAPHY

1. Biffl WL, Spain DA, Reitsma AM, et al. Responsible development and application of surgical innovations: a position statement of the Society of University Surgeons. *J Am Coll Surg* 2008;206:1204-1209.
   Suggests criteria for when surgical innovation should be peer reviewed and require informed consent from the patient.
2. Langerman A. Concurrent surgery and informed consent. *JAMA Surg* 2016;151:601-602.
   Mello MM, Livingston EH. The evolving story of overlapping surgery. *JAMA* 2017;315:1563-1564.
   Thoughtful analyses of ethical issues regarding concurrent surgery.
3. McAlister C. Breaking the silence of the switch—increasing transparency about trainee participation in surgery. *N Engl J Med* 2015;372:2477-2479.
   Argues that teaching hospitals should proudly and transparently discuss the role of surgical residents, together with details about how surgical competency is developed and how teaching institutions are committed to quality improvement.

CHAPTER

Ethical Issues in Obstetrics and Gynecology

INTRODUCTION

Obstetrics poses ethical dilemmas because care for a pregnant woman and her fetus are inextricably linked. Gynecologic care and sexuality and reproduction involves intimate and private topics that are often socially contested.

WHY ARE ETHICAL ISSUES IN OBSTETRICS AND GYNECOLOGY SO DIFFICULT?

People Have Divergent Personal Core Beliefs

Many women want control of their reproductive decisions and have strong preferences in family planning and childbirth. Many believe that society and physicians exercise inappropriate control over women through policies regarding reproductive health care. Some women also believe that pregnancy and childbirth have become overly technologic and medicalized. For example, continuous electronic fetal monitoring for all pregnant women is widely used even though evidence shows that there is no benefit but significant harm, including increased surgical births (1). At the same time, many people reaffirm attitudes toward the role of women, reproduction, and sexuality on the basis of traditional or religious beliefs, and seek public policies that embody those views, even for women who strongly disagree (2). Discussions of reproductive health in the United States, particularly discussions regarding abortion, are polarized and often fail to take into account that the United States is a pluralistic society in which people hold different core values and religious beliefs.

Philosophic Quandaries That Science Cannot Resolve

Decisions about reproduction inevitably raise philosophic or religious questions that science cannot resolve.

- Do women have an ethical right to reproductive liberty that encompasses a right to contraception and abortion?
- When does personhood begin: at conception, viability, birth, or some other time?

Theologians, philosophers, public officials, and the public have debated these conundrums without reaching agreement or common ground. Indeed, polarization has increased, and public policies need to be developed despite deep disagreements in US society.

Intertwined Interests of the Pregnant Woman and Fetus

Everyone hopes that children will be born healthy. It is tragic when a child is born with a serious preventable illness or congenital anomaly. The pregnant woman who decides to carry a fetus to term has a responsibility to take reasonable steps to reduce harm and provide benefit to the child who will be born (3). Physicians have a responsibility to represent the interests of such future children, who cannot represent themselves. Doctors should recommend interventions that will provide important benefits to the fetus without unacceptable risk to the pregnant woman, after taking the time to educate the woman about the risks and benefits of intervention, understand her concerns and objections, and try to negotiate a mutually acceptable plan of care. In this book, the term *children who will be born* always refers to cases in which the pregnant women has decided to carry the fetus to term; it does not imply a belief that the fetus is a person with rights (3).

Fetal movements and heartbeat can be visualized with ultrasound and other imaging techniques. Doctors can diagnose many conditions in utero, such as congenital abnormalities or fetal distress. Furthermore, physicians can treat the fetus through interventions on the mother, such as prenatal vitamins, tocolytic agents in premature labor, corticosteroids in prematurity, and fetal blood transfusion for Rh isoimmunization. In light of this ability to diagnose, prevent, and treat fetal disorders, some people consider the fetus a patient, along with the pregnant woman, once she decides to carry the fetus to term and presents for prenatal care (3). Thinking of the fetus as a patient helps prevent inadvertent injury to the fetus by reminding physicians and pregnant women to consider how care for the woman might affect the fetus. However, the idea that the fetus is a patient is also flawed and incomplete because interventions directed to the fetus are also interventions on the pregnant woman that might cause her unacceptable adverse effects or disrupt other important aspects of her life (4). For example, in premature labor, terbutaline causes tremors and anxiety in the pregnant woman. Long-term bed rest for premature labor might prevent the pregnant woman from caring for her other children or working at a job that supports her family. Most pregnant women accept considerable side effects, inconvenience, and disruption of their life for the sake of the fetus. Pregnant woman need not accept every intervention that might benefit the fetus, however, regardless of the degree of benefit, risks, or impact on her life. The pregnant woman herself is a patient with needs, interests, and rights (4). The requirement of informed consent cannot be abolished just because a woman is pregnant. Responsibilities to a fetus who will become a child have limits; logically they should not exceed responsibilities that parents have to living children (2). Parents are not obligated to provide all potentially beneficial interventions to children after birth or to minimize all harms to them.

INFORMED CONSENT IN OBSTETRICS AND GYNECOLOGY

Several situations in obstetrics and gynecology raise particular ethical issues regarding consent. With increasing attention to patient autonomy in modern medicine, the informed preferences of the pregnant woman must be given appropriate respect.

Information About Family Planning and Abortion

Without adequate information about medical options, patients cannot make informed decisions, and physicians have an obligation to provide information to patients they need for informed consent. Some physicians who have strong personal moral and religious objections to these interventions believe it would violate their conscience to write a prescription for birth control or perform an abortion. Institutions should make reasonable accommodations to conscientious objections, but also provide patients the information they need to make informed decisions (*see* Chapter 24 for more discussion of conscientious objection). If an institution determines that it will not provide certain services or information, such restrictions should be transparent to potential patients when they choose a health insurance plan or seek an appointment for care, so that they can seek alternative arrangements.

Reproductive Health for Adolescents

Girls below 18 years of age, who are often sexually active, might seek care for contraception, sexually transmitted diseases, or pregnancy. Many people believe that allowing minors to obtain such care without parental consent undermines family values or encourages promiscuity and irresponsibility.

Most adolescents, however, present for reproductive care after they have already been sexually active, decided to do so, or become pregnant. In most states, adolescents may legally seek reproductive health care without parental consent. The rationale is that it is preferable for adolescents to have access to such care rather than to forego it because they are reluctant or unable to obtain parental approval (*see* Chapter 37). Usually, it is in the adolescent's best interest to involve their parents in their care, and physicians generally should encourage them to do so. In some cases, however, adolescents might have compelling reasons for not involving parents—for example, in cases of domestic violence or incest.

Elective Cesarean Delivery on Maternal Request

The discussion on this issue has shifted from the pregnant woman's autonomy to schedule the date of delivery to the physician's responsibility to inform woman about the risks and benefits of elective Cesarean (C-section) delivery, keeping in mind the limitations of evidence (5). For the neonate, elective C-section at term reduces birth injuries but increases rare but serious complications, including neonatal respiratory morbidity. For the woman, elective C-section avoids rare but serious complications of labor. Long-term maternal outcomes are similar for elective C-section and vaginal delivery. However, the risk of serious placental abnormalities in subsequent pregnancies is increased. In informed consent discussions, the obstetrician should ascertain the reasons for the request and try to address them, for example, responding to concerns about pain of vaginal delivery by discussing epidural anesthesia (5)

Obstetric Emergencies

Some obstetric decisions need to be made in crisis situations. An uncomplicated pregnancy at term might unexpectedly and rapidly become an emergency if severe fetal distress develops or if the umbilical cord is wrapped around the fetus's neck. A C-section might need to be carried out immediately to prevent severe, irreversible harm to a child. As with any emergency situation, the informed consent process may be truncated if delaying care to obtain consent would cause serious harm, and most patients would agree to the intervention if fully informed. In an emergency, a C-section may be performed on the basis of the pregnant woman's assent rather than informed consent. That is, the patient agrees to the doctor's recommendations without being informed of all the risks and benefits of the procedure. Almost all pregnant women agree to recommended emergency C-sections (6).

Compelled Treatment of Pregnant Women

In a number of cases, the courts have ordered pregnant women who have decided to carry the fetus to term to be jailed or undergo C-section deliveries or blood transfusions over their objections, allegedly to protect serious harms to the child who will be born (7). Women have been charged with refusing physician's recommendations for bed rest or C-section, or with child endangerment, drug possession, or drug delivery to the fetus (7). These rulings, however, have been sharply criticized for violating the woman's bodily integrity and right of self-determination, for disproportionately singling out women who are poor or members of minority groups, as well as for problematic clinical reasoning in the particular case about the actual risk to the to-be-born child (4) and violations of due process. In many cases, these detentions and forced interventions were rejected by appellate courts (7). If such interventions are justified, they should be a last resort after addressing the woman's concerns and needs, trying to persuade, providing supportive services, and following due process (8).

Sterilization

Sterilization without a woman's consent is a grave violation of her autonomy. In the early 1900s, nonvoluntary eugenic sterilization was carried out in the United States on women who had mental retardation, resided in psychiatric institutions, and were prisoners (9). African American women were disproportionately subjected to nonvoluntary sterilization. In response to these abuses, many states have enacted procedural requirements, such as waiting periods, to ensure that sterilization decisions are voluntary and informed (10).

On the other hand, restrictions on sterilization to prevent coercion and undue influence may have unintended adverse effects on women who have completed their family and wish to be sterilized during the same hospitalization as the last delivery. Medicaid requirements for a waiting periods between consent and the sterilization procedure and federally mandated consent forms have been criticized as restrictions that violate rather than promote informed decisions by the woman and lead to unintended pregnancies (11).

Sterilization is often considered for severely mentally disabled persons. It might be in the best interests of a person who will never have the capacity to make informed reproductive decisions or to provide basic care for a child (12). Generally, a court hearing is required to sterilize a woman who is not capable of giving informed consent (10).

MATERNAL–FETAL MEDICINE

Disparities in Maternal and Fetal Outcomes of Pregnancy

Death rates for US women during pregnancy or shortly after delivery have been rising for two decades and are higher than in other advanced countries, where maternal mortality has been dropping (13). Women who are poor, rural residents or African American are at even greater risk (13). In infant mortality, the United States lags all other developed countries and has the same rate as Serbia and a rate greater than Greece, Slovakia, or Hungary (14). Again, African American infants have double the infant mortality rate as other US children. There are multiple causes for such disparities, including poor access to care, inadequate health insurance, unaddressed social and economic determinants of health, lack of quality-improvement programs, and racism. Such disparities are a compelling ethical problem.

Prenatal Testing

During pregnancy, women routinely have screening tests for rubella, syphilis, gonorrhea, Rh type, diabetes, and HIV infections. In many prenatal blood tests, the patient usually assents rather than gives full informed consent. The physician does not discuss the risks, benefits, and alternatives of each test, and testing is carried out unless the patient objects. Another way to describe routine testing is that women may opt out of testing but do not need to give affirmative consent.

Going beyond routine testing, most states require mandatory prenatal testing for syphilis (15). The ethical justifications for routine and mandatory prenatal screening tests are prevention of serious harm to children who will be born, the poor uptake of voluntary testing, and the judgment that the infringement of the woman's autonomy is acceptable relative to the high likelihood of significant benefit.

Technical advances have dramatically changed balance of benefits and risks of prenatal screening. The noninvasive combination of serum biochemical markers in the mother's blood plus fetal ultrasound have been shown to be effective and safe. It is now recommended that the various options for screening for chromosomal abnormalities be offered to all pregnant women receiving prenatal care, regardless of age (16). Cell-free fetal DNA can be detected in maternal blood, allowing noninvasive prenatal screening for birth defects early in pregnancy (17). Genomic sequencing of fetal DNA fragments allows multiple tests for genetic abnormalities to be run on a single maternal blood sample. Because the testing is noninvasive, there is no risk of miscarriage. The significance of many genomic variants identified will be unclear or unknown. If multiplex testing raises is carried out as a "routine test," pregnant women will not appreciate the possibility of uninterpretable or uncertain results; after receiving such results, they might wish they did not have such knowledge (18). Pregnant women who receive computer-based interactive decision support have greater understanding of pregnant women about the benefits and risks of prenatal tests and are less likely to agree to multiplex testing than patients who receive standard care (18).

Women vary in their desire for information regarding the risk of fetal abnormalities. Some women might place a high value on information about the fetus, earlier ability to treat the fetus for problems such as Rh incompatibility prenatally, the option of pregnancy termination, and reassurance that the pregnancy is progressing normally (19). Moreover, some women might want to know of congenital abnormalities even though they would still carry the fetus to term. Furthermore, women's values regarding prenatal testing may differ from those of physicians. In accordance with the principle of respect for patient autonomy, the indications for screening for chromosomal abnormalities have broadened to include the pregnant woman's informed preferences. Obstetricians and nurse midwives need to help pregnant women understand the decisions they may face after multiplex prenatal testing, help secure access to validated decision support tools, help the woman deliberate about the decision, and communicate that foregoing such testing is a reasonable choice (18).

Care of Pregnant Women with Other Medical Problems

Physicians and pregnant women are understandably concerned about the risks that medical treatments for the mother pose to the fetus. However, such concern must not lead to inappropriately withholding effective therapies for conditions from the pregnant woman (2). Physicians and pregnant women often overestimate the risks and underestimate the risks of untreated serious medical illness during pregnancy (20). In conditions such as depression or epilepsy, aggressive treatment for the pregnant woman promotes the physical health of the child who will be born as well as the health of the woman. Furthermore, it will be in the child's best interests for the mother to be healthy. Women commonly experience depression during pregnancy and the postpartum period. The teratogenic risks of antidepressants are outweighed by the benefits to the fetus from better control of maternal major depression. Physicians need to help the woman understand the benefits of taking medications regularly, in conjunction with talk therapy and support, identify barriers to compliance, and work with her to address them, as with any patient. The pregnant woman should make informed decisions about the care of her medical problems and about what risks to the fetus are acceptable in view of the intervention's overall benefits. It is inappropriate if physicians either withhold effective interventions from the mother or exert undue influence on an informed and competent patient to take medications against her objections.

Substance and Alcohol Abuse During Pregnancy

Many states have enacted laws to try to prevent harm to the fetus caused by prenatal substance abuse. About one half of the states permit involuntary civil commitment of pregnant women who use certain illegal drugs (21). In a few states, drug abuse during pregnancy triggers child abuse laws (21-22). No state mandates drug screening for all pregnant women. Use of criminal sanctions against pregnant substance abusers is ethically problematic. Physicians and hospitals may not conduct drug testing of pregnant women for criminal prosecution without a warrant or explicit consent (22). Except in South Carolina, courts have refused to apply existing criminal laws on child endangerment or delivery of drugs to a minor to drug-using pregnant women. Criminal charges are disproportionately brought against poor women of color (27). There is some evidence that punitive approaches to drug and alcohol abuse during pregnancy are counterproductive, deterring women from seeking prenatal care or being candid with physicians (23). Focusing on high-quality substance abuse treatment is more likely than criminal punishment to benefit the health of the fetus and the mother (23, 24).

Home Births

Some pregnant women desire a more natural, less technologic childbirth and want to deliver at home. They and the midwife may ask a physician to serve as backup in case complications occur. Physicians should help women understand that the risk of perinatal mortality is higher for intended home deliveries than planned hospital births. Doctors should respect women's informed choices regarding site of delivery, even if contrary to their recommendation, and to use their expertise to minimize risks that might otherwise occur with home births (25).

ABORTION

Debates over abortion in the United States are highly contentious and polarized. Prolife advocates contend that the fetus is a person with a right to live and that abortion is murder. Prochoice advocates claim that women have a right to control their bodies and their reproductive choices and generally contend that a fetus becomes a person only after birth. Disagreements over abortion are associated with different views on women's roles and the meaning of their lives (26).

The Supreme Court has made several important rulings on abortion. In *Planned Parenthood v. Casey* (1992), the Supreme Court affirmed the landmark 1973 *Roe v. Wade* decision, which protected a woman's right to choose to abort her fetus. In *Casey,* the court held that states may ban abortion after fetal viability, as long as exceptions were made to protect the woman's health or life and as long as the restriction's "purpose or effect [was not] to place substantial obstacles in the path of a woman seeking an abortion before the fetus attains viability" (27). Many states require parental notification if a minor seeks an abortion; these states must have a procedure for adolescents to seek judicial authorization for the procedure instead of parental notification. Physicians need to understand the laws in their state. Many states have enacted increasingly stringent restrictions on abortion, which are then litigated in the courts. Opponents of abortion are hoping the Supreme Court will reverse *Roe v. Wade.*

Some requests for abortion are particularly problematic (28). For example, a pregnant woman might seek an abortion because of the sex of her fetus even though there is no increased risk of sex-linked genetic disease. The parents might desire a son or daughter to balance their family. Some cultures or religions prize male children more than females, and some parents and doctors may want to respect those norms. There are strong ethical objections, however, to selecting the sex of a fetus (29). The practice reflects and contributes to discrimination against women. Furthermore, some critics argue that sex selection violates the proper parental role and expectations. In this view, children should be unconditionally accepted, not regarded as products made to the parents' specifications.

ASSISTED REPRODUCTIVE TECHNOLOGIES

Because physicians take an active and essential role in assisted reproductive technologies (ARTs), they feel a responsibility for the well-being of the child who might be born (30). Many physicians would hesitate to provide infertility treatments to women with drug addiction, serious developmental delay, or severe psychiatric illness whom they believe would not be a good parent. Other physicians might be reluctant to assist single, unmarried, or lesbian women because they believe that only married women should be parents.

Concern for the well-being of children who will be born is laudable. Physicians should help women and couples who seek ARTs appreciate the difficulties of infertility treatments and childrearing. The physician might also make recommendations on the basis of the patient's situation, needs, and goals. Furthermore, it would be irresponsible for physicians to provide ARTs to women who are incapable of giving informed consent or who have abused their children. However, physicians should distinguish concerns that are based on sound clinical evidence from their personal views of parenthood and family. Some characteristics, such as marital status, poorly predict good parenting (31). Many married couples fail as parents, and many persons who are single or in nontraditional relationships are successful parents.

Some women post menopause seek infertility treatments (31). Many are committed to raising a child, have strong social support, and have carefully considered their decision. However, some writers believe that the natural span of childbearing years should be respected (32). Because having a child is such a private decision, it is ethically problematic for third parties to impose their personal views of who is worthy of being a parent.

ARTs allow pregnancy to occur in unprecedented ways. With ARTs and gamete donation, different persons can fill the roles of genetic, gestational, and childrearing parents. Dramatic dilemmas have arisen over the disposition of frozen embryos after a couple has separated and "surrogate motherhood," in which the gestational mother has no genetic link with the fetus and will not raise the child after birth. Such dilemmas force people to reconsider fundamental, often unspoken beliefs about parental responsibility and roles.

SUMMARY

1. Obstetrics and gynecology raise ethical issues that may be particularly controversial.
2. Doctors need to appreciate that the patient's values might differ from their own, try to understand how the woman's decision might make sense from her perspective, and negotiate a mutually acceptable plan for care.

References

1. Mullins E, Lees C, Brocklehurst P. Is continuous electronic fetal monitoring useful for all women in labour? *BMJ* 2017;359:j5423.
2. Lyerly AD, Mitchell LM, Armstrong EM, et al. Risk and the pregnant body. *Hastings Cent Rep* 2009;39:34-42.
3. Chervenak FA, McCullough LB, Brent RL. The professional responsibility model of obstetrical ethics: avoiding the perils of clashing rights. *Am J Obstet Gynecol* 2011;205:315.e1-5.
4. Minkoff H, Marshall MF, Liaschenko J. The fetus, the "potential child," and the ethical obligations of obstetricians. *Obstet Gynecol* 2014;123:1100-1103.
5. Ecker J. Elective cesarean delivery on maternal request. *JAMA* 2013;309:1930-1936.
6. Lescale KB, Inglis SR, Eddleman KA, et al. Conflicts between physicians and patients in non-elective cesarean delivery: incidence and adequacy of informed consent. *Am J Perinat* 1996;13:171-176.
7. Paltrow LM, Flavin J. Arrests of and forced interventions on pregnant women in the United States, 1973-2005: implications for women's legal status and public health. *J Health Polit Policy Law* 2013;38:299-343.
8. Deshpande NA, Oxford CM. Management of pregnant patients who refuse medically indicated cesarean delivery. *Rev Obstet Gynecol* 2012;5:e144-150.
9. ACOG Committee Opinion. Number 371. July 2007. Sterilization of women, including those with mental disabilities. *Obstet Gynecol* 2007;110:217-220.
10. Committee Opinion No. 695: Sterilization of Women: Ethical Issues and Considerations. *Obstet Gynecol* 2017;129:e109-e116.
11. Borrero S, Zite N, Potter JE, et al. Medicaid policy on sterilization—anachronistic or still relevant? *N Engl J Med* 2014;370:102-104.
12. Caralis D, Kodner IJ, Brown DE. Permanent sterilization of mentally disabled individuals: a case study. *Surgery* 2009;146:959-963.
13. Molina RL, Pace LE. A renewed focus on maternal health in the United States. *N Engl J Med* 2017;377:1705-1707.
14. Central Intelligence Agency. *The World Factbook: Infant Mortality Rate. 2017.* Available at: https://www.cia.gov/library/publications/the-world-factbook/rankorder/2091rank.html. Accessed June 21, 2018.
15. Acuff KL. Prenatal and newborn screening: state legislative approaches and current practice standards. In: Faden RR, Geller G, Powers M, eds. *AIDS, Women and the Next Generation.* New York: Oxford University Press; 1991:121-165.
16. Sharma G, McCullough LB, Chervenak FA. Ethical considerations of early (first vs. second trimester) risk assessment disclosure for trisomy 21 and patient choice in screening versus diagnostic testing. *Am J Med Genet C Semin Med Genet* 2007;145:99-104.
17. Greely HT. Get ready for the flood of fetal gene screening. *Nature* 2011;469:289-291.
18. Johnston J, Farrell RM, Parens E. Supporting women's autonomy in prenatal testing. *N Engl J Med* 2017;377:505-507.
19. Kuppermann M, Learman LA, Gates E, et al. Beyond race or ethnicity and socioeconomic status: predictors of prenatal testing for Down syndrome. *Obstet Gynecol* 2006;107:1087-1097.
20. Kalfoglou AL. Ethical and clinical dilemmas in using psychotropic medications during pregnancy. *AMA J Ethics* 2016;18:614-623.
21. Jos PH, Perlmutter M, Marshall MF. Substance abuse during pregnancy: clinical and public health approaches. *Journal of Law, Medicine & Ethics* 2003;31:340-350.
22. Harris LJ, Paltrow L. The status of pregnant women and fetuses in U.S. criminal law. *JAMA* 2003;289:1697-1699.
23. ACOG Committee Opinion No. 422: at-risk drinking and illicit drug use: ethical issues in obstetric and gynecologic practice. *Obstet Gynecol* 2008;112:1449-1460.
24. Armstrong EM. Drug and alcohol use during pregnancy: we need to protect, not punish, women. *Women's Health Issues* 2005;15:45-47.

25. Greene MF, Ecker JL. Choosing benefits while balancing risks. *N Engl J Med* 2015;373:2681-2682.

26. Murray TH. *The Worth of a Child*. Berkeley, Los Angeles, London: University of California Press; 1996:96-114.

27. Planned Parenthood of Southeastern Pennsylvania v. Casey. 112 US 674 (1992).

28. Harris LH, Cooper A, Rasinski KA, et al. Obstetrician-gynecologists' objections to and willingness to help patients obtain an abortion. *Obstet Gynecol* 2011;118:905-912.

29. The President's Council on Bioethics. *Beyond Therapy: Biotechnology and the Pursuit of Happiness. 2003.* Available at: http://bioethics.georgetown.edu/pcbe/reports/beyondtherapy/. Accessed September 12, 2012.

30. The New York State Task Force on Life and the Law. *Assisted Reproductive Technologies*. New York: The New York State Task Force on Life and the Law; 1998:177-213.

31. Fisseha S, Clark NA. Assisted reproduction for postmenopausal women. *Virtual Mentor* 2014;16:5-9.

32. The President's Council on Bioethics. *Reproduction and Responsibility: The Regulation of New Biotechnologies. 2004.* Available at: http://bioethics.georgetown.edu/pcbe/reports/reproductionandresponsibility/. Accessed September 12, 2012.

ANNOTATED BIBLIOGRAPHY

1. Chervenak FA, McCullough LB, Brent RL. The professional responsibility model of obstetrical ethics: avoiding the perils of clashing rights. *Am J Obstet Gynecol* 2011;205:315.e1-5.
   Minkoff H, Marshall MF, Liaschenko J. The fetus, the "potential child," and the ethical obligations of obstetricians. *Obstet Gynecol* 2014;123:1100-1103.
   Two analyses of the obstetrician's responsibilities to the fetus who is being carried to term.

2. Ecker J. Elective cesarean delivery on maternal request. *JAMA* 2013;309:1930-1936.
   Emphasizes obstetrician's responsibility to ensure that the patient is informed of the risks and benefits of elective cesarean delivery.

3. Committee Opinion No. 695: Sterilization of Women: Ethical Issues and Considerations. *Obstet Gynecol* 2017;129:e109-e116.
   Discusses clinical and ethical issues regarding sterilization of women.

4. Johnston J, Farrell RM, Parens E. Supporting women's autonomy in prenatal testing. *N Engl J Med* 2017;377:505-507.
   Discusses ethical and policy issues regarding multiplex prenatal testing.

5. ACOG Committee Opinion #321: maternal decision making, ethics, and the law. *Obstet Gynecol* 2005;106:1127-1137.
   Argues against punitive and coercive approaches to protecting the fetus, which violate the woman's right to informed consent, are often based on unsound clinical judgments and are selectively applied to the most vulnerable women.

Ethical Issues in Psychiatry

INTRODUCTION

Some patients with severe psychiatric illness might seriously harm themselves or others. Treating their psychiatric illness might restore their decision-making capacity and their control over their actions. To protect them from the grave consequences of nonautonomous decisions and actions, physicians might need to restrict their freedom temporarily. Involuntary legally sanctioned interventions raise ethical concerns because they deprive patients of liberty. In the past, many psychiatric patients were subjected to extreme nonvoluntary measures, such as lengthy confinement in inhumane institutions and psychosurgery.

HOW ARE ETHICAL ISSUES IN PSYCHIATRY DIFFERENT?

Severe Psychiatric Illness Might Impair Autonomy

Severe psychiatric illness might hinder patients from making informed decisions; distinguish right from wrong; appreciate the consequences of their actions; control their thoughts, impulses, and actions; or care for themselves. When such patients are severely symptomatic, they might have different values, preferences, and judgments than when their illness is in remission.

Treatment Might Restore the Patient's Autonomy

Treating the underlying psychiatric illness can restore the patient's decision-making capacity and ameliorate psychiatric symptoms. Thus, a short-term infringement on the patient's freedom, such as court-ordered treatment, might restore the patient's autonomy in the long term.

Physicians Can Prevent Serious Harm

Physicians are in a unique position to identify patients who are rendered nonautonomous by psychiatric illness and to prevent serious harm. Society, therefore, has authorized physicians to restrict such patients' liberty in certain circumstances. Recent mass shootings by psychologically troubled individuals has increased concern for identifying such persons and intervention before they harm others.

Psychiatric Therapies Change Thoughts and Feelings

Psychiatric medications can alter how people think and feel. Many patients believe that effective psychiatric therapies restore their true self by removing delusions, disturbed thinking, and mood disorders. However, other patients object that medication transforms them into a different person or alters their thought processes, mental state, and essential characteristics in unacceptable ways.

Confidentiality Encourages Care for Mental Illness

During therapy, patients reveal their innermost emotions, fears, and fantasies. Maintaining confidentiality respects the personal and sensitive nature of such information, encourages patients to seek mental health care and to be candid with physicians, and protects patients from stigma and discrimination. Recent federal privacy regulations, as well as some state laws, give special protection to psychotherapy notes by requiring specific patient authorization to disclose them. Dilemmas arise because protecting severely impaired psychiatric patients or third parties may require confidentiality to be overridden.

Strict confidentiality might be harmful to patients in some situations. Without permission from the patient, physicians do not disclose to family members if a patient is becoming seriously depressed or delusional, although family members may be in a position to persuade the patient to take medications or provide emotional support, shelter, or food and have moral responsibility for doing so. One approach to this dilemma is to ask a patient during remission to give the physician permission to contact designated family members if a serious psychiatric relapse occurs.

Access to Psychiatric Care

Despite efforts to achieve insurance parity for medical and psychiatric conditions, many patients have inadequate access to mental health care. Health insurers often restrict the availability, frequency, or duration of mental health services. Many patients with severe psychiatric illness are uninsured, and public mental health services are severely underfunded. Many patients have additional problems, including homelessness, alcoholism, or substance abuse, which further complicate access to care.

INVOLUNTARY PSYCHIATRIC COMMITMENT

Involuntary commitment is a dramatic exception to the ethical guideline of respecting people's liberty. Because it infringes on freedom so profoundly, it must be carefully justified.

Rationale for Involuntary Commitment

Intervention is warranted to prevent patients who lack the capacity to make informed decisions from causing serious harm to themselves or to others. Depriving them of liberty for a short time might allow treatment to restore their autonomy (1). After depression, bipolar disorder, or schizophrenia is treated, most patients no longer choose to kill themselves or harm others. In contrast, persons who are likely to harm others but are not mentally ill may not be detained against their will unless they have committed a crime.

Standards for Involuntary Commitment

States have different criteria for involuntary commitment, but typically require that because mental illness patients are (2):

- dangerous to themselves, for example, suicidal
- unable to care for themselves, for example, unable to provide food, clothing, and shelter
- dangerous to others, for example, threatening, attempting, or committing violence
- (in some states) at high risk of deteriorating to the point where they will require involuntary commitment.

Procedures for Involuntary Commitment

Physicians need to be familiar with the law in their state. On an emergency basis, patients typically may be held against their will for brief periods (usually a few days). During an emergency, patients may also be treated against their will to prevent serious physical injury to themselves or others or, in some states, to prevent an irreversible deterioration of their condition. A court hearing must be held to determine whether the patient may be confined for a longer period.

Legal hearings are time-consuming, and many physicians believe that they are an unwarranted intrusion of the legal system into medical practice. However, the public demands rigorous safeguards because involuntary psychiatric hospitalization is a serious deprivation of liberty and has been abused in the past.

Outpatient Commitment and Involuntary Treatment

Outpatient commitment may be considered in several situations. First, outpatient commitment may be instituted on the basis of advance directives from the patient. While in remission, a patient may indicate that he or she would want outpatient commitment if his or her condition deteriorated so that inpatient commitment was highly likely. The patient may, therefore, direct physicians and surrogates to override his or her refusal of treatment to avoid more severe impairment and involuntary hospitalization.

Second, outpatient commitment may be a less restrictive alternative to inpatient commitment to prevent serious harm to self or others or to prevent a deterioration that would require a more restrictive alternative of involuntary inpatient commitment. Almost all states allow involuntary outpatient commitment (3). Some states require that the patient have a history of noncompliance with treatment for mental illness that led to a hospitalization or a history of serious violent behavior toward self or others. Procedures to issue such orders often may be started by relatives or roommates of the patient, as well as by mental health, medical, or social service providers or probation or parole officers. These involuntary outpatient commitment laws have been criticized because they do not address the underlying problem of poor access to underfunded mental health services, because less restrictive alternatives such as peer counseling and street outreach are not considered, and because the laws may not require enhanced services and care coordination to patients who are committed. Although outcomes studies are controversial, real-world quasi-experimental designs show reduced psychiatric hospitalizations and arrests and increased use of mental health services and psychiatric medications (4, 5).

Other situations in which involuntary outpatient commitment is employed are controversial. Some patients accept outpatient commitment as a condition of receiving social services, such as subsidized housing, or to receive probation rather than a prison sentence after a conviction or guilty plea for a minor crime. Critics charge that such leverage is coercive and therefore unethical. However, offering outpatient commitment as an alternative to a prison sentence is more accurately characterized as an offer that makes the person making the choice better off, not as a threat to make him or her worse off (6).

Mitigating Adverse Consequences

Psychiatric patients who are hospitalized involuntarily have certain legal rights (1), including a right to treatment and a right to the least restrictive alternative, as well as rights of visitation, communication, privacy, and freedom of movement, subject to legitimate restrictions.

After patients are involuntarily hospitalized, they might view the physicians as adversaries who can no longer be trusted. Such feelings might make subsequent psychiatric care difficult. Physicians should try to stress shared therapeutic goals and concern. An experienced psychiatrist has suggested saying, "It would be a shame if you killed yourself while your depression clouded your judgment."

SUICIDAL PATIENTS

When patients attempt or threaten suicide, physicians have an ethical obligation to intervene.

Rationale for Suicide Intervention

The ethical justification for suicide intervention is to prevent serious, irreversible harm to persons who lack decision-making capacity. Suicidal patients are almost always impaired by severe depression or other severe mental illness. Their actions do not result from autonomous choices. Interventions to prevent suicide provide time to treat the underlying mental illness or let it enter a remission, thereby restoring the patient's autonomy. Empirical studies show that suicide prevention prevents people from killing themselves. After persons are prevented from committing suicide, only about 10% to 20% subsequently kill themselves (7).

Some suicidal threats, although representing a "cry for help," might not warrant involuntary commitment and might be treated through less restrictive measures, such as arranging for voluntary psychiatric treatment, mobilizing assistance from family and friends, removing the means of suicide, and getting patients to promise to call for help. Imposing involuntary commitment is a last resort and should be continued only as long as necessary to protect the nonautonomous patient. In contrast, it is ethically problematic to restrict the liberty of autonomous persons to protect them. Some patients with terminal illnesses with decision-making capacity might make a deliberate decision to end their lives. The ethics of physician-assisted suicide is controversial (*see* Chapter 19).

When Is a Patient Suicidal?

When patients are severely depressed or mention suicide, physicians should ask specific questions to determine the likelihood of a serious suicide attempt. Fears that raising or probing the topic of suicide will suggest or even encourage it are unfounded and deter physicians from gathering crucial information and initiating effective treatment. Many depressed patients feel relieved to discuss suicide with a caring and nonjudgmental physician.

PATIENTS WHO ARE DANGEROUS TO OTHERS

Widely publicized recent cases of mass shootings by persons with severe psychological disorders have focused attention on the physician's obligation to prevent patients from killing third parties. Patients with serious psychiatric illnesses might disclose to physicians plans to kill or injure third parties, actual attempts, or overt acts of harm. Thus, the physician might be in a unique position to prevent serious harm to potential victims. Social norms and criminal sanctions might not deter psychiatric patients who cannot control their violent impulses. In this situation, the landmark Tarasoff case established that confidentiality should be overridden to prevent serious harm to third parties (8).

CASE 40.1	**The Tarasoff case and the duty to prevent harm**

A university student, Prosenjit Poddar, confided to his psychologist that he was planning to kill a woman, readily identifiable as Tatiana Tarasoff, who had rejected him romantically. The therapist and his superiors at the student health service decided that Poddar should be committed involuntarily and asked the campus police to detain him. The police did so but released him because he appeared rational. The director of psychiatry ordered no action to place Poddar under involuntary detention. Subsequently Poddar went to Tarasoff's home and stabbed her to death.

Most states now require therapists to protect identifiable persons threatened with serious violence by psychiatric patients (8, 9). Generally, the duty is limited to serious and imminent harms, identifiable victims, and actual threats. The federal HIPAA privacy regulations allow an exception to confidentiality to "prevent or lessen a serious and imminent threat to the health and safety of a person or the public" (9). Although therapists initially feared that the decision would deter patients from seeking mental health services and disclosing their violent thoughts, this has not occurred.

Steps to Prevent Harm

The duty to prevent harm to potential victims of psychiatric patients requires several steps. First, the physician needs to evaluate the threat of violence. Asking about violence does not give patients the idea of harming others or encourage them to do so.

Predictions of violence by physicians are not very accurate. In one study, 53% of psychiatric patients whom physicians predicted would be violent in fact committed violent acts over the subsequent 6 months; in comparison, 36% of psychiatric patients whose psychiatrists had no concerns about violence committed violent acts (10). Research decision tools for predication of violence might provide better discrimination (11). Doctors need to do the best they can within the limits of clinical judgment. The standard of care is what a reasonable physician would do under the circumstances.

After determining that the threat of violence is severe and probable, the physician must decide how to respond. A number of actions might protect the victim, such as changing the patient's medications, increasing the frequency of therapy sessions, having the patient give up weapons, hospitalizing the patient voluntarily, committing the patient involuntarily, and notifying the police (12). With recent mass shootings, some states are enacting laws to allow guns to be removed from persons with severe mental illness who are a threat to others.

The law in many states specifically requires warning the threatened victim. Such warning does not replace steps to reduce the risk of violence. Physicians should notify patients before they override confidentiality and explain why they are required to do so (12). Patients might agree with warning the threatened person. Many patients are ambivalent about violence and welcome help with expressing their emotions or dealing with interpersonal conflicts. When beginning therapy with patients who have a history of violence, physicians should discuss the situations in which confidentiality may be overridden (1).

REFUSAL OF PSYCHIATRIC TREATMENT

Patients who are involuntarily committed may have a right to refuse psychiatric treatment. The rationale is that confinement without treatment can sometimes accomplish the goal of preventing nonautonomous patients from seriously harming themselves or others (1). Moreover, administering medications to competent patients against their will violates their liberty and bodily integrity. It is intrusive, inhumane, and impractical in the long run. Even if psychiatric medications can be forcibly administered to inpatients, patients can (and often do) discontinue them after discharge.

On the other hand, confining patients, but not treating them with effective medications has been criticized as letting people "rot with their rights on." To critics, it is cruel and pointless to withhold from severely impaired patients the very treatments that are likely to restore their autonomy and well-being. In this view, short-term involuntary treatment for the underlying psychiatric illness is a lesser infringement on the patient's freedom than prolonged involuntary hospitalization without treatment.

Because competency is determined with regard to specific tasks, a patient who is not competent to refuse commitment may still be competent to refuse psychiatric medications. Patients often view the risks and benefits of psychiatric therapies differently from physicians. Many psychiatric patients refuse drugs because they have experienced unacceptable side effects or changes in their thinking and personality (13). Assessing the patient's decision-making capacity can be challenging. People with major depression might underestimate the benefits of treatment and overestimate the risks. They might be convinced that the treatment will fail or that they will experience a serious side effect of therapy. Similarly, manic patients might believe that nothing is wrong with them and, therefore, they do not need treatment.

Most refusals of inpatient treatment are resolved in a few days. In one study, only 7% of inpatients refused antipsychotic medication for longer than 24 hours (14). Common reasons for refusal were psychotic or idiosyncratic thought processes, side effects of medications, denial of mental illness, and alleged ineffectiveness of medications. Cases were resolved in several ways. In 50% of cases, patients eventually took medication voluntarily, after nursing staff, psychiatrists, or family reassured, coaxed, or persuaded them. In 23% of cases, the psychiatrist discontinued antipsychotic drugs, or the patient was discharged without them—that is, the physician ultimately did not consider these medications essential. Finally, in 18% of cases the psychiatrists obtained a court order for involuntary administration of the medication. In all of the cases that went to court, the judge authorized involuntary treatment.

Physicians should anticipate the possibility of a recurrence of psychosis or severe depression and discuss with patients how it should be managed when they are still in remission (13). Statements that the patient would not want medication need to be discussed further in terms of specific scenarios, such as attacking family members or requiring long-term involuntary hospitalization (13). See Case 6.2 for how such advance planning might be helpful in the care of a psychiatric patient.

REFUSAL OF MEDICAL TREATMENT

Patients with serious psychiatric illness might refuse recommended therapy for concurrent medical problems. As with any patient refusal, the first step is to ask whether the patient lacks decision-making capacity (*see* Chapter 9). A psychiatric diagnosis *per se* does not imply that a patient lacks the capacity to make an informed decision about medical treatment. A competent patient's refusal should be respected if attempts at persuasion are unsuccessful. If the patient lacks decision-making capacity, decisions should be based on advance directives or made by surrogates (*see* Chapters 11 and 12).

Dilemmas arise if psychiatric patients who lack decision-making capacity actively resist medical treatment that is clearly in their best interests. Family and friends may be able to persuade or cajole the patient into accepting treatment, or they might authorize administering it covertly in the patient's food, preferably on the basis of the patient's previously stated preferences (*see* Chapter 6). Resorting to physical force or deception is ethically troubling and may seem inhumane. Forced treatment might also undermine the doctor–patient relationship and is impossible in the long term because the patient can discontinue medicines after discharge.

PSYCHOTROPIC DRUGS IN LESS SEVERE CONDITIONS

Selective serotonin reuptake inhibitors (SSRIs) are effective not only in major depression, but also in other conditions, such as dysthymia or social anxiety. Some patients with these conditions report that SSRIs make them feel better than they normally do. Their mood brightens, and anxiety, social inhibition, obsession, compulsion, and fear diminish. Some patients report that such medications allow them to become themselves again, gain their true identity for the first time, or function in social situations where they previously felt extreme anxiety or inhibitions.

Critics object to the use of psychoactive medications in persons with "merely melancholy or inhibited temperaments" (15). In their view, using medications in this context is not a proper goal of medicine (15). From their perspective, people should achieve a more flourishing life through self-examination and arduous effort, not through brain-altering medications. Furthermore, from their viewpoint, some negative feelings should not be blunted; it is part of the human condition to experience sadness or outrage.

Such broad philosophical objections, however, overlook severe symptoms and functional impairment that people with these conditions might experience. Generalized social anxiety disorder is much more severe than shyness or performance anxiety; people with it avoid or fear most social and work situations and experience distress and functional impairment. Clinical trials show that both cognitive-behavioral therapy and pharmacologic therapy with SSRIs are effective for this condition (16).

Furthermore, these critics present a problematic view of the physician's role and responsibilities. Discounting the patient's experience and distress is disrespectful. Also, critics need to examine empirical evidence. Is exhorting patients to greater efforts at self-improvement effective when patients are impaired by intrusive feelings and thoughts that they cannot control? Omitting the option of medications that have been shown to be effective is inconsistent with the ethical ideal that physicians should act in the best interests of the patient, as defined by the patient's values. Finally, it is questionable whether physicians should try to impose their view of the good life on their patients who have not selected them for that view.

SUMMARY

1. When psychiatric patients are suicidal, unable to care for themselves, or are dangerous to others, physicians have ethical and legal obligations to prevent harm.
2. These obligations may override respecting patient autonomy and maintaining confidentiality.
3. In fulfilling this duty, physicians also need to use their clinical skills and judgment to encourage effective treatment for the underlying psychiatric disorders.

References

1. Appelbaum PS, Gutheil TG. *Clinical Handbook of Psychiatry and the Law*. 4th ed. Philadelphia: Lippincott Williams & Wilkins; 2007.
2. The Policy Surveillance Program. *Long-Term Involuntary Commitment Laws*. Available at: http://lawatlas.org/datasets/long-term-involuntary-commitment-laws. Accessed November 12, 2018.
3. Rowe M. Alternatives to outpatient commitment. *J Am Acad Psychiatry Law* 2013;41:332-336.
4. Swartz MS. Introduction to the special section on assisted outpatient treatment in New York State. *Psychiatr Serv* 2010;61:967-969.
5. Swanson JW, Swartz MS. Why the evidence for outpatient commitment is good enough. *Psychiatr Serv* 2014;65:808-811.
6. Monahan J. Mandated community treatment: applying leverage to achieve adherence. *J Am Acad Psychiatry Law* 2008;36:282-285.
7. Miller RD. Need-for-treatment criteria for involuntary civil commitment: impact in practice. *Am J Psychiatry* 1992;149:1380-1384.
8. Rothstein MA. Tarasoff duties after newtown. *J Law Med Ethics* 2014;42:104-109.
9. National Conference of State Legislators. *Mental Health Professionals' Duty to Warn. 2015*. Available at: http://www.ncsl.org/research/health/mental-health-professionals-duty-to-warn.aspx. Accessed November 12, 2018.
10. Lidz C, Mulvey EP, Gardner W. The accuracy of predictions of violence to others. *JAMA* 1993;269:1007-1011.
11. Monahan J, Steadman HJ, Robbins PC, et al. An actuarial model of violence risk assessment for persons with mental disorders. *Psychiatr Serv* 2005;56:810-815.
12. Anfang SA, Appelbaum PS. Twenty years after Tarasoff: reviewing the duty to protect. *Harv Rev Psychiatry* 1996;4:67-76.
13. Sabin J. Medication refusal in schizophrenia: preventive and reactive ethical considerations. *AMA J Ethics* 2016;18:572-578.
14. Hoge SK, Appelbaum PS, Lawlor T. A prospective, multicenter study of patients' refusal of antipsychotic medication. *Arch Gen Psychiatry* 1990;47:949-956.
15. The President's Council on Bioethics. *Beyond Therapy: Biotechnology and the Pursuit of Happiness. 2003*. Available at: http://bioethics.georgetown.edu/pcbe/reports/beyondtherapy/. Accessed September 12, 2012.
16. Schneier FR. Social anxiety disorder. *N Engl J Med* 2006;355:1029-1036.

ANNOTATED BIBLIOGRAPHY

1. Sabin J. Medication refusal in schizophrenia: preventive and reactive ethical considerations. *AMA J Ethics* 2016;18:572-578.
   Astute analysis of a case of medication refusal by a patient with relapsed schizophrenia and his proxy. Physicians should carry out advance planning on how to manage a severe recurrence with patients when they are in remission.
2. Appelbaum PS, Gutheil TG. *Clinical Handbook of Psychiatry and the Law*. 4th ed. Philadelphia, PA: Lippincott Williams & Wilkins; 2007.
   Discusses ethical and legal issues regarding psychiatric patients. Contains practical clinical advice on managing patients with severe psychiatric disorders.
3. Swartz MS. Introduction to the special section on assisted outpatient treatment in New York State. *Psychiatr Serv* 2010;61:967-969.
   Lucid overview of involuntary outpatient commitment and its rationale and outcomes. Other articles in this issue present outcomes research regarding the New York policy.
4. Rowe M. Alternatives to outpatient commitment. *J Am Acad Psychiatry Law* 2013;41:332-336.
   Critique of outpatient commitment policies.

Ethical Issues in Organ Transplantation

INTRODUCTION

Transplantation saves lives and allows many recipients with end-stage illness to resume active lives. Organ donors undergo interventions in order to benefit the recipient. The ethical concern is that the donor's well-being might be compromised to benefit someone else. Thus, informed and voluntary consent for donation and minimization of harm to donors are essential to maintain public trust.

The need for organ transplantation far exceeds the supply of donated organs. As of April 2018, about 75,000 persons were on the active waiting list for a transplant in the United States. In 2017, around 25,000 transplants were performed. On average, around 20 people die each day because a transplant is not available. Many proposals have been made to narrow the gap between the number of donated organs and the need for transplantation; each presents additional ethical issues that must be addressed. In addition, difficult decisions need to be made regarding the allocation of donated organs. Patients on the waiting list and potential donors need to believe that allocation procedures are fair and trustworthy.

ETHICAL GUIDELINES IN ORGAN TRANSPLANTATION

Minimize Harm to Donors

When transplantation was initiated, concerns were raised that cadaveric organ transplantation hastened or caused the donor's death. More generally, the best interests of organ donors should not be compromised to retrieve organs and benefit the recipient. Donation from living donors raises heightened concerns about harm because donors face operative risks but have no prospect of medical benefit.

Respect Donors

Informed and voluntary consent from donors respects their autonomy. If people do not want to be organ donors, their wishes must be respected. Although donors who are dead cannot be harmed medically, they still deserve respect. The decedent's wishes regarding donation must be respected, as well as the sensitivities of survivors (1). Novel proposals to increase cadaveric organ donation raise concerns that invasive procedures to increase the viability of the organ may harm or disrespect donors.

Eliminate or Manage Conflicts of Interest

Decisions about the potential donor's care must be separate from and take priority over decisions about procurement and transplantation (2). The potential donor's physicians may not be part of the transplantation team. Other conflicts of interest arise because transplant surgeons and centers have an interest in building their reputation by carrying out transplants. However, outcomes in low-volume centers are inferior to outcomes at high-volume programs.

Justice

In the United States and almost all other countries, payments to organ donors are prohibited to prevent abuse and exploitation of potential donors. Although some have advocated a regulated market in organ donation, serious abuse and exploitation of low-income, disadvantaged donors have been well documented. Black markets flourish in some countries, even though payment of donors is illegal.

Payment for organs should be distinguished from reimbursement of living donors for their out-of-pocket expenses associated with donation, which has been advocated to make donation financially neutral, compared with not donating (3).

Justice is also important in the allocation of cadaveric organs: fair allocation is crucial to public trust in the transplantation system and willingness to be a donor. Organs are allocated on the basis of a publicly known computerized scoring system.

DONATION OF CADAVERIC ORGANS

The Current System for Cadaveric Donation

The United States has a voluntary system for organ donation. The Uniform Anatomical Gift Act allows people to use an organ donor card to donate their organs for transplantation after death. This card is usually part of a person's driver license. However, many supporters of organ transplantation have not signed such cards. Some fear that if they agree to organ donation, they will receive suboptimal care (1).

Donation After Brain Determination of Death

All states have laws that permit organs to be harvested from persons who have been declared dead by brain criteria for death. Chapter 21 discusses some of the current controversies surrounding the concept and implementation of brain criteria for death. After death is determined, life-sustaining interventions are continued until the organs are harvested; this ongoing perfusion and ventilation reduces warm ischemia time and improves transplantation outcomes.

Under existing state laws, organs may be retrieved from people who had signed donor cards even if the next of kin does not agree. Ethically, such a practice is consistent with respecting patient autonomy. As a practical matter, however, objections from family members are honored because of concerns about adverse publicity that might undermine public trust in the transplantation system.

Only about 50% of relatives of patients with brain death give permission for organ donation (1). Many families do not understand the concept of brain death, and some perceive the organ procurement process as insensitive (1). Some cultural beliefs pose barriers to organ donation (4). For instance, many Asian or Latino families believe that bodies must be buried whole or else spirits will suffer after death.

Proposals to Increase DBDD

Many proposals have been made to increase cadaveric organ donation (1, 5). However, some proposals that have been adopted in other countries have not been adopted in the United States because they might undermine public trust in transplantation and make people less willing to donate.

Mandated Choice

Persons would be required to state their preferences about organ donation when renewing driver licenses or filing income taxes, rather than merely given the opportunity to declare their preferences on a donor card or registry. In surveys, most Americans support this policy.

Presumed Consent

Currently, organs are harvested only if the patient or family has given explicit consent. Under this proposal, organs would be harvested unless the patient or family specifically objects. Although this approach has been adopted in some countries, many people in the United States find this unacceptable (1).

Donors Who Are Physiologically Marginal

Donors who are older or have a history of hypertension or very mild renal insufficiency are currently excluded as cadaveric donors, because their organs may have a shorter graft survival. However, although such organs would not be suitable for young recipients with long life expectancies, they might be acceptable for older recipients who have shorter expected survival. Such organs might be offered to older recipients, who could either accept the organ or choose to remain on the waiting list (6).

Donation After Circulatory Determination of Death

Most cadaver donors are declared dead by brain criteria and have effective circulation until the organs are harvested. However, the vast majority of deaths are declared on the basis on circulatory criteria. After persons are declared dead by circulatory and respiratory criteria (*see* Chapter 21), organ retrieval may be attempted with appropriate consent. This practice is also called donation after circulatory death. During the time between withdrawal of life-sustaining interventions and declaration of death, organs are damaged by hypoxia and hypotension and transplantation outcomes are worsened.

Donation after circulatory determination of death (DCDD) therefore raises several ethical concerns (7, 8). First, how long after the development of asystole should death be declared? Death should be declared only if circulation cannot be spontaneously restored by auto-resuscitation. Typically 2 to 5 minutes are allowed to elapse after the development of asystole. On the one hand, the longer the time from asystole to the declaration of death, the more certainty that circulation cannot resume. However, the longer the duration of nonperfusion, the greater the deterioration of organ function. On the other hand, if the time between asystole and declaration of death is shorter, recipient outcomes are improved, but it might be questioned whether the donor is really dead. Thus, there is a tension between certainty that the patient is dead and greater risk of decreased organ function and transplantation outcomes.

Second, interventions can maintain organ function during the time between asystole and declaration of death, as discussed in more detail below. If initiated before death, such interventions are clearly not for the benefit of the donor but may cause medical complications and discomfort or may be inconsistent with the patient's hopes for a good death (9). Respect for donors requires that explicit permission be obtained for such interventions (10). If such interventions are initiated after death is declared, there still may be concerns about respect for the deceased person.

Controlled Donation after Declaration of Cardiac Death (cDCDD)

After the patient or surrogate decides to withdraw life-sustaining interventions and donate organs, life support is withdrawn in the operating room. The patient and family need to understand that he or she will die in the operating room on invasive interventions, away from the family (11). If after withdrawal of life-sustaining interventions the patient does not die before unacceptable deterioration in organ function occurs, no organs are harvested, and the patient is returned to a hospital room to die. This occurs in about one quarter of cases in which cDCDD is planned. cDCDD raises several particular ethical concerns.

Perfusion of organs to be transplanted. After death declared by circulatory criteria, perfusion is restored to maintain organ function. Large-bore catheters are inserted for cold perfusion or for extracorporeal membrane oxygenation (ECMO). As noted, specific consent for these procedures should be obtained from the patient or surrogate. Institution of ECMO after DCDD might restore perfusion to the brain and heart and reanimate them, negating the declaration of death. To address this concern, ECMO procedures are modified to block circulation to these organs.

Emotional stress in family and heath care workers. Families report that return of the patient from the operating room after unsuccessful cDCDD disrupted their ability to find something positive in the patient's death, failed to honor the donor's memory and character through donation, and disrupted their grieving. Health care workers may experience distress in transitioning from caring for the patient to harvesting organs, rather than transitioning to palliative care, as usually occurs after life-sustaining interventions are withdrawn. Such distress might be more pronounced if no usable organs are retrieved. Other adverse consequences of unsuccessful cDCDD include waste of hospital resources.

Acceptability of DCDD. There are racial differences in acceptance of donation after cardiac death (12). White family decision makers who had been asked to consent to organ donation after the death of a loved one were equally likely to agree to DCDD as donation after brain determination of death (DBDD). However, Black family decision makers were less likely than White family decision makers to agree to organ donation after brain death, and even less likely to consent to donate after cardiac death.

Donation before life support is withdrawn. It has been proposed that organ donors from whom life-sustaining interventions will be withdrawn be offered the opportunity to serve as a living donor of nonvital organs before life support is withdrawn (13). After donation, the patient is returned to a hospital room, where life support is withdrawn and the patient dies surrounded by family. This proposal has been criticized because proposals do not specify who would be eligible to donate, because it may be uncertain that such donation is consistent with the patient's values, and because donation might hasten or cause the donor's death, thereby undermining public trust.

Donation of vital organs by living donors. A more radical proposal to increase the number of organs for transplant is to allow donation of vital organs from patients from whom withdrawal of life support is planned (14). The rationale is that "patients whose death is imminent because life-sustaining interventions will be foregone cannot be harmed if they choose to donate vital organs." Abolishing the so-called dead donor rule, that organs may only be retrieved from persons who have died, would require revision to homicide laws.

Opponents of this proposal argue that although some informed patients would accept donation that leads to their death, this practice would lead to loss of trust in physicians and in the organ donation system (15). Another objection is the impact of the death of a living donor on a transplant team and program, because deaths of living donors trigger intense scrutiny and suspension of the program.

Uncontrolled Donation after Declaration of Cardiac Death (uDCDD)

Protocols have been devised to retrieve organs from patients who die after resuscitation efforts have failed (16). Invasive interventions to restore circulation and preserve organ function need to be continued or started after the declaration of death.

Informed consent. uDCDD differs so markedly from usual clinical practice after unsuccessful CPR that consent cannot be inferred from an organ donor card. Patients did not consider the scenario of uDCDD when completing the card. Next-of-kin therefore should give consent for interventions to preserve organs.

Difficulties with implementation. The actual yield of transplantable organs from uDCDD is much lower than projections. A multiyear program in New York City to initiate uDCDD failed to yield any usable organs.

ORGANS FROM LIVING DONORS

Transplantation of kidneys and portions of liver and lung from living donors is increasing. Most living donors have a preexisting emotional relationship with the recipient, such as relatives, friends, and coworkers. A few donors are "Good Samaritans" who have no previous relationship with the recipient. Donation from persons who are not genetically related is feasible because human leukocyte antigen (HLA) compatibility does not enhance outcomes in liver and lung transplants and is less important in living kidney transplants than cadaveric transplants. The quality of organs from live donors is higher because of more thorough medical screening and shorter ischemia time compared with cadaveric donors. Transplants from living donors do not delay transplants to other patients on the waiting list because the total number of donors is increased.

Ethical Issues Regarding Live Donation

Harm to Donors

Surgeons violate the guideline of "do no harm" when they operate on a healthy person, exposing the patient to operative risk to benefit another person. A highly publicized death of a living liver donor in 2002 led to a decline in live donations. Other risks to donors include pain, postoperative complications, and lost income (17). For living kidney donation, the risk of end-stage renal disease is slightly increased, although the absolute risk is low.

To minimize risks, persons may not serve as living donors if they have medical conditions that significantly increase operative risk or if they already have abnormal organ function. To further reduce risk of living liver donation, some have advocated that it be carried out only at experienced, high-volume centers.

Motives of Donors

Donation to relatives and friends is understandable because people want to help and care for persons they have close relationships with. Donating to a stranger, however, raises ethical concerns (18). On the one hand, donating to a stranger in need can be an extraordinary expression of altruism and humanitarianism. On the other hand, it can also be driven by a desire for publicity, financial gain, or internal psychological conflicts. Thus, offers by strangers to donate should be carefully reviewed.

Consent from Donors

Because a live donor undergoes serious risks to benefit another person, it is essential that the decision to donate be free and informed. Many live donors choose to donate immediately before they learn of the risks of donation. Altruism does not fit a model of rational utilitarian deliberation about risks and benefits. People commonly base important decisions on emotion rather than reason. However, donors should be able to explain their decision to donate in a coherent manner, even though they might give less weight than most people to the possibility of a serious risk. The donor's decision should remain stable after the donor receives more information and has time to reflect.

After the death of a live donor of part of a liver, the consent process was modified to provide every living donor with an advocate, independent of the transplant team, whose role is to ensure that consent is informed and voluntary (19). Some in the transplant community believe that the independent advocates should have veto power over donation if they believe the consent is inadequate.

Consent should be voluntary as well as informed (20). A patient's relative might feel family pressure to donate. Doctors may offer a general excuse that someone is not a suitable donor, without specifying why. However, it would be ethically problematic for a physician to provide a false medical reason as an excuse (21), as with any deception by a physician (*see* Chapter 6).

Children as Living Donors

Use of children as donors raises particular ethical concerns because they cannot give consent for themselves and depend on others to protect their interests. Although adults may make extraordinary sacrifices for others, they may not require children to do so. Hence, children should be live donors only as a last resort if no suitable adult donor can be identified, if the recipient is a close family member, and if the child assents (22). To assure that a child donor's interests are protected, approval from a donor advocacy team should be obtained.

Payment to Donors

Paying living donors of unpaired organs and setting up a regulated market has been proposed to increase the number of organs for transplantation. However, it is unlikely that black markets for organs can be prevented. Exploitation, coercion, and abuse of paid donors have been well documented (23). It is questionable whether informed and voluntary consent for organ donation can be obtained from persons with poor education, low literacy and health literacy, and low income, particularly those residing in resource-poor countries. Finally, commodification of organ donation might reduce altruistic donations, perhaps causing an overall reduction in the number of organs available for transplantation. In the United States as well as almost all other countries, buying and selling of organs is illegal.

Reimbursement for Donors

Proposals have been made to give living donors reimbursement of out-of-pocket expenses such as expenses for travel and lodging for evaluation and surgery, lost wages, and the costs of caring for their dependents during the period of donation and recovery.

Such reimbursement would not result in a net financial gain for donors. To further mitigate the risks borne by living donors, they should also receive free medical care for complications of donation, and high priority for transplantation should they need it (3). These financial incentives can be distinguished from payments because they simply return donors to the position they would have been in had they not donated their organs. As a matter of fairness, there is a strong case for making donation financially neutral for live donors, who undergo the pain and risk of surgery compared with not donating.

Confidentiality of Recipient

The recipient might have a medical condition that might reduce the potential donor's willingness to donate. For example, the recipient might have cancer that might recur and reduce the likelihood of long-term success. Moreover, some donors may not want to help patients with alcoholic liver disease or HIV infection, whose illness they regard as caused by the recipient's choices and actions. According to the principle of informed consent, prospective living donors should receive information that is pertinent to their decision to donate. Because confidentiality is also important, potential recipients must give permission to disclose such information to potential donors (24).

Paired Donation

Paired kidney donations overcome incompatibilities between donors and their intended recipients. A living donor directs the donated organ to a compatible recipient, while another donor donates to the first donor's recipient (25). Chain exchanges extend this approach by including additional pairs of donors and recipients. Although such donations increase the number of people who receive transplants, they also raise ethical concerns (25). First, pressure on potential donors may increase, because incompatibility is no longer a contraindication to donation. Second, no pair should give a kidney but fail to receive one. Carrying out all operations simultaneously precludes this possibility, but logistics make long chains difficult. Donor chains that are initiated by a non-directed donor address this problem: a transplant candidate receives an organ before his or her partner donates an organ.

SELECTION OF RECIPIENTS

Because the number of people needing transplants far exceeds the number of donated organs, difficult allocation decisions must be made.

Historical Background

When dialysis was developed in the 1960s, few dialysis machines were available and committees ranked candidates according to their perceived social worth (26). Responding to concerns that selection was based on prejudice and unwarranted value judgments, Congress funded dialysis for all patients with end-stage renal disease. In transplantation, however, allocation decisions cannot be avoided because of a shortage of organs.

Because people donate cadaveric organs without knowing who will receive them, a fair allocation procedure is essential to maintain public willingness to donate organs (27). Moreover, it is unfair to ask people to donate if there is no likelihood they would receive a transplant if they needed it.

The following section discusses general ethical principles for allocating organs. Specific selection criteria are too detailed to be discussed here but can be found at www.unos.org. Different considerations receive priority for different organs (27).

Beneficence

From a utilitarian perspective, scarce organs should go to those patients who will receive the greatest net medical benefit (27). Relevant outcomes include the likelihood and duration of recipient survival and quality of life, compared to not receiving a transplant. Although this criterion appears objective, it involves complex value judgments.

An increasing number of elderly patients are placed on transplant waiting lists. If they receive an organ from a younger cadaveric donor, they might die years before the graft is projected to stop functioning. Younger transplant candidates would have more years of use from such an organ. Thus, it has been proposed to match cadaveric kidneys with better projected graft survival to recipients with longer estimated survival. The specifics of these proposals, however, are controversial and unproven (6).

Justice

The guideline that scarce resources should be distributed fairly or equitably is indisputable in the abstract but difficult to specify. Several approaches to operationalize equity have been considered (27, 28).

Time on the Waiting List

The precept of "first-come, first-served" seems intuitively fair if there are no other compelling reasons to distinguish among candidates. However, time on the waiting list can be manipulated by placing patients on the waiting list earlier in the course of illness or on several regional transplantation networks. Better-educated and wealthier patients are more likely to take advantage of these possibilities. To make time on the waiting list fairer, only patients meeting minimum clinical criteria may be placed on the list.

Medical Need

To assist those in greatest need, in liver and heart transplantation patients who would die soon without transplantation are given priority over more stable patients. Cadaveric livers are assigned according to the Model for End-Stage Liver Disease system, a severity of illness score based on laboratory tests, which predicts the risk of death while on the waiting list. Significant geographical disparities remain, however, with sicker patients in larger organ-procurement areas waiting longer for transplants than patients in smaller organ-procurement areas (29, 30).

Geographic Location

Waiting times for liver transplantation vary up to fivefold among various geographical regions, even among sickest candidates who are most likely to die without transplantation (30). To reduce these disparities in waiting times, it has been suggested that the United States allocate organs on a regional or national basis to those with the greatest medical need, with less emphasis on keeping organs in the geographic area in which they are donated (29, 30). This policy is justified by the idea that organs belong to the nation as a whole and that where a person resides or is on the waiting list is not a morally relevant allocation criterion. This proposed change would provide more organs to large referral centers, which transplant sicker patients and have better outcomes. Opponents object that such redistribution penalizes states that try to increase donations and might worsen outcomes by increasing cold ischemia time.

Ability to Pay

Transplantation is generally performed only on patients who can pay for it. Medicare covers kidney transplantation for all Americans. Most private insurers and state Medicaid programs cover liver and heart transplantation. Americans who lack health insurance must raise money for transplantation of these organs, for example, through public appeals.

Although allocating organs by ability to pay is routinely practiced, it has been strongly criticized (27). It seems unfair to ask all people, rich and poor alike, to be organ donors if the poor or uninsured would not be eligible recipients.

Previous Transplantation

Outcomes for transplanting a second organ after one has failed are substantially lower than in first-time transplants (31, 32). The guideline of promise keeping or loyalty is often used to justify retransplantation; having made a commitment to the patient, the surgeons cannot now abandon him or her. Critics contend, however, that retransplantation might violate duties of stewardship over scarce resources.

Citizenship

Should people who are not long-term US residents receive cadaveric organs in the United States? Particular objections have been directed at foreigners who come to the United States specifically to obtain a transplant (33). It seems unfair, however, to exclude foreign nationals who contribute to the US economy and who would be asked to serve as organ donors.

Ethnic Background

Even though African Americans are more likely than Caucasians to develop chronic renal failure, they are less likely to receive a kidney transplant: they are less likely to be evaluated for transplantation, to be placed on waiting lists, and to find a donor (34). Also, they have longer waiting times on transplantation lists (35).

The United Network for Organ Sharing (UNOS) runs the US system for matching organ donors and recipients. UNOS policy forbids explicit consideration of gender, race, or social factors, such as wealth or celebrity status in allocating cadaveric organs. However, adjustments have been made in the scoring for assigning priority on the waiting list because of implicit bias in the scoring. The point system for prioritizing cadaveric kidneys gives priority to HLA matching, which improves graft and patient survival. Because the prevalence of ABO and HLA antigens differs among ethnic groups, African Americans are less likely to find a highly matched Caucasian donor. Most donors are Caucasian. Thus, allocation rules that optimize graft survival disadvantage African Americans. Changing the point system to decrease the importance of HLA matching improved access of African Americans to renal transplants, while decreasing average graft survival only slightly (34).

Differences in Allocating Various Organs

The ethical guidelines of beneficence and justice are balanced differently for different organs (27). For renal failure, dialysis is an effective alternative to transplantation and the level of HLA matching is a predictor of cadaveric graft survival. Hence, urgency is not considered, and HLA matching is taken into account. In contrast, in liver failure, there is no alternative to transplantation. Highest priority is given to patients in the most critical condition. HLA matching is not considered because it has little impact on outcomes. Different ethical considerations might conflict. For example, liver recipients with the most urgent need have worse outcomes and greater costs than more stable patients.

Patient Behaviors That Cause Disease

Transplantation to persons with alcoholic liver disease has been controversial (36). Earlier concerns that outcomes were worse, in part because of poor adherence to post-transplant care, have not been substantiated. Patients with alcoholic liver disease selected for liver transplantation have outcomes similar to recipients with other liver conditions. However, objections persist that patients should be held responsible for repeatedly and knowingly putting in jeopardy a scarce, lifesaving resource (37). In this view, patients who develop end-stage liver disease "through no fault of their own" should have higher priority than persons with alcoholism (38).

Many physicians object to transplanting a scarce organ that is likely to be rejected because of recipient nonadherence, for example, because of active injection drug use or alcoholism. Critics, however, contend that these judgments might "cloak biases about race, class, social status, and other factors that, if stated openly, would not be tolerated" (39). Furthermore, obstacles to adherence might be overcome with rehabilitation and psychosocial support.

Restrictions on liver transplantation for alcoholics might be considered unfair (36). Alcoholism has genetic and environmental components that are beyond the person's control. Moreover, criteria for disqualification are inconsistent and arbitrary, requirements for 6 months of abstinence are not strongly evidence-based, and treatment for alcohol dependence after the transplant may not be offered (36). Furthermore, judgments of moral responsibility are not made for other illnesses requiring transplantation.

Selected patients with alcoholic liver disease have liver transplant survival rates comparable to those of patients with other liver diseases (40). Most transplant centers require a period of abstinence from alcohol and adherence to medical care for patients with alcoholic liver disease as a surrogate for their post-transplant behavior. Such abstinence may also permit the liver to recover, so that transplantation may no longer be needed. Similarly, substance abusers must undergo drug testing to document abstinence. Patients also should receive referrals for counseling and rehabilitation.

Directed Donation to Strangers

CASE 41.1 | Public solicitation of organs

In 2004, Mr. K, a 32-year-old newlywed man with advanced liver cancer, placed an ad on billboards: "I need a liver. Please help save my life." The next month he received a cadaveric liver that was donated specifically to him. Seven months later he died. It was not known whether his death was due to recurrent liver cancer, complications of transplantation, or other causes.

Cadaveric organs, as well as organs from living donors, may be donated to a specific individual. Most commonly, relatives, friends, or colleagues donate organs. Some donated organs, however, result from solicitations on social networks, websites, or advertisements. The directed donation in Case 41.1 was severely criticized as unfair (41). Some patients with localized liver cancer are given higher priority to increase their chances of transplant before widespread metastases develop. In Case 41.1, because Mr. K already had advanced disease and a poor prognosis, he was low on the waiting list. Advertisements portray a transplantation candidate as deserving an exception to usual allocation criteria. Everyone on the waiting list, however, has powerful stories of why he or she needs a transplant. Advertisements allow wealthy and well-educated persons to jump ahead of people who are higher on the list because they are more likely to die without a liver transplant (42). Organ donation depends on a public perception of fairness, that no candidate is favored because of social standing, fame, or wealth. There are also concerns about whether consent is informed. Potential donors need to be informed of other options, including donating to someone with greater medical need, entering paired exchange program, and not donating. The transplant center and the living donor advocate have an obligation to assure that the potential donor is informed, has no realistic expectations for publicity or monetary gain, and has a full evaluation.

SUMMARY

1. Although transplantation can return patients with end-stage illness to active lives, it raises difficult issues of informed choice, acceptable risk in donation, and fair allocation.
2. Living donation presents particular ethical challenges because healthy donors undergo risks to benefit others and because consent needs to be both informed and free.
3. Transparency and accountability in the transplantation process are essential to maintain public willingness to donate organs.

References

1. Committee on Increasing Rates of Organ Donation. *Organ Donation: Opportunities for Action*. Washington, DC: National Academies Press; 2006.
2. DeVita MA, Caplan AL. Caring for organs or for patients? Ethical concerns about the Uniform Anatomical Gift Act (2006). *Ann Intern Med* 2007;147:876-879.
3. Delmonico FL, Martin D, Dominguez-Gil B, et al. Living and deceased organ donation should be financially neutral acts. *Am J Transplant* 2015;15:1187-1191.
4. Hippen BE. A modest approach to a new frontier: commentary on Danovitch. *Transplant* 2007;84:464-466.
5. Childress JF. How can we ethically increase the supply of transplantable organs? *Ann Intern Med* 2006;145:224-225.
6. Hippen BE, Thistlethwaite JR, Jr., Ross LF. Risk, prognosis, and unintended consequences in kidney allocation. *N Engl J Med* 2011;364:1285-1287.
7. Steinbrook R. Organ donation after cardiac death. *N Engl J Med* 2007;357:209-213.
8. Miller FG, Truog RD. *Death, Dying, and Organ Transplantation*. New York, NY: Oxford University Press; 2012.
9. Dalle Ave AL, Shaw DM, Gardiner D. Extracorporeal membrane oxygenation (ECMO) assisted cardiopulmonary resuscitation or uncontrolled donation after the circulatory determination of death following out-of-hospital refractory cardiac arrest-An ethical analysis of an unresolved clinical dilemma. *Resuscitation* 2016;108:87-94.
10. Overby KJ, Weinstein MS, Fiester A. Addressing consent issues in donation after circulatory determination of death. *Am J Bioeth* 2015;15:3-9.
11. Dalle Ave AL, Shaw DM. Controlled donation after circulatory determination of death. *J Inten Care Med* 2017;32:179-186.
12. Siminoff LA, Alolod GP, Wilson-Genderson M, et al. A comparison of request process and outcomes in donation after cardiac death and donation after brain death: results from a national study. *Am J Transplant* 2017;17:1278-1285.
13. Lee GS, Potluri VS, Reese PP. The case against imminent death donation. *Curr Opin Organ Transplant* 2017;22:184-188.
14. Truog RD, Miller FG, Halpern SD. The dead-donor rule and the future of organ donation. *N Engl J Med* 2013;369:1287-1289.
15. Bernat JL. Life or death for the dead-donor rule? *N Engl J Med* 2013;369:1289-1291.
16. Hart JL, Halpern SD. Between a rock and a hard place: terminating cardiopulmonary resuscitation and preserving opportunities for organ donation. *Ann Intern Med* 2016;165:820-821.
17. Poggio ED, Reese PP. The quest to define individual risk after living kidney donation. *Ann Intern Med* 2018;168:296-297.
18. Neuberger J. Making an offer you can't refuse? A challenge of altruistic donation. *Transpl Int* 2011;24:1159-1161.
19. Hays RE, LaPointe Rudow D, Dew MA, et al. The independent living donor advocate: a guidance document from the American Society of Transplantation's Living Donor Community of Practice (AST LD-COP). *Am J Transplant* 2015;15:518-525.
20. Biller-Andorno N. Voluntariness in living-related organ donation. *Transplantation* 2011;92:617-619.
21. Ross LF. What the medical excuse teaches us about the potential living donor as patient. *Am J Transplant* 2010;10:731-736.
22. Ross LF, Thistlethwaite JR, Jr. Minors as living solid-organ donors. *Pediatrics* 2008;122:454-461.
23. The Declaration of Istanbul on organ trafficking and transplant tourism. *Transplant* 2008;86:1013-1018.
24. Roland ME, Lo B, Braff J, et al. Key clinical, ethical, and policy issues in the evaluation of the safety and effectiveness of solid organ transplantation in HIV-infected patients. *Arch Intern Med* 2003;163:1773-1778.
25. Wallis CB, Samy KP, Roth AE, et al. Kidney paired donation. *Nephrol Dial Transplant* 2011;26:2091-2099.
26. Fox RC, Swazey JP. The *Courage to Fail: A Social View of Organ Transplants and Dialysis*. 2nd ed. Chicago, IL: University of Chicago Press; 1978.
27. Childress JF. Putting patients first in organ allocation: an ethical analysis of the U.S. debate. *Camb Q Healthc Ethics* 2001;10:365-376.
28. Stegall MD. The development of kidney allocation policy. *Am J Kidney Dis* 2005;46:974-975.
29. Washburn K, Pomfret E, Roberts J. Liver allocation and distribution: possible next steps. *Liver Transpl* 2011;17:1005-1012.

30. Committee on Organ Procurement and Transplantation Policy. *Organ Procurement and Transplantation: Assessing Current Policies and the Potential Impact of the HHS Final Rule.* Washington, DC: National Academy Press; 1999.
31. Biggins SW. Futility and rationing in liver retransplantation: when and how can we say no? *J Hepatol* 2012;56:1404-1411.
32. Ubel PA, Arnold RM, Caplan AL. Rationing failure: the ethical lessons of the retransplantation of scarce organs. *JAMA* 1993;270:2469-2474.
33. Hartsock JA, Ivy SS, Helft PR. Liver allocation to non-U.S. citizen non-U.S. residents: an ethical framework for a last-in-line approach. *Am J Transplant* 2016;16:1681-1687.
34. Danovitch GM, Cecka JM. Allocation of deceased donor kidneys: past, present, and future. *Am J Kidney Dis* 2003;42:882-890.
35. Hall YN, Choi AI, Xu P, et al. Racial ethnic differences in rates and determinants of deceased donor kidney transplantation. *J Am Soc Nephrol* 2011;22:743-751.
36. Singhvi A, Welch AN, Levitsky J, et al. Ethical considerations of transplantation and living donation for patients with alcoholic liver diseases. *AMA J Ethics* 2016;18:163-173.
37. Brudney D. Are alcoholics less deserving of liver transplants? *Hastings Cent Rep* 2007;37:41-47.
38. Moss AH, Siegler M. Should alcoholics compete equally for liver transplantation? *JAMA* 1991;265:1295-1298.
39. Robertson JA. Patient selection for organ transplantation: age, incarceration, family support, and other social factors. *Transplant Proc* 1989;21:3431-3436.
40. Bathgate AJ. Recommendations for alcohol-related liver disease. *Lancet* 2006;367:2045-2046.
41. Steinbrook R. Public solicitation of organ donors. *N Engl J Med* 2005;353:441-444.
42. Fortin MC, Buchman D, Wright L, et al. Public solicitation of anonymous organ donors: a position paper by the Canadian society of transplantation. *Transplantation* 2017;101:17-20.

ANNOTATED BIBLIOGRAPHY

1. Committee on Increasing Rates of Organ Donation. Organ Donation: *Opportunities for Action.* Washington, DC: National Academies Press; 2006.
   Consensus report recommending greater use of donation after circulatory determination of death to decrease the gap between the need for transplants and the supply of organs.
2. Childress JF. Putting patients first in organ allocation: an ethical analysis of the U.S. debate. *Camb Q Healthc Ethics* 2001;10:365-376.
   Washburn K, Pomfret E, Roberts J. Liver allocation and distribution: possible next steps. *Liver Transpl* 2011;17:1005-1012.
   Ethical analysis of organ allocation options and application to liver transplantation.
3. Delmonico FL, Arnold R, Scheper-Hughes N, et al. Ethical incentives—not payment—for organ donation. *N Engl J Med* 2002;346:2002-2005.
   Argues that modest financial incentives to reward organ donation are ethically defensible, whereas payment for organs is not.
4. Bakdash T, Scheper-Hughes N. Is it ethical for patients with renal disease to purchase kidneys from the world's poor? *PLoS Med* 2006;3:e349.
   Pro and con debate over paying renal donors.
5. Dalle Ave AL, Shaw DM. Controlled donation after circulatory determination of death. *J Inten Care Med* 2017;32:179-186.
   Analyzes growing approach to increasing the supply of organs for transplantation.
6. Fortin MC, Buchman D, Wright L, et al. Public solicitation of anonymous organ donors: a position paper by the Canadian society of transplantation. *Transplantation* 2017;101:17-20.
   Analysis of ethical concerns solicitation of stranger donors by patients needing a transplant.

Ethical Issues at the Intersection of Public Health and Clinical Medicine

INTRODUCTION

Traditionally, public health has focused on communicable diseases that can be transmitted from an infected patient to someone else. Recently, public health officials have addressed preventing threats to the health of populations resulting from noncommunicable conditions, such as natural disasters and mass shootings. Public health emergencies have required physicians, the public, and public health officials to consider how the doctor–patient relationship may change during a public health emergency. Grave threats to public health may require mandatory public health interventions and raise dilemmas about how to protect the public health, while still respecting individual freedom and treating different groups equitably (1).

This chapter addresses situations where physicians in clinical practice confront ethical dilemmas because some patients might disagree with public health measures. Although there are many difficult ethical issues that public health officials face in their routine work (2), they are beyond the scope of this book.

RECENT PUBLIC HEALTH EMERGENCIES

Inhalational Anthrax from Bioterrorism

In October 2001, Congressional staff who were exposed to anthrax contained in a letter were offered prophylactic antibiotics within hours. In contrast, prophylactic antibiotics for postal workers were delayed, even after several workers were hospitalized with what was found to be anthrax pneumonia. Concerns were raised that predominantly African American postal workers received less timely attention than predominantly Caucasian Congressional staff. As seasonal upper respiratory infections peaked, prescriptions for ciprofloxacin, the recommended drug for inhalational anthrax, increased so much that a shortage was feared. These anthrax outbreaks illustrate how knowledge about an outbreak is incomplete and evolving, that public health measures may be perceived as unfair, and how people may request measures that are not recommended by public health officials.

Severe Acute Respiratory Distress Syndrome

In 2002–2003, the severe acute respiratory distress syndrome (SARS) epidemic illustrated how emerging infections may spread rapidly through international airplane travel. Although quarantine and isolation were widely instituted, their implementation varied markedly in different nations. In China, officials locked patients and health care workers in hospitals that experienced many cases of SARS. In Canada, in contrast, exposed persons were quarantined in their homes.

Extremely Drug-Resistant Tuberculosis

In March 2007, a US citizen with extremely drug-resistant tuberculosis (XDR-TB) flew from the United States to travel to Europe for his wedding and honeymoon, although public health officials recommended that he not travel (3). At the end of his return flight, a federal isolation order was issued. Public health officials in several countries had to contact hundreds of airline passengers who might have been exposed to XDR-TB. The case illustrates how procedures for mandatory public health measures should to be in place before the need for them arises.

Ebola Virus Disease

In 2014–2016, an unprecedented outbreak of Ebola occurred in West Africa, with high fatality rates and widespread public fears because protective measures did not prevent health care workers caring for patients from getting infected, including two highly publicized cases in the United States. When medical personnel who had volunteered to work on the epidemic returned to the United States, states enacted various isolation and quarantine measures, as discussed further in Case 42.1.

HOW DO ETHICAL ISSUES IN PUBLIC HEALTH DIFFER?

Public health differs from clinical practice in several important ethical ways. In clinical practice, physicians are guided by the well-being of individual patients and their informed consent. During a public health emergency, the government may institute mandatory interventions, such as surveillance, testing, quarantine, isolation, and directly observed treatment, which infringe on the liberty and autonomy of individuals.

Focus on Population Outcomes

Public health focuses on the benefits and risks to a population, rather than to individual patients. The goal is to improve aggregate measures of community health, such as reducing the incidence and mortality of SARS, XDR-TB, pandemic influenza, or Ebola. Achieving public health goals may require measures that are not in the best interests of individual persons.

Individual Liberty and Autonomy May Be Overridden

Government officials have the authority to restrict individual liberty in response to a serious, probable threat to the public that the governor declares to be a public health emergency. *Quarantine* restricts the movement of persons who have been exposed or might have been exposed to a communicable disease. The goal is to prevent transmission of infection during the incubation period. Historically, quarantine separated and detained travelers before they were allowed to enter a country. *Isolation* separates persons known to have a communicable disease from other people, during the period when they can communicate the disease to others. These measures place heavy burdens on those who are detained, restricting freedom, violating privacy, disrupting work, child care, and daily activities, and putting them at risk for economic losses and stigmatization (4). Other mandatory medical interventions may also be imposed, such as testing, vaccination, and treatment.

Such mandatory public health measures contrast with ordinary clinical practice, where the patient decides whether to accept or decline an intervention. The ethical tension between the interests of the individual and the well-being of the public should be acknowledged and addressed in public health programs.

Ethical Guidelines for Public Health Restrictions on Liberty

Public officials should follow several requirements when imposing public health interventions that restrict individual liberty (1):

* The threat to public health must be serious and likely.
* The intervention should be effective in addressing the threat.
* The intervention should be the *least restrictive alternative* that addresses the threat.

- *Procedural due process* should be available to persons deprived of their liberty autonomy, including the right to an open, impartial, and timely appeal of their case.
- Policies should be *implemented equitably*. The benefits and burdens of the intervention should be equitably distributed across society, consistent with the epidemiologic features of the threat. In the past, public health measures were sometimes applied in a discriminatory manner, and persons and groups affected by epidemics often were stigmatized (1). Any perception that some groups are being treated unfairly will undermine public support for compulsory measures.

These requirements assure that the balance of benefits to harm in overriding individual autonomy is acceptable and that violations on individual liberty are minimized.

Public health officials may enforce public health mandates through the state's police powers. Public health measures, however, usually require the cooperation of affected persons. The use of force may undermine cooperation. Because isolation and quarantine raise social, financial, and logistical challenges, public health officials generally invoke compulsory measures only as a last resort, after less restrictive measures have failed. It is not necessary to have complete enforcement of isolation or quarantine to stem an outbreak (5).

Change in the Physician's Role

The physician has less decision-making power in a public health emergency. Public health policies during an emergency are set by public health officials, not by individual clinicians, and may be enforced by the state's police powers. Physicians should presume that public measures are reasonable and fair if they are developed through appropriate decision-making procedures. If doctors have questions or disagreements, then they should raise them with officials, rather than try to override guidelines on a case-by-case basis (6).

Weaker Evidence Base

The evidence base for interventions in public health emergencies often is weaker than the evidence base for clinical practice. Knowledge about new conditions is incomplete and increases over the course of an emergency. Public health officials, however, may need to act quickly despite uncertain and incomplete information.

REFUSAL OF PUBLIC HEALTH INTERVENTIONS

During a public health emergency, physicians can expect to encounter patients requesting to be exempted from public health restrictions.

CASE 42.1	Patient who wants to avoid quarantine

Ms. J is a 42-year-old lawyer returned from trip to a West African country where she was far from the region where cases of Ebola virus disease have been identified. The state policy is that all travelers returning from a country where Ebola cases have been recently reported must be medically evaluated by a physician and, if they develop a fever or symptoms, be quarantined for 21 days. Ms. J had a fever of 99.1, which she said was due to a runny nose she had developed just before leaving the country and was almost completely resolved. She had no headache, muscle aches, vomiting, abdominal pain, or diarrhea, the usual symptoms of Ebola. Ms. J asked her physician not to record that she had fever, lest she be placed in quarantine. "I have a lot of meetings that I can't do over the phone. I can postpone them for a few days until I'm completely recovered, but I can't put them off for 21 days. My clients will suffer and my business would go down the tubes if I were put in quarantine. I'm willing to report my condition as often as I need to, and I'll call you immediately if any symptoms develop."

In clinical practice, when patients refuse recommended interventions, their informed wishes are respected. In public health emergencies, however, individual autonomy is not paramount. Compulsory measures such as isolation or quarantine may be imposed to prevent transmission to others and to control an outbreak of a serious infection.

Follow Public Health Guidelines

Physicians need to be clear about the limits of their discretion in public health emergencies. In some situations, doctors may have little control over public health measures. Reporting of emerging infections or infections related to bioterrorism may be mandatory and done directly by hospitals or clinical laboratories, rather than individual physicians. In other situations, isolation and quarantine may be voluntary rather than mandatory.

During the Ebola outbreak of 2014, US public health departments were criticized for enacting isolation and quarantine policies that were not medically or ethically sound. Some individuals whose liberty were restricted were not at risk, because they had no contact with persons who could have been exposed to Ebola. The least restrictive means of isolation or quarantine were not always employed (7). Furthermore, procedural due process, including the opportunity to appeal restrictions on freedom, was lacking (7). Persons subject to isolation or quarantine may need assistance with problems caused by the public health restrictions, such as obtaining food, diapers, or medicine, paying rent or utilities, losing income, or overcoming isolation and stigma (4). In retrospect, some public health measures may have been driven more by public alarm over a new, potentially fatal threat and by political factors, rather than by sound public health advice (7).

Act in the Best Interests of the Patient

Advocate for Changes in Guidelines or Exceptions

Doctors should communicate any disagreements with public health guidelines to responsible officials (6). For example, a policy of quarantine for all persons who have traveled to a particular country may not be warranted if cases of the disease have been reported only from a well-defined area of a large country. Justifications for exceptions need to have a sound public health basis. It would be ethically inappropriate to argue that all people who would suffer economic losses should be exempted from home quarantine.

Establish Common Ground with the Patients

When patients refuse public health measures, physicians can try to find areas of agreement (6). For example, most patients do not want to infect their family and friends. Also, people may suffer greater harm to reputation and business relationships if they flout public health measures and others are infected as a result. Furthermore, cooperating with public health officials may enable patients to have access to special tests or treatments that are not otherwise available.

Mitigate the Risks of Mandatory Public Health Interventions

Physicians can assuage the adverse psychosocial consequences of quarantine or isolation by keeping in telephone contact with patients, addressing their feelings of isolation, and connecting patients with social services agencies and legal assistance as needed.

Avoid Deception

Patients might ask doctors to intentionally misrepresent their condition to exempt them from public health policies. Such deception is ethically problematic for physicians (*see* Chapter 6). Moreover, the harms of such deception outweigh the benefits when potential adverse consequences to other patients and the public health are taken into account.

REQUESTS FOR INTERVENTIONS THAT ARE NOT RECOMMENDED

In public health emergencies, some patients request interventions that are not recommended in public health guidelines. In usual clinical practice, when patients request interventions that are not indicated, physicians attempt to persuade the patient that they are unnecessary (*see* Chapter 32) but generally accede to such requests if the intervention does not present undue risk to the patient. In contrast, during a public health emergency, medically needed interventions may be in short supply and thus not available for persons outside of public health criteria (6).

Protect the Public Health

During public health emergencies, all citizens, including physicians, have a new primary obligation—to act for the common good. Physicians need to consider how a decision for one patient may impact on the spread of an epidemic, on public trust, and on perceptions of fairness.

Follow Public Health Guidelines for Allocation

If effective interventions will be in short supply during severe public health emergencies, allocation and triage will be unavoidable. During an influenza pandemic, the need for triage should be anticipated, as the following case illustrates (8).

CASE 42.2 **Vaccination early in an influenza pandemic**

An influenza pandemic is expected to occur. Vaccine against a pandemic strain are in short supply because it can be manufactured only after an outbreak begins and the specific viral antigens causing the pandemic are known. Moreover, the influenza vaccine manufacturing process is complex, and only a few companies are capable of producing it.

During an outbreak of pandemic influenza, a healthy 67-year-old businessman, who has no chronic illness, asks his primary care physician for vaccination. "We've just bought a new apartment in a senior community and had our first grandchild. I can't afford to get sick, and my family can't afford to lose me." Public health guidelines for vaccination during a pandemic give low priority to healthy people of this age.

Guidelines for influenza vaccine give first priority to persons needed to respond to the pandemic (such as workers in vaccine manufacturing plants and essential medical personnel) and then to those at highest risk for influenza-associated hospitalization and death (9). For example, people 6 months to 64 years of age with two or more high-risk conditions are in the second highest priority group. In a lower priority level are healthy people 65 years and older, who have lower mortality rates due to influenza. These priorities have the utilitarian rationale of saving the greatest number of lives by giving priority to those at highest risk of dying. Scarce resources are allocated to those in greatest need. All human lives are valued equally in this context. In addition, groups who have a poor response to influenza vaccine receive lower priority, such as nursing home residents and patients with severe immunodeficiency. Once the supply of vaccines is adequate, all patients who request a vaccine can receive it.

Other ethical principles, however, may be more appropriate for allocating scarce resources during a public health emergency (10). Some propose a life-cycle allocation procedure (11): every person should have an opportunity to live through all the stages of life. Under this principle, children would have priority over elderly persons. This principle is consistent with the common belief that the death of a child or young adult is more tragic than the death of an elderly person who has already had the opportunity to have a family and career and grow old.

Perceptions of Fairness

Public acceptance of priorities for allocating scarce resources during a public health emergency will be greater if the policies are implemented fairly. If many patients receive interventions even though they are not in high-priority groups, people may conclude that the guidelines are unsound or are being unfairly implemented or that the threat is greater than officials acknowledge. Any perception that public health measures are worsening existing health disparities will undermine willingness to accept restrictions.

Act in the Best Interests of the Patient

Insofar as it is possible, physicians should maintain their usual role of acting in the best interests of the patient after respecting public health guidelines.

Advocate for Appropriate Exceptions to Restrictions

A particular case may be a justified exception to public health policies. An exception should be fair in the sense that it would be appropriate for all patients in a similar clinical situation, not just the particular patient.

Elicit and Address Patient Concerns and Emotions

Physicians should acknowledge that fear and a sense of loss of control are natural human reactions to public health emergencies. Trying to reassure people by telling them not to worry is unlikely to be effective. Patients may be more willing to pay attention to public health after their own needs are acknowledged. It also might be possible to address the patient's concerns and needs without violating public health guidelines.

CASE 42.2 | *Continued*

The physician should try to respond to the patient's concerns through empathic listening and by reminding him of measures that he can take to reduce his risk of being infected, such as social distance. To avoid this scenario, public health officials might limit the number of doses available to physicians' offices, instead distributing most doses through vaccination clinics. This would reduce the need for treating physicians to deny vaccinations to patients with whom they have an ongoing relationship.

CRISIS STANDARDS OF CARE

In disasters, such as natural disasters, pandemics, or bioterrorism, the need for medical care might overwhelm the supply of health care workers, hospital beds, medicines, and critical care equipment and personnel. Scarce life-saving resources might need to be allocated according to emergency public health directives. Ethical norms would not change; health care workers would need to provide the best care they reasonably can under the circumstances. However, legal standards of care may change (12). Emergency care might be triaged, some services might be relocated from emergency departments and hospitals to alternate facilities, and licensing, certification, and credentialing might be altered.

If an influenza pandemic occurs, allocation decisions will also need to be made for antiviral therapy and for mechanical ventilation for persons who develop respiratory failure. Triage of patients with respiratory failure will be particularly difficult because some persons will die because life-sustaining treatment is withheld (10). Chapter 32 discusses the related topic of allocation of resources in ordinary clinical care.

REFUSAL TO CARE FOR CONTAGIOUS PATIENTS

During epidemics, physicians and other health care workers may be at increased risk for contracting the disease. During the SARS epidemic of 2002–2003, a disproportionate percentage of cases and deaths occurred among physicians and nurses caring for hospitalized patients with SARS. During an influenza pandemic, despite receiving vaccines, health care workers are likely to also be at increased risk. Some health care workers might refuse to care for patients because of fears of contracting a fatal illness, uncertain knowledge about how an emerging infection is transmitted, and lack of proven protective equipment. Chapter 24 discusses such refusal to care for patients.

CONTROVERSIES OVER VACCINATIONS

Day-to-day clinical practice also presents public health ethical dilemmas. Although vaccines sharply reduce the mortality and morbidly of childhood contagious diseases such as polio, pertussis, diphtheria, measles, mumps, and rubella, they still raise controversies.

Childhood Immunizations

Some parents object to childhood immunizations because of religious beliefs, concerns about side effects, or opposition to modern medicine. Concerns about adverse effects persist even though scientific studies show no association with vaccines (13). The original study that alleged a link between vaccination and autism was falsified and retracted, and the physician who published the study had his medical license revoked (14). Immunizations are required for children entering school, although many states allow parents to refuse on the basis of religious or personal objections or do not enforce requirements (15). Two states allow exemption only for valid medical reasons and may require a physician to certify the exemption. As discussed in Chapter 6, physicians should not misrepresent the medical condition of the patient, particularly during an outbreak.

If the number of unimmunized children is small and herd immunity exists, physicians should try to understand the parents' concerns, acknowledge that vaccines have risks, and try to persuade them that the benefits outweigh the risks (16, 17). Unvaccinated children, however, can transmit infection to children who cannot be vaccinated (e.g., because of very young age or medical contraindications such as leukemia or cancer) or who have failed to develop an immune response.

Immunizations During an Outbreak

During an outbreak of measles or meningococcal disease, vaccination can reduce the risk of further transmission and protect persons who have a medical contraindication to vaccination. Public health officials may order mandatory vaccination to unvaccinated children who were exposed to an infected person.

Human Papilloma Virus Vaccine

Human papilloma virus (HPV) vaccine dramatizes controversies over the role of adolescents and parents in decisions regarding medical care related to risky behaviors (18–20).

CASE 42.3 | **HPV vaccine**

The HPV vaccine is more than 90% effective in preventing new infections and precancerous cervical lesions caused by the HPV types that it covers. The vaccine is expected to prevent cervical cancer through preventing sexual transmission of HPV types that cause it. Because the vaccine must be given before HPV infection is acquired, the Centers for Disease Control and Prevention recommends routine vaccination for 11- and 12-year-old girls and boys. "Routine" means that the vaccine is administered without extensive discussion or expressed consent unless the parent or child objects.

Proposals for mandatory HPV vaccination as a condition of entry into middle school were driven by a vaccine manufacturer and by advocacy groups funded by it (21). Strong objections were raised to requiring mandatory vaccination for infections that could not be communicated by casual contact in the classroom, because such a policy would undermine parental choice, raise the topic of sexuality before parents thought it was appropriate, and allegedly promote sexual promiscuity (18, 19, 21). Some opponents rejected childhood vaccinations because they mistrusted government requirements. Although the HPV vaccine raises some similar issues as abortion, it need not be as contentious. Unlike abortion, HPV vaccine cannot be considered morally wrong *per se*: its long-term goal is cancer prevention, an undisputable benefit.

Mandatory public health policies can be ethically justified if voluntary measures have failed, no less coercive alternatives exist, the scientific rationale is compelling, and the general public is unknowingly at risk (1). HPV vaccine does not meet these criteria.

How can doctors respond to adolescents and parents who refuse recommendations for HPV vaccination? When disagreements arise in other clinical situations, physicians are encouraged to understand the perspective of patients (in this case, parents) and to respond to their concerns. Such a patient-centered approach might also be useful regarding the HPV vaccination (22).

Some parents question the need for vaccination because they believe their children are not sexually active. Physicians should acknowledge that the HPV vaccine is not needed until shortly before sexual activity starts. It is also not unreasonable to delay vaccination because of uncertainty about long-term effectiveness and rare adverse effects that may not have been identified. Doctors need to help parents consider a different perspective: many children become sexually active before parents would like or approve. By age 14 to 15, 28% of US girls are sexually active. It is understandable that parents fear that children grow up too quickly in the 21st century. Once parents have their underlying concerns acknowledged, they might be more willing to listen to evidence that sexual activity is not greater or earlier in individuals who have received HPV vaccine.

Some adolescents might want to be vaccinated against HPV even though their parents object, and they also might not want to discuss their sexuality candidly with their parents. Adolescents who know they are likely to become sexually active should have the opportunity to benefit from the HPV vaccine. Most states allow adolescents to obtain care for sexually transmitted infections, contraception, and pregnancy care without parental consent (*see* Chapter 37). The ethical rationale is that reducing serious harms to adolescents and respecting their emerging independence outweigh parental interests in control over their children in these situations. Similarly, adolescents should be permitted to receive HPV vaccination without parental permission.

SUICIDE AND SHOOTINGS BY PERSONS WITH SEVERE PSYCHIATRIC ILLNESS

Deaths due to suicide and shootings, carried out by individuals with severe psychiatric illness, have increased recently. Suicides increased significantly in the United States between 1999 and 2016, when nearly 45,000 people took their own lives; firearms accounted for about one half of suicides (23). Since 2007, 173 people have been killed in mass shootings in the United States with firearms similar to military assault weapons. The victims died in schools and public places in locations including Newtown, Connecticut; Las Vegas; San Bernardino, California; and Parkland, Florida (24). In evaluating patients with severe psychological disorders or extreme stress, physicians have an ethical and legal duty to assess and respond to the risk that the patient may inflict serious imminent harm on themselves or other persons (*see* Chapter 40). Physicians may be concerned that asking whether the patient has access to firearms may violate the patient's (or parent's) Second Amendment right to keep and bear arms or contravene federal or state statues restricting required collection of information about firearms. However, there is no legal barrier against physicians asking about firearms when in their professional judgment the question is relevant to the safety of the patient or other people (25). Experienced clinicians recommend helpful approaches and words to use in these discussions, which respect the competent patient's autonomy to choose a safe option for storing guns (26, 27).

SUMMARY

1. In public health emergencies, time for physicians to deliberate about a particular case may be limited.
2. Before a crisis occurs, physicians should think through in advance how they would respond to foreseeable dilemmas arising when patients disagree with public health recommendations or requirements.

References

1. Gostin LO, Wiley LF. *Public Health Law: Power, Duty, Restraint.* 3rd ed. Berkeley, CA: University of California Press; 2016.
2. Barrett DH, Ortmann LW, Dawson A, et al, eds. *Public Health Ethics: Cases Spanning the Globe.* New York: Springer Open; 2016. Available at: https://link.springer.com/book10.1007%2F978-3-319-23847-0.
3. Markel H, Gostin LO, Fidler DP. Extensively drug-resistant tuberculosis: an isolation order, public health powers, and a global crisis. *JAMA* 2007;298:83-86.
4. Smith CL, Hughes SM, Karwowski MP, et al. Addressing needs of contacts of Ebola patients during an investigation of an Ebola cluster in the United States–Dallas, Texas, 2014. *MMWR Morb Mortal Wkly Rep* 2015;64:121-123.
5. Centers for Disease Control and Prevention. *Community Containment Measures, Including Isolation and Quarantine.* 2004. Available at: http://www.cdc.gov/ncidod/sars/quarantine.htm. Accessed May 5, 2008.
6. Lo B, Katz MH. Clinical decision making during public health emergencies: ethical considerations. *Ann Intern Med* 2005;143:493-498.
7. Rothstein MA. Ebola, quarantine, and the law. *Hastings Cent Rep* 2015;45:5-6.
8. Fidler DP, Gostin LO, Markel H. Through the quarantine looking glass: drug-resistant tuberculosis and public health governance, law, and ethics. *J Law Med Ethics* 2007;35:616-628, 512.
9. US Department of Health and Human Services. *NVAC/ACIP Recommendations on Use of Vaccines and NVAC Recommendations on Pandemic Antiviral Drug Use.* 2005. Available at: http://www.hhs.gov/pandemicflu/plan/appendixd.html. Accessed June 2, 2008.
10. White DB, Katz MH, Luce JM, et al. Who should receive life support during a public health emergency? Using ethical principles to improve allocation decisions. *Ann Intern Med* 2009;150:132-138.
11. Emanuel EJ, Wertheimer A. Who should get influenza vaccine when not all can? *Science* 2006;312:854-855.
12. Altvogel B, Stroud C, Hanson SL, et al. *Guidance for Establishing Crisis Standards of Care for Use in Disaster Situations.* 2009. Available at: http://www.nap.edu/catalog.php?record_id=12749&m=0003000740. Accessed June 25, 2018
13. Committee to Review Adverse Effects of Vaccines. *Adverse Effects of Vaccines: Evidence and Causality.* Washington, DC: National Academies Press; 2012.
14. Godlee F, Smith J, Marcovitch H. Wakefield's article linking MMR vaccine and autism was fraudulent. *BMJ* 2011;342:c7452.
15. Opel DJ, Kronman MP, Diekema DS, et al. Childhood vaccine exemption policy: the case for a less restrictive alternative. *Pediatrics* 2016;137:pii: e20154230.
16. Omer SB, Salmon DA, Orenstein WA, et al. Vaccine refusal, mandatory immunization, and the risks of vaccine-preventable diseases. *N Engl J Med* 2009;360:1981-1988.
17. Healy CM, Pickering LK. How to communicate with vaccine-hesitant parents. *Pediatrics* 2011;127: S127-S133.
18. Lo B. HPV vaccine and adolescents' sexual activity. *BMJ* 2006;332:1106-1107.
19. Charo RA. Politics, parents, and prophylaxis–mandating HPV vaccination in the United States. *N Engl J Med* 2007;356:1905-1908.
20. Gostin LO, DeAngelis CD. Mandatory HPV vaccination: public health vs private wealth. *JAMA* 2007;297:1921-1923.
21. Colgrove J, Abiola S, Mello MM. HPV vaccination mandates–lawmaking amid political and scientific controversy. *N Engl J Med* 2010;363:785-791.
22. Lo B. Human papilloma virus vaccination programmes. *BMJ* 2007;335:357-358.
23. Stone DM, Simon TR, Fowler KA, et al. Vital signs: trends in state suicide rates–United States, 1999-2016 and circumstances contributing to suicide - 27 States, 2015. *MMWR Morb Mortal Wkly Rep* 2018;67:617-624.

24. Chivers CJ. *With AR-15s, Mass Shooters Attack With the Rifle Firepower Typically Used by Infantry Troops.* New York Times. February 28, 2018. Available at: https://www.nytimes.com/interactive/2018/02/28/us/ar-15-rifle-mass-shootings.html. Accessed June 26, 2018.

25. Wintemute GJ, Betz ME, Ranney ML. Yes, you can: physicians, patients, and firearms. *Ann Intern Med* 2016;165:205-213.

26. Betz ME. Firearms and suicide: finding the right words. *Acad Emerg Med* 2018;25:605-606.

27. Barnhorst A, Wintemute G, Betz ME. How should physicians make decisions about mandatory reporting when a patient might become violent? *AMA J Ethics* 2018;20:29-35.

ANNOTATED BIBLIOGRAPHY

1. Barrett DH, Ortmann LW, Dawson A, et al, eds. *Public Health Ethics: Cases Spanning the Globe.* New York: Springer Open; 2016. Available at: https://link.springer.com/book10.1007%2F978-3-319-23847-0. Presents an ethical framework for public health policies.

2. Gostin LO, Wiley LF. *Public Health Law: Power, Duty, Restraint.* 3rd ed. Berkeley: University of California Press; 2016. Comprehensive treatise on public health law and policy.

3. Altevogt B, Stroud C, Hanson SL, et al, eds. *Guidance for Establishing Crisis Standards of Care for Use in Disaster Situations.* Washington, DC: The National Academies Press; 2009. http://www.nap.edu/catalog.php?record_id=12749&m=0003000740. Accessed December 9, 2011. Consensus recommendations for modifying legal standards of care in disasters where the need for care overwhelms available resources.

4. Lo B, Katz MH. Clinical decision-making during public health emergencies: ethical considerations. *Ann Intern Med* 2005;143:493-498. Analyzes ethical dilemmas that frontline clinicians face during public health emergencies.

5. White DB, Katz MH, Luce JM, et al. Who should receive life support during a public health emergency? Using ethical principles to improve allocation decisions. *Ann Intern Med* 2009;150:132-138. Analyzes the allocation of scarce ICU beds during an influenza pandemic, highlighting the changes from ordinary clinical care.

6. Rothstein MA. Ebola, quarantine, and the law. *Hastings Cent Rep* 2015;45:5-6. Concise review of the legal and ethical issues regarding quarantine, focusing on the 2014 Ebola cases in the United States.

7. Wintemute GJ, Betz ME, Ranney ML. Yes, you can: physicians, patients, and firearms. *Ann Intern Med* 2016;165:205-213. Argues that the Second Amendment and federal and state laws do not bar physicians from asking about firearms when a patient behaviors indicate an increased risk of violence.

8. Betz ME. Firearms and suicide: finding the right words. *Acad Emerg Med* 2018;25:605-606. A physician describes how working with gun owners helped her learn how to ask suicidal patients about their access to guns.

Ethical Issues in Caring for Diverse Populations

INTRODUCTION

The ethnic and cultural backgrounds of US patients are becoming increasingly diverse. The Census Bureau projects that by 2044 non-Hispanic Caucasians will no longer be a majority of the population. Thus, physicians across the country increasingly will care for patients from many cultural heritages.

Previous chapters discussed specific ethical dilemmas in which culture influences patients' values and medical decisions, including the disclosure of a serious diagnosis (*see* Chapter 6), surrogate decision-making (*see* Chapter 12), and insistence on life-sustaining interventions (*see* Chapter 14). Those chapters focused on how to resolve the specific ethical issue. In this chapter, we address two cross-cutting questions: First, what can physicians be expected to know about the cultural issues that are salient in an ethical dilemma? Second, how can physicians respond to these cultural issues in an ethically appropriate manner?

THE IMPACT OF CULTURE ON CLINICAL CARE

Physicians need to appreciate how a patient's cultural background impacts on how he or she views ethical dilemmas and how they should be resolved.

Understand How Culture Influences Patients

Culture molds a patient's values, beliefs, and expectations about health, medical care, the doctor–patient relationship, and decision-making style (1). It shapes what concerns patients express to physicians and how they describe their symptoms. Patients draw upon cultural values when they weigh risks and benefits and make health care decisions. In many cultures, for example, individual patient autonomy is less important than protecting patients from distress and fulfilling obligations to family members.

Physicians should be familiar with cultures to which many of their patients belong and how these cultures view common ethical dilemmas. Doctors, however, cannot be expected to have in-depth knowledge of every culture. To obtain more information, physicians need to consult the literature and knowledgeable colleagues and cultural interpreters, such as religious leaders. As with other aspects of medicine, training cannot provide physicians all the information they will need during their career.

Avoid Cultural Stereotyping

Physicians must not make assumptions about an individual patient's values on the basis of his or her cultural heritage (1, 2). Culture is not homogeneous or monolithic. Individuals and subgroups within a culture vary in their attitudes and values. In addition to culture, education, socioeconomic status, and many other factors also shape preferences for decision-making and care. Furthermore, cultures change over time, and immigrants typically acculturate to the United States.

Elicit Information About a Patient's Culture

To respect the patient's values and preferences, physicians need to understand how an individual patient is shaped by his or her culture. Open-ended questions help the doctor to do this, regardless of the patient's background (2).

DISCLOSURE OF A SERIOUS DIAGNOSIS TO THE PATIENT

In Chapter 6, Case 6.1 presented a Chinese American patient whose family did not want her to be told she had carcinoma of the colon. In that chapter, the focus was on disclosing and misrepresenting the patient's diagnosis. In this chapter, we present a similar case, involving a patient from a different cultural background, but we focus on the cultural issues in the case.

CASE 43.1	Family requests not to tell the patient he has cancer

> Mr. Z, a 70-year-old Spanish-speaking man with a change in bowel habits and weight loss, is found to have colon cancer. His daughter and son ask the physician not to tell their father he has cancer. Mr. Z lived in Mexico most of his life, where people in his generation are not told they have cancer. His children fear if Mr. Z is told he will lose hope.

What Should a Physician Know About Cultural Issues?

In many cultures, patients traditionally are not told a diagnosis of cancer or other serious illness. In an older study, 87% of European American patients and 89% of African American patients wanted to be told if they have cancer, compared with 65% of Mexican Americans and 47% of Korean Americans (3). In some cultures, disclosure of a grave diagnosis is believed to cause patients to suffer, whereas withholding the diagnosis allows serenity, security, and hope (4). Communicating the diagnosis directly and explicitly might be considered insensitive and cruel. Families might try to protect the patient by communicating the diagnosis nonverbally or indirectly or by taking on the decision-making responsibility (5, 6). They may mistrust or get angry at physicians who tell the patient his or diagnosis.

Traditional cultures reluctant to disclose serious diagnoses may be changing. Attitudes change. On a questionnaire carried out in 2009 in China, 44% of family members of cancer patients said that patients should be told the truth (7). In another study in China, over two thirds of cancer patients said they knew their cancer diagnosis immediately upon diagnosis, and almost half said patients should be told before their family members (8). Of note, studies show that one half or more of patients found out their diagnosis themselves (7, 8). In the United States, physicians should appreciate that patients from traditional cultures may acculturate to prevalent US beliefs about disclosure of diagnoses (9).

How Should Physicians Respond to Cultural Issues?

Regardless of the percentage of persons in a culture who do not want to be told they have cancer, the key ethical issue for doctors is whether the individual patient wants to know the diagnosis (10).

Chapter 6 gives more specific suggestions regarding how to disclose a grave diagnosis to patients (10, 11). It may be appropriate to disclose the diagnosis indirectly and to determine the degree of disclosure the patient desires.

END-OF-LIFE DECISION-MAKING

The following case was discussed in Chapter 13 as Case 13.2, where the focus was on resolving persistent disagreements between health care providers and family (12). In this chapter, we revisit the case from the perspective of race, ethnicity, and culture.

CASE 43.2	**Family insistence that everything is to be done**

Bishop P is a 60-year-old African American man with diabetes, quadriplegia, and refractory infections. He was hospitalized with urosepsis from *Enterobacter cloacae* complicated by hypotension, respiratory failure, renal failure, stroke, and seizures. He required mechanical ventilation and dialysis. Despite multiple courses of antibiotics, his blood cultures remained positive for *E. cloacae*, resistant to all antibiotics. A drug reaction caused a total body rash, and his skin sheared away around his bandages and electrocardiographic leads. The physicians believed that further interventions would be inhumane and disfiguring, that he would not survive the hospitalization, and that attempts at CPR would be futile.

Bishop P's Pentecostal church emphasizes faith healing. Bishop P was obtunded and could not state his preferences for care. His family insisted that everything be done because he believed that all life was sacred.

What Should a Physician Know About Cultural Issues?

African Americans complete advance directives and forego life support less frequently than other patients (13, 14). Physicians need to understand how these decisions are based on cultural values and religious beliefs. For many African Americans, spiritual beliefs provide comfort and a way to cope with illness (13). Many African Americans believe that God is ultimately responsible for health, that the physician is God's instrument, and that prayer can promote healing. Because only God has power to decide life and death, human beings must preserve life until God determines its end. Many African Americans also believe in divine intervention and miracles (15). They may also view illness as something to endure or as a test of their faith. These beliefs tend to make African American patients desire life support (13).

Inequalities and discrimination in health care have shaped the beliefs of many African American patients about end-of-life decisions (16). Many African Americans worry that a Do Not Attempt Resuscitation order or an advance directive might lead to withholding of needed care. African Americans have lower use of hospice services, are more likely to die in the hospital, and are more likely to receive intensive care in the last 6 months of life, compared with Whites (17).

How Should Physicians Respond to Cultural Issues?

Whenever the physician disagrees with a patient or family over care, it is crucial to understand their concerns and values and to identify cultural or religious values that influence their decisions (Table 43-1). Open-ended questions are particularly helpful, no matter what the patient's culture.

Empirical studies suggest how doctor–patient communication affects patient trust.

African Americans are less satisfied with the quality of communication and how health care workers listen and share information compared with Whites (17).

Studies of conversations show that African American patients and patients whose race differs from their physician receive less information from physicians and play a less active role in decisions (18). There might be a vicious cycle in which such patients do not prompt doctors to provide more

TABLE 43-1. Caring for patients from different cultures
Understand the concerns and values of the patient and family.
Use open-ended questions.
Show you understand their perspective through empathic comments.
Summarize what the patient or family has said, and check that it is correct.
Seek help from cultural and religious leaders or cultural interpreters, including caregivers who have experienced caring for similar patients.
Find common ground, such as providing the best care possible and forging an ongoing partnership.

information and doctors, in turn, provide less information. Furthermore, African American patients perceive their physicians as less informative, less partnering, and less supportive than Caucasian patients consider their physicians, and these perceptions are associated with lower trust in physicians (19).

Respond to Religious or Spiritual Statements by Patients and Surrogates

Over three quarters of surrogate decision makers report religion or spirituality as fairly or very important in their life. However, discussion of religious or spiritual considerations occurred in only 16% of family conferences (20). Most often surrogates raised the issue however, physicians generally failed to try to understand surrogates' beliefs, for example, by asking questions about the patient's religion (20). Support for terminally ill patients' spiritual needs by the medical team is associated with greater hospice utilization and less aggressive care at the end of life (21).

CASE 43.2 *Continued*

Knowing that religion is important to Bishop P, the physicians can ask open-ended questions to better understand how religious beliefs impact on his and his family's medical decisions. "How does religion or spirituality play a role in your life?" (11, 22, 23). "In your religion or culture, is there anything that should be done now?"

With an African American family, the physician might also ask open-ended questions focused on mistrust of the medical system. "Many African Americans are concerned that they will not receive the care they need. I wonder what stories you might have heard?" Asking the question with regard to "stories" rather than a patient's personal experience might be useful because people may be deeply influenced by stories about people like them (24). After listening to a family's concerns, physicians should acknowledge that mistrust is an understandable reaction. The physician might say, "I've heard stories like that too." or "I think it would be hard for me to trust doctors and hospitals if I heard stories like that." Physicians should not try to reassure the family immediately that they will provide all appropriate care (25). Premature reassurance might be ineffective or counterproductive, deterring patients from disclosing their concerns and emotions in enough detail that they feel understood (26).

The physician should try to find common ground, for example, by acknowledging that religion is an important source of comfort for patients and their families and that the physicians and nurses are also hoping for a miracle (27).

An innovative program has been developed to address spiritual needs when patients die in critical care units and to humanize their death (28). The Three Wishes program asks the patient, family, and clinicians what they wish for and implements those wishes. Most commonly the wishes were for comfort and peace, connections and reconnections, personal tributes, and spiritual rituals and practices (29). These wishes can be readily implemented.

ADVANCE CARE PLANNING

In some cultures advance care planning is viewed with skepticism.

CASE 43.3 **Reluctance to discuss advance care planning**

Mrs. W is a 73-year-old woman with congestive heart failure who was hospitalized a month ago with a severe exacerbation, which almost required intubation and mechanical ventilation. Mrs. W emigrated from China 30 years ago and speaks Cantonese at home. To try to ascertain her preferences for life support if she suffered another severe exacerbation, the physician tries to raise the topic of advance directives. Mrs. W smiles politely and says simply, "Thank you." When pressed further, she says, "My children will know what to do." Similar attempts to engage in advance planning have also been unproductive in the past.

What Should a Physician Know About Cultural Issues?

Because posthospitalization visits provide an opportunity to discuss advance care planning with patients with congestive heart failure (30), Mrs. W's physician feels frustrated. Physicians need to understand that there may be strong cultural reasons why some patients are reluctant to do so.

Traditional Chinese Americans may prefer discussions of end-of-life care to be indirect and informal (31). For example, they may prefer to express their preferences as a comment on the death of others and in casual family conversations. The culture encourages avoiding topics that make people feel negative. Some believe that talking about death is inauspicious and brings bad luck. Moreover, some may believe that giving explicit directives or designating one person as surrogate might imply that the family cannot be trusted to make the right decisions and might cause the patient and family to lose face. In addition, children's filial responsibility and respect for parents might lead them to insist on maximal life-sustaining interventions to prolong her life. Of course, patients and families vary in their willingness to discuss advance care planning, and this may be related to acculturation.

How Should Physicians Respond to Cultural Issues?

Physicians need to respect the family's sense of responsibility, while ascertaining whether limiting some life-sustaining interventions is consistent with that responsibility as well as the patient's goals and preferences. Once the family realizes that the doctor understands their values, they may be more willing to consider limiting life-sustaining interventions. Conversely, physicians who understand the family's perspective may be more flexible regarding life-sustaining interventions.

Physicians also need to pay attention to ethical issues surrounding the decision to use a professional translator rather than a bilingual health care worker or a family member (32). The decision to call a professional interpreter should depend on the clinical situation, degree of language gap, available resources, and patient preference. Alternatives to professional translators have disadvantages and risks. Although bilingual staff may be convenient and available, their skill at medical translation might be inadequate and not formally assessed. Having family members serve as interpreters may be congruent with patient preferences and cultural expectations. Relatives may also serve as patient advocates and participate in decisions regarding a patient's care. Family members, however, often have inadequate language skills and may interpret selectively to fit their own beliefs. Physicians should offer patients with low English proficiency a professional interpreter at each encounter; this can be carried out through telephone access to translators if in-person translation is not available. Many patients may not appreciate that they have the right to translation services, without charge. Physicians should ensure that patients understand the advantages of professional interpreters and not assume that patients prefer to have family members interpret. Informed patients should decide the type of interpreter.

CASE 43.3 *Continued*

With any patient, it is useful for the physician to summarize what the patient has said and check that it is accurate. "I want to make sure I understand what you want. You want your children to make medical decisions for you if you were too sick to talk to me directly. But rather than talk with them about what kinds of care you want or not want, you trust them to make decisions. Have I understood you correctly?" The doctor might later ask, "Have you talked with your children about how you felt about how a relative or friend died?"

If the physician infers that the children's sense of responsibility to parents is important, she could ask more focused but still open-ended questions: "Some Chinese Americans feel that to respect their parents, they must do all life-sustaining interventions. Have you ever felt like that?" The physician might say later, "No one could be a better daughter than you."

RESPONDING TO CULTURAL PREFERENCES ABOUT CARE

Some patients have culturally based preferences regarding who may provide medical care.

CASE 43.4 | **Request for a Muslim physician**

Mrs. K is a 62-year-old woman who presented to the emergency department (ED) the day after a fall on her back. She has dull low back pain and shooting pains down her right leg, as well as an inability to urinate. An hour ago, she developed substernal chest pain and shortness of breath. Mrs. K was born in Pakistan and has lived in the United States for 15 years. She is a devout Muslim. The ED physician assigned to her care is male.

Mrs. K refuses a physical examination, but is eventually persuaded to allow her heart and lungs to be examined. She refuses a back examination. After coaxing, she allows the physician to examine her spinal column with gloves on. There is spinal tenderness. She adamantly refuses a rectal examination. Because of her chest pain, Mrs. K is placed on a cardiac monitor and bed rest. She becomes agitated and refuses a bedpan and bedside commode. Later, a nurse allows Mrs. K to walk to the bathroom, where she has a large bowel movement. Her workup is negative for spinal or cardiac disease. The following morning her symptoms have greatly improved, and she is discharged.

What Should a Physician Know About Cultural Issues?

In Case 43.4, Mrs. K had strong preferences regarding caregivers, which complicated her care. Many Muslims prefer a Muslim physician of the same gender, or at least a non-Muslim physician of the same gender (33). In Muslim culture, separation of genders is important (34). With a male clinician, Muslim women might object to making direct eye contact, answering direct questions, undressing for examinations, being touched, or removing their headscarves (33). Care from a male physician is not strictly banned because medical necessity allows "things that are ordinarily forbidden to be permissible" (33). Theological debates, however, are not appropriate or constructive at the bedside. Mrs. K refused a bedpan and commode because of her modesty and privacy, which are highly valued in Muslim culture (33). Standards of modesty and privacy vary across cultures (35). In a patient with possible cardiac ischemia, both the exertion of going to the bathroom and the stress of not having a bowel movement might be dangerous. In this case, given Mrs. K's distress, overriding the routine ED procedures to allow her to walk with assistance to the bathroom was appropriate.

How Should Physicians Respond to Cultural Issues?

There are good reasons to accommodate a patient's preferences regarding the type of physician. The doctor–patient relationship is highly personal, and trust is important. Since 9/11, many Muslims report they have faced stereotyping, stigma, and discrimination and have refrained from seeking care (34, 36). Trying to meet Mrs. K's preferences respects her as a person and her cultural heritage and fosters better health outcomes.

The legal concept of reasonable accommodation provides a helpful conceptual framework. Physicians should take reasonable steps to accommodate Mrs. K's preferences regarding a female physician, even if standard hospital procedures need to be modified.

The suggestions in Table 43-1 can help physicians understand the patient's concerns and develop practical plans to address them.

CASE 43.4 *Continued*

Physicians who have little experience with Muslim patients might not anticipate Mrs. K's prefer-ences for a female Muslim physician or the importance of toilet privacy. After seeing that she is refusing routine medical procedures, the physician should try to elicit the reasons for her refusal through open-ended questions: "I want to try to take care of your medical problems. Is there any-thing I need to know to give you the best care we can?" Open-ended questions to elicit the patient's expectations and concerns are an effective communication technique, regardless of the patient's cultural background.

After learning of Mrs. K's strong preference for a female physician, the doctors might informally agree among themselves to accommodate her wishes. If there is a female physician working in the ED that shift, she could take over Mrs. K's care with little burden on the ED and its staff. If a female physician is not available, then the treating physician should explain the situation and ask the pa-tient and family how the patient would like to proceed. The physician might also ask permission to talk with the patient's imam for suggestions. Such joint problem-solving helps build a partnership to care for the patient. The patient or family may offer suggestions, such as perhaps having the physician wear gloves or placing her behind a drape during an examination. These measures to ac-commodate Mrs. K's preferences place only small burdens on the ED staff. There are limits, however, on what physicians or a hospital could reasonably be asked to do. The ED is not required to call in a female physician from home or from another service or disrupt the care of other patients in ways that place them at serious risk or inconvenience.

Racist Requests by Patients

Some requests for a specific type of health care worker may be ethically problematical (37). Racist and demeaning comments by patients may be increasing in recent years as such behavior has become more common in US society in general.

CASE 43.5 **Racist refusal of a physician**

Mr. D is a 52-year-old Caucasian man who came to the ED because of crushing substernal chest pain and is found to have ST elevation in the lateral leads. He will be admitted to the cardiac care unit (CCU). The CCU physician, an African American woman, comes to the ED to admit him. He refuses to allow her to care for him, calling her insulting terms that are racially and sexually offensive and loudly declaring his white supremacist beliefs.

Patients have health care needs that physicians and hospitals are in a unique position to address. Because patients depend on them, the professional ideal is that physicians should care for patients in medical need and place the patient's best interests ahead of their own interests. For example, in wartime, military physicians are expected to attend to the medical needs of enemy combatants, even those who espouse and articulate offensive ideologies. Hospitals have an obligation to stabilize pa-tients who present to their ED with an emergency condition.

Patients have the right to refuse care from a physician they do not want. Case 43.5 raises the issues of the medical risk to a patient who refuses care from a specific physician because of offensive racist and sexual stereotypes and whether a hospital should call in a physician who is acceptable to the patient.

Physicians and other health care workers have rights as well. Race, color, religion, and national origin are protected under the US Constitution, and from an ethical perspective health care workers should not be discriminated against because of these characteristics. Furthermore, health care work-ers who are caring for difficult patients should not be subjected to degrading verbal or physical abuse in their workplace (37). Patients should not insult or disparage health care workers who are trying to care for them. Health care workers may decide among themselves to trade patient assignments, but the hospital should not require them to do so. The physician in Case 43.5 should make sure that the patient understands the urgency of the situation and the need for timely care. She should also present the options the patient may choose, while also setting limits on unacceptable behavior and words (37). Later, the physician should offer to help transfer the patient after he is stabilized and to try to accommodate the request if possible the next day.

Health care institutions should set limits on unacceptable patient conduct, although patients are free to hold whatever beliefs they wish. Even if a different physician is available and willing, such limits should be set. This is usually best done by a hospital administrator, the chief of service, or the attending physician. The institution also should provide support for staff who are the targets of racist or sexual comments, particularly trainees.

CASE 43.5 | *Continued*

The CCU physician might say, "I am the doctor on call tonight in the CCU. You may be having a heart attack and you need treatment immediately. If you want to be treated in this hospital tonight, I have to ask you not to use that kind of language. I can try to transfer you to another heart doctor tomorrow if you wish. If you want to leave this hospital and seek care elsewhere, you are free to do so, but delaying care would put you at serious medical risk." The ED physician or hospital administrator on call should reinforce these conditions, particularly if Caucasian or male. If Mr. D agrees to receive treatment, the physician should strive to provide high-quality and compassionate care (38).

Some requests for physician reassignment may be clinically and ethically appropriate (37). Requests by patients from minority groups for a physician of similar ethnic background and language may promote greater trust and satisfaction. Some veterans with posttraumatic stress disorder may refuse treatment by a physician of the same ethnic background as former enemy combatants.

Many physicians would seek to accommodate Mrs. K, the Muslim patient in Case 43.4, but not Mr. D, the white supremacist patient in Case 43.5. Can these cases be ethically distinguished? Physicians should not try to judge the sincerity or validity of a patient's beliefs or determine if some beliefs are more deserving of respect. Physicians should focus on actions and words. Mrs. K in Case 43.4 does not insult or disparage non-Muslim physicians. However, had she framed her refusal of care in terms of a hatred of infidels and used racial insults to the staff, the situation would be similar to Case 43.5.

Female Genital Cutting

Ritual genital cutting of female minors (a more neutral term than female genital mutilation) is widely practiced in Africa and the Middle East (39). The term refers to a range of procedures, including excision of the clitoris and labia minora and infibulation, in which labial surfaces are stitched together to cover the urethra and vaginal introitus. Parents believe that it will integrate their daughter's into their culture, protect her virginity and family honor, and make her more desirable a wife. Serious complications include infection, painful intercourse, infertility, prolonged labor, and difficult delivery (40). In the United States, some parents ask physicians to perform female genital cutting using sterile conditions and anesthesia, perhaps making a ritual minimal incision. Otherwise, they might have the procedure done in their native country or by someone without medical training.

The issue is controversial because it raises issues of moral relativism, cultural imperialism, the role of women in society, the impracticality of putting on children and adolescents the burden of saying no, and the challenges of changing broadly accepted cultural practices. Discussions are heated, with critics calling the practice a human rights violation and defenders saying that charges are hyperbolic and sensationalized (41). Moreover, some question why circumcision on male infants for cultural or religious reasons is widely accepted while the arguably analogous procedure on girls is not.

Under US federal law, all types of female genital cutting on minors are prohibited as a criminal offenses. In declining these procedures, physicians should express respect for parents and their cultural, religious, and ethnic traditions (39). Cessation of this practice will likely require community educational programs led by immigrant women (42).

SUMMARY

1. Physicians should be sensitive to how culture may influence a patient's values and decisions.
2. Physicians can use open-ended questions to elicit from patients how their cultural backgrounds influence their expectations and values regarding ethical dilemmas.
3. Doctors should then address cultural differences in a respectful manner.

References

1. Kleinman A, Benson P. Anthropology in the clinic: the problem of cultural competency and how to fix it. *PLoS Med* 2006;3:e294.
2. Betancourt JR. Cultural competence and medical education: many names, many perspectives, one goal. *Acad Med* 2006;81:499-501.
3. Blackhall LJ, Murphy ST, Frank G, et al. Ethnicity and attitudes toward patient autonomy. *JAMA* 1995;274:820-825.
4. Gordon DR, Paci E. Disclosure practices and cultural narratives: understanding concealment and silence around cancer in Tuscany, Italy. *Soc Sci Med* 1997;46:1433-1452.
5. Surbone A. Truth telling to the patient. *JAMA* 1992;268:1661-1662.
6. Surbone A. Telling the truth to patients with cancer: what is the truth? *Lancet Oncol* 2006;7:944-950.
7. Wang DC, Peng X, Guo CB, et al. When clinicians telling the truth is de facto discouraged, what is the family's attitude towards disclosing to a relative their cancer diagnosis? *Support Care Cancer* 2013;21:1089-1095.
8. Huang B, Chen H, Deng Y, et al. Diagnosis, disease stage, and distress of Chinese cancer patients. *Ann Transl Med* 2016;4:73-82.
9. Smith AK, Sudore RL, Pérez-Stable EJ. Palliative care for Latino patients and their families: Whenever we prayed, she wept. *JAMA* 2009;301:1047-1057.
10. Kagawa-Singer M, Blackhall LJ. Negotiating cross-cultural issues at the end of life: "You got to go where he lives." *JAMA* 2001;286:2993-3001.
11. Barclay JS, Blackhall LJ, Tulsky JA. Communication strategies and cultural issues in the delivery of bad news. *J Palliat Med* 2007;10:958-977.
12. Alpers A, Lo B. Avoiding family feuds: responding to surrogates' demands for life-sustaining treatment. *Journal of Law, Medicine & Ethics* 1999;27:74-80.
13. Johnson KS, Elbert-Avila KI, Tulsky JA. The influence of spiritual beliefs and practices on the treatment preferences of African Americans: a review of the literature. *J Am Geriatr Soc* 2005;53:711-719.
14. Raghavan M, Smith AK, Arnold RM. African Americans and end-of-life care #204. *J Palliat Med* 2010;13:1382-1383.
15. Widera EW, Rosenfeld KE, Fromme EK, et al. Approaching patients and family members who hope for a miracle. *J Pain Symptom Manage* 2011;42:119-125.
16. Crawley LM, Marshall PA, Lo B, et al. Strategies for culturally effective end-of-life care. *Ann Intern Med* 2002;136:673-679.
17. Johnson KS. Racial and ethnic disparities in palliative care. *J Palliat Med* 2013;16:1329-1334.
18. Gordon HS, Street RL, Jr., Sharf BF, et al. Racial differences in doctors' information-giving and patients' participation. *Cancer* 2006;107:1313-1320.
19. Gordon HS, Street RL, Jr., Sharf BF, et al. Racial differences in trust and lung cancer patients' perceptions of physician communication. *J Clin Oncol* 2006;24:904-909.
20. Ernecoff NC, Curlin FA, Buddadhumaruk P, et al. Health care professionals' responses to religious or spiritual statements by surrogate decision makers during goals-of-care discussions. *JAMA Intern Med* 2015;175:1662-1669.
21. Balboni TA, Paulk ME, Balboni MJ, et al. Provision of spiritual care to patients with advanced cancer: associations with medical care and quality of life near death. *J Clin Oncol* 2010;28:445-452.
22. Lo B, Ruston D, Kates LW, et al. Discussing religious and spiritual issues at the end of life: a practical guide for physicians. *JAMA* 2002;287:749-754.

23. Lo B, Kates LW, Ruston D, et al. Responding to requests regarding prayer and religious ceremonies by patients near the end of life and their families. *J Palliat Med* 2003;6:409-415.
24. Holloway KFC. *Passed On: African American Mourning Stories.* Durham, NC: Duke University Press; 2003.
25. Lo B, Quill T, Tulsky J. Discussing palliative care with patients. *Ann Intern Med* 1999;130:744-749.
26. Maguire P, Faulkner A, Booth K, et al. Helping cancer patients disclose their concerns. *Eur J Can* 1996;32A:78-81.
27. Cooper RS, Ferguson A, Bodurtha JN, et al. AMEN in challenging conversations: bridging the gaps between faith, hope, and medicine. *J Oncol Pract* 2014;10:e191-195.
28. Cook D, Swinton M, Toledo F, et al. Personalizing death in the intensive care unit: the 3 Wishes Project: a mixed-methods study. *Ann Intern Med* 2015;163:271-279.
29. Swinton M, Giacomini M, Toledo F, et al. Experiences and expressions of spirituality at the end of life in the intensive care unit. *Am J Respir Crit Care Med* 2017;195:198-204.
30. Rogers JG, Patel CB, Mentz RJ, et al. Palliative care in heart failure: the PAL-HF randomized, controlled clinical trial. *J Am Coll Cardiol* 2017;70:331-341.
31. Yonashiro-Cho J, Cote S, Enguidanos S. Knowledge about and perceptions of advance care planning and communication of Chinese-American older adults. *J Am Geriatr Soc* 2016;64:1884-1889.
32. Schenker Y, Lo B, Ettinger KM, et al. Navigating language barriers under difficult circumstances: a conceptual and practical approach for clinicians. *Ann Int Med* 2008;149:264-269.
33. Padela AI. Can you take care of my mother? Reflections on cultural competency and clinical accommodation. *Acad Emerg Med* 2007;14:275-277.
34. Inhorn MC, Serour GI. Islam, medicine, and Arab-Muslim refugee health in America after 9/11. *Lancet* 2011;378:935-943.
35. Fiester A. What "patient-centered care" requires in serious cultural conflict. *Acad Med* 2012;87:20-24.
36. Samari G, Alcala HE, Sharif MZ. Islamophobia, health, and public health: a systematic literature review. *Am J Public Health* 2018;108:e1-e9.
37. Paul-Emile K, Smith AK, Lo B, et al. Dealing with racist patients. *N Engl J Med* 2016;374:708-711.
38. Tweedy DS. A case of racism and reconciliation. *Ann Intern Med* 2012;156:246-247.
39. Committee on Bioethics, Davis DS. Ritual genital cutting of female minors. *Pediatrics* 2010;125:1088-1093.
40. Berg RC, Underland V, Odgaard-Jensen J, et al. Effects of female genital cutting on physical health outcomes: a systematic review and meta-analysis. *BMJ Open* 2014;4:e006316.
41. Public Policy Advisory Network on Female Genital Surgeries in Africa. Seven things to know about female genital surgeries in Africa. *Hastings Cent Rep* 2012;42:19-27.
42. Appiah KA. *The Honor Code.* New York: W.W. Norton; 2010.

ANNOTATED BIBLIOGRAPHY

1. Schenker Y, Lo B, Ettinger KM, et al. Navigating language barriers under difficult circumstances: a conceptual and practical approach for clinicians. *Ann Int Med* 2008;149:264-269.
   Analyzes ethical and practical dilemmas regarding translation services.
2. Swinton M, Giacomini M, Toledo F, et al. Experiences and expressions of spirituality at the end of life in the intensive care unit. *Am J Respir Crit Care Med* 2017;195:198-204.
   Asking patients dying in critical care units, their family, and clinicians what they wish for and implementing those wishes addresses spiritual needs and humanizes their deaths.
3. Paul-Emile K, Smith AK, Lo B, et al. Dealing with racist patients. *N Engl J Med* 2016;374:708-711.
   Suggests how health care workers should respond when a patient refuses care from an individual physician for racial, ethnic, or cultural reasons.
4. Inhorn MC, Serour GI. Islam, medicine, and Arab-Muslim refugee health in America after 9/11. *Lancet* 2011;378:935-943.
   American Academy of Pediatrics Board of Directors. Ritual genital cutting of female minors. *Pediatrics* 2010;126:191.
   Thoughtful articles that illustrate the value of search for articles in the medical literature on specific ethical dilemmas in cross-cultural care.

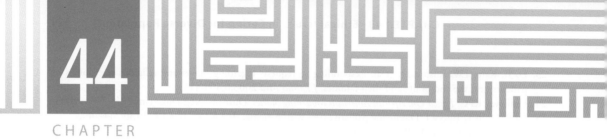

Ethical Issues with Digital Health Information

INTRODUCTION

Digital technologies offer the promise of more efficient and higher quality health care. Electronic health records (EHRs), e-mail, the Internet, and social media are increasingly common in medicine, as in other areas of life. These digital technologies open the possibility of using big data and artificial intelligence to improve health outcomes (*see* Chapter 46).

OVERARCHING ETHICAL FRAMEWORK FOR DIGITAL HEALTH INFORMATION

Several guiding principles can help physicians use digital health information appropriately (1).

First, physicians should balance the benefits and risk of digital health information and take steps to enhance the benefits and minimize the risks.

Second, physicians should respect patients and their autonomy. Physicians should respond constructively and supportively to patients using digital information and applications and use them to strengthen the doctor—patient relationship and improve health outcomes.

A particularly important aspect of respecting patients is protecting their privacy and confidentiality. Breaches of digital health information usually involve more patients and larger amounts of personal information than breaches of paper records. The HIPAA Health Privacy Rule protections do not apply to many organizations that collect, store, use, and share individualized health information, including Internet providers, search engines, and websites; e-mail, social networking, mobile health, and recreational and ancestry genomics applications; credit card companies; and retail stores, including pharmacies (2). For example, purchases of health products, Internet searches on health topics, and posts regarding health on Facebook leave a digital trail linked to the individual. Users agree to a company's privacy policies using a click-through button as a condition of using an application, product, service, or website without charge. Typically these policies allow companies to collect, use, and share information, for example, to send individualized advertisements or to sell data to data mining companies. Some companies now allow users take some steps to opt out of such tracking. But even if these companies collect, store, and share data without explicit identifiers, it is straightforward, with enough computing power, to reidentify individuals by combining data from additional sources (3).

Third, physicians should work toward distributing the benefits of digital health information more equitably and overcome the "digital divide" that may worsen health disparities. For example, Latino and African American patients reported barriers to using a patient portal to access their electronic health records, including a preference for in-person, caring interactions with a physician, as well as a lack of technical proficiency and medical literacy (4). Addressing these barriers requires physicians to work toward organizational changes.

ELECTRONIC HEALTH RECORDS

EHRs, which are increasingly used in clinical medicine, can improve care by making a patient's medical information immediately available to physicians and enabling quality-of-care initiatives.

Security of EHRs

Large security breaches, in which unencrypted personal information has been compromised, have been reported at health care organizations, other businesses, and Internet providers. There is a tradeoff between data security and access by health care workers to clinical information needed to provide care. Off-site access to EHRs facilitates convenience and continuity of care but also poses risk if physicians' unencrypted laptops and mobile devices are lost or stolen. Data that have been encrypted according to federal standards is presumed to be unreadable, unusable, and undecipherable. Security measures are intended to increase patient trust in EHRs and willingness to allow information in EHRs to be shared with other providers and used for other purposes, such as research and quality improvement.

Patient Restrictions on Access to EHR Information

EHRs can be configured to give health care workers different levels of access to patient information. Administrative and billing personnel do not need access to clinical information to do their tasks. Furthermore, EHRs can also block certain health information from physicians and nurses or reveal it only to certain health care workers (5). Patients may want to restrict access to personal health information that they consider very sensitive or not relevant to the problem at hand, for example, information regarding alcohol, marijuana, or substance use, mental health, or a previous abortion. Alternatively, they may disclose information to a physician orally but ask them not to place it in the medical record.

When patients request that information not be shared with other providers, the physician and health care system need to balance respect for patient autonomy to control information about intimate aspects of their life with protecting the patient from unintended harm (6). The doctor should make sure the patient appreciates how omitting information from the EHR might compromise care (6, 7). For example, doctors, nurses, and pharmacists caring for the patient need to know all of the patient's medications or previous test results. Failure to have such information may result in suboptimal care, including delays or errors in diagnosis, unnecessary repetition of tests, trials of therapies that have already failed, or adverse drug interactions. Knowing a patient's psychiatric medicines, for example, will help physicians evaluate apparently unrelated complaints such as palpitations, fatigue, or gastrointestinal distress. Not duplicating previous imaging studies avoids unnecessary risks of contrast media or radiation exposure. The doctor should also explain confidentiality protections that are in place, for example, restricting access to health care workers who need to know a patient's personal health information. Usually, the patient then agrees to share his or her information after such discussions.

If patients decide to restrict access to some information in the EHR, they assume responsibility for the consequences of their choices and the risk of substandard care resulting from the lack of information that they decided to hide or omit from the EHR (7).

Some EHRs allow providers to activate a "Break the Glass" button to override patients' restrictions on information, with an audit trail of the information obtained (5). In one system, the most common reason for overriding restrictions on information was concern about opioid use disorder when prescribing opioids.

Sharing Electronic Patient Information Among Providers

Different doctors and hospitals caring for a patient need to share information to coordinate care. HIPAA allows the use and disclosure of personal health information for the purposes of treatment, billing, and administration without patient authorization (8). When a doctor or hospital shares information about a patient with another treatment provider, patient permission is commonly requested as a matter of respect or defensive medicine, but it is not required.

Electronic health information exchanges are agreements among health care providers to exchange health care information electronically. Health information exchanges enhance coordination of care, for example, between acute care hospital and home care services or long-term care, reduce duplicative care by allowing access to records, including imaging studies, from another health care system where the patient received care, and are more efficient than photocopying, faxing, or mailing medical records (9).

In health information exchanges, shared information might also be used for quality improvement, research, or public health. Serious adverse events identified after the drug was approved for market led the FDA to withdraw approval of rofecoxib. The FDA also created the Sentinel program to use data from medical records to investigate postmarketing adverse events (10). Rather than centralizing patient-specific data, Sentinel uses a distributed data network. Each hospital or health care plan retains its own data and respond to specific data queries by analyzing their data and submitting their de-identified results.

Personal Health Records

Personal health records (PHRs) are controlled by the patient rather than by the physician, clinic, or hospital. They are also known as patient-controlled health records. Patients assemble their health information from the physicians, clinics, and hospitals that have cared for them, add patient-measured outcomes (such as home blood pressure and glucose measurements, functional status, and quality of life), and determine what information they wish to share with various providers.

PHRs have several potential advantages (11). They are more comprehensive than the information held by a single health care provider. They enhance patient autonomy by giving patients more information, responsibility, and control over their health care. By including patient-generated data, PHRs focus physicians on patient-centered outcomes. However, PHRs have not been widely accepted by patients.

HEALTH INFORMATION ON THE INTERNET

Patients commonly use the Internet for information related to their health issues. Physicians need to keep in mind the benefits and risks of such information.

Prospective Benefits

The Internet makes health information searchable and accessible to patients at any time. After obtaining information on the Internet, patients generally feel more knowledgeable, in control, confident, and willing to ask questions (12, 13). Furthermore, social networking sites organized around specific conditions may provide psychosocial support to patients and help them learn how to cope with their illness.

Risks and Burdens

Inaccurate or Misleading Information

Medical information and advice on the Internet is not screened, edited, curated, or rated for accuracy; physicians find such information is of variable quality. It is difficult for patients to judge the quality of medical websites or the information presented (14). Furthermore, patients may have difficulty putting information into the context of their individual clinical situation. Personal narratives and dramatic cases on the Internet may lead patients to overestimate the frequency of rare events.

Medical Risks

Some physicians fear that Internet information will lead patients to request medical interventions that are not indicated. However, in one study 71% of patients who brought information from the Internet to physicians did so simply to obtain the physician's opinion, not to insist on a test, medication, or referral (13). Whether or not patients received the requested intervention did not affect their rating of the doctor–patient relationship (13). Thus, at the point of clinical services, most patients accept the physician's recommendations.

Impact on the Doctor–Patient Relationship

Patients are concerned about how physicians will react to the knowledge they acquired through the Internet (12): patients were afraid doctors would feel challenged if they directly revealed their on-line findings to them. Generally patients feel that bringing health information from the Internet to the physician had a positive impact on the doctor–patient relationship, provided the physician had communication skills and did not appear challenged (13). From the perspective of physicians, those doctors who perceived that the patient was challenging their authority were more likely to believe the doctor–patient relationship had deteriorated (15).

Recommendations for Physicians

Doctors should promote the benefits of these information innovations and minimize their risks and burdens (1).

Promote Informed Decision-Making by Patients

Physicians and health care organizations should encourage patients to seek information about their condition, help them assess the quality of medical information on the Internet, put it in context, and recommend reliable websites.

Recognize and Minimize Counterproductive Reactions

Doctors need to recognize that they might feel threatened when patients bring them health in-formation from the Internet. Physicians should not let their own emotions compromise patient care. In other situations, doctors learn not to overreact and to form alliances with patients rather than polarize the situation (*see* Chapter 14). If a patient requests a medically inappropriate in-tervention because of information from the Internet, the physician should explore the concerns underlying the request, explain why it is not appropriate, and negotiate a mutually acceptable plan of care.

E-MAIL COMMUNICATION PATIENTS

E-mail allows patients and physicians to communicate asynchronously outside of clinic hours and avoid "telephone tag." Patients can ask questions, report their condition, and request appointments, referrals, and medication refills. Doctors can communicate with patients, write orders, and route messages to other staff without interrupting their workflow. If the e-mail platform is linked to an EHR, doctors can document their actions. However, e-mail communication with patients also pres-ents risks and challenges, as the following case illustrates.

CASE 44.1 | **New chest pain**

A 63-year-old woman e-mailed her physician, "I was awakened this morning with persistent dis-comfort in the middle of my chest (which I had once a few years ago). It has since gone away. Given the fact that my brother had to get five stents last year, I wonder if I should be evaluated. I am hop-ing to be seen today." The message was not opened until 2 hours after it was sent.

In responding to e-mails, physicians should follow the same clinical and ethical guidelines that they follow in face-to-face visits, taking into account the characteristics of the medium.

First, physicians should respect patients by ascertaining their concerns and needs, educating them, forming a mutually acceptable plan of care, and protecting their privacy and confidentiality.

Second, doctors should act in the patient's best interests. Some clinical situations require real-time conversation and attention to the patient's emotions and are better handled through phone calls or face-to-face conversations than through e-mail. An example is telling a patient that an imaging study shows probable cancer. In conversations, nonverbal communication such as the tone and loudness of voice, pauses, and interruptions can transmit valuable information. In face-to-face or video meetings, facial expression, eye contact, body position, and head nods convey meaning and emotion.

CASE 44.1 | *Continued*

Because this patient may have new-onset coronary artery disease, she needs to be triaged to a possible paramedic call, emergency department visit, or same-day clinic visit. When her e-mail was not answered promptly, the patient phoned the clinic and was connected with the nurse, who determined that she could be scheduled for an appointment for that afternoon. At that visit, the physician determined that the pain was not typical of angina, confirmed that the EKG was normal, and ordered an urgent treadmill test.

The clinic realized it needed to set up procedures to screen e-mails in real time, identify urgent messages, and respond to them promptly. Also, it began to send automated e-mail responses to patients telling them when to expect a reply and explaining how to communicate urgent concerns.

Despite their use of text messaging and social media, patients prefer not to use these tools for communicating with their physicians regarding test results or discussing goals such as an exercise plan. As an alternative to face-to-face meeting, almost one half of respondents supported using email for these purposes, but preferred phone calls even more (16).

PHYSICIAN USE OF SOCIAL MEDIA

Physicians post information on social media, including blogs, websites, and social networks at similar rates as the general population. Medical students and residents use social media more than older physicians. Some materials that physicians post violate professional and ethical standards, for example, because they breach patient confidentiality, use offensive or discriminatory language regarding patients, and picture the physician intoxicated, using illegal drugs, or in sexually suggestive poses (17). Postings that contain sufficient detail to identify a patient or allow others to infer patient identify violate confidentiality; they should be "never" events (18). Furthermore, physicians might use online dating sites where they reveal highly personal information that would be considered inappropriate in face-to-face or telephone encounters. On social media, however, people may be less inhibited.

Physicians should keep in mind the following guidelines (17, 18). First, online postings on the Internet and social networking sites are accessible to the public and patients unless physicians consistently use highly restrictive privacy settings. Physicians should expect some patients to Google them and forward information to others. Once posted, online materials are public and permanent (18). Second, behaviors and words that are inappropriate in face-to-face encounters should also be avoided on the Internet. Patients and potential patients who view problematic materials might question the physician's judgment, common sense, or character.

LEARNING HEALTH SYSTEMS

In learning health systems, the large amounts of clinical, administrative, and billing data that are collected routinely in the delivery of health care are analyzed to improve the quality, value, and efficiency of care (19, 20). These data can be analyzed in real time. In learning health systems, the care of one patient is informed by the care of similar patients in the past, and in turn the patient's care feeds into a system of improving the care of future patients (20).

Activities of Learning Health Systems

Learning health systems can address a variety of questions, such as (19):

- What is the prevalence of undiagnosed diabetes, central-line blood infections, unvaccinated patients at risk for influenza, or patients who have not had recommended cancer screening?
- Does the rate of meeting evidence-based practice guidelines for treatment or prevention vary at different sites in the system? How do these rates compare with those of peers? Is it decreasing or increasing?
- Can interventions be implemented to improve the quality of care, for example, to bring management of chronic conditions such as diabetes or asthma in accordance with evidence-based practice guidelines? Similarly, what interventions can improve the rate of recommended cancer screening?

To address these questions, learning health systems use a variety of study designs, including observational studies, comparative effectiveness studies, pragmatic clinical trials, and cluster randomized trials. To set up a learning health system, organizations need to commit resources for data collection and analytics, an institutional culture that prizes quality of care and change, and support for specific projects.

Ethical Issues in Learning Health Systems

Learning health care systems raise several ethical issues (21).

Notification About Learning Health Systems

What should patients be told about how routinely collected patient-level data are used to improve the quality of care? In the spirit of transparency and patient engagement, patients should be informed that such activities are carried out. Most patients are likely to support the goal of improving care, which, after all, is in their own best interest. However, some patients may raise concerns or objections, for example, about confidentiality. Although some analyses may be carried out using de-identified data, individual patients are identified and targeted in other projects. Furthermore, there may be concerns about sharing of data outside the health system. The health care organization should set up a process to respond to patient questions and concerns.

Informed Consent for Learning Health System Activities

Should patients be asked to consent to having data collected during their care used in a learning health system (22)? Should requirements for consent depend on the nature of the specific activity?

First, learning health system activities differ from both clinical care and research. Unlike clinical care, the goal of learning health care activities is not to benefit the individual patient but to benefit the group of patients receiving care in the health care system. However, learning health care activities also differs from clinical research in that there is generally a much tighter connection between projects and the implementation of changes to improve care. Although the goal of research is generalizable new knowledge, the goal of learning health system activities is to improve care with a health care system or a unit of the health care system. The findings of a learning health care activity may not be applicable to other health care organizations or even to other sites within a large health care system.

Second, although research is considered an optional activity, carrying out studies to improve the quality of patient care is increasingly recognized as a core professional obligation of physicians. Although research is desirable, it is optional in the sense that without International Review Board (IRB) approval and the determination that the risks are proportionate to the expected benefits, it may not proceed. In contrast, quality-improvement activities commonly are aimed at bringing the level of care up to a professionally determined standard. Physicians have an ethical obligation to act in the best interests of patients, which includes providing care that is consistent with evidence-based practice guidelines.

Third, the risk of learning health system activities is often very low. Many learning health care activities are exempt from federal requirements for IRB review and informed consent because they analyze previously collected data that have been de-identified. Furthermore, there are risks to not carrying out quality-improvement activities because patients will continue to receive care that does not meet evidence-based consensus recommendations. In addition, even interventional studies to improve the quality of care may present very low risk. Many of the interventions have minimal if any risk to patients, for example, having providers complete a checklist and take a time out before a surgical procedure, having reminders in the EHR about overdue vaccinations and screening tests, or providing additional outreach to coordinate care for complex patients. If the component interventions have been shown to be effective in other institutions and are widely employed, it can be argued that the organization is merely providing services that it arguably should have been providing already, but determining how to do so most effectively and efficiently in their particular organizational and clinical setting (23).

Fourth, in comparative effectiveness trials that compare two management strategies that are already widely used in practice, the risks of being in a trial are no greater than receiving ordinary clinical care. The only difference may be to receive care on the basis of randomization, often in a cluster-randomized design, rather than by the decision of the attending physician. In ordinary practice the attending physician often does not offer patients alternatives to the plan for care proposed. In this line of thinking, informed consent and IRB review are not needed for cluster-randomized trials that involve interventions already shown to be effective, even for trials that employ randomization (24, 25). However, some IRBs may not agree with this approach to comparative effectiveness trials. Moreover, there may be a mismatch between, on the one hand, the professional imperative for physicians and health care organizations to improve the quality of clinical care, and on the other hand, the federal regulations on human participants research and their interpretation by institutional review boards (26).

Fifth, do learning health systems take into account social determinants of health that are linked to poor outcomes? To raise the quality-of-care and health outcomes, learning health systems may need to address social determinants of health, for example, targeting interventions to patients with low health literacy, poor insurance coverage, and limited financial resources to cover copayments and deductibles. Furthermore, some patients face structural barriers to improving health outcomes. Some patients with diabetes may have no grocery stores in their neighborhoods that offer fresh vegetables and no safe areas for walking and other exercise. Some health care systems have tried to address these issues directly, for example, setting up farmers markets at clinic sites and providing community access to exercise facilities for employees and students.

SUMMARY

1. Digital information technologies not only offer unprecedented opportunities to improve the quality and efficiency of medical care but also pose novel ethical concerns, particularly regarding confidentiality, consent, and justice, which need to be addressed.

References

1. Lo B, Parham L. The impact of web 2.0 on the doctor–patient relationship. *J Law Med Ethics* 2010;38:17-26.
2. Cohen IG, Mello MM. HIPAA and Protecting Health Information in the 21st Century. *JAMA* 2018;320:231-232.
3. Gymrek M, McGuire AL, Golan D, et al. Identifying personal genomes by surname inference. *Science* 2013;339:321-324.
4. Lyles CR, Allen JY, Poole D, et al. "I want to keep the personal relationship with my doctor": understanding barriers to portal use among African Americans and Latinos. *J Med Internet Res* 2016;18:e263.
5. Leventhal JC, Cummins JA, Schwartz PH, et al. Designing a system for patients controlling providers' access to their electronic health records: organizational and technical challenges. *J Gen Intern Med* 2015;30:S17-S24.
6. Meslin EM, Schwartz PH. How bioethics principles can aid design of electronic health records to accommodate patient granular control. *J Gen Intern Med* 2015;30:S3-S6.
7. Blumenthal D, Squires D. Giving patients control of their EHR data. *J Gen Intern Med* 2015;30:S42-S43.

8. Rothstein MA. The end of the HIPAA privacy rule? Currents in contemporary bioethics. *J Law Med Ethics* 2016;44:352-358.

9. Mello MM, Adler-Milstein J, Ding KL, et al. Legal barriers to the growth of health information exchange—boulders or pebbles? *Milbank Q* 2018;96:110-143.

10. Behrman RE, Benner JS, Brown JS, et al. Developing the sentinel system—a national resource for evidence development. *N Engl J Med* 2011;364:498-499.

11. Telenti A, Steinhubl SR, Topol EJ. Rethinking the medical record. *Lancet* 2018;391:1013.

12. Tan SS, Goonawardene N. Internet health information seeking and the patient–physician relationship: a systematic review. *J Med Internet Res* 2017;19:e9.

13. Murray E, Lo B, Pollack L, et al. The impact of health information on the internet on the physician–patient relationship: patient perceptions. *Arch Intern Med* 2003;163:1727-1734.

14. Wald HS, Dube CE, Anthony DC. Untangling the web—the impact of Internet use on health care and the physician–patient relationship. *Patient Education and Counseling* 2007;68:218-224.

15. Murray E, Lo B, Pollack L, et al. The impact of health information on the Internet on health care and the physician–patient relationship: national U.S. survey among 1,050 U.S. physicians. *J Med Internet Res* 2003;5:e17.

16. Jenssen BP, Mitra N, Shah A, et al. Using digital technology to engage and communicate with patients: a survey of patient attitudes. *J Gen Intern Med* 2016;31:85-92.

17. Koo K, Bowman MS, Ficko Z, et al. Older and wiser? Changes in unprofessional content on urologists' social media after transition from residency to practice. *BJU Int* 2018.

18. Attai DJ, Anderson PF, Fisch MJ, et al. Risks and benefits of Twitter use by hematologists/oncologists in the era of digital medicine. *Semin Hematol* 2017;54:198-204.

19. Stoto M, Oakes M, Stuart E, et al. Analytical methods for a learning health system: 1. Framing the research question. *EGEMS (Wash DC)* 2017;5:28.

20. Abernethy AP. Demonstrating the learning health system through practical use cases. *Pediatrics* 2014;134:171-172.

21. Morain SR, Kass NE. Ethics issues arising in the transition to learning health care systems: results from interviews with leaders from 25 health systems. *EGEMS (Wash DC)* 2016;4:1212.

22. Faden RR, Kass NE, Goodman SN, et al. An ethics framework for a learning health care system: a departure from traditional research ethics and clinical ethics. *Hastings Cent Rep* 2013;Spec No:S16-S27.

23. Whicher DM, Kass NE, Audera-Lopez C, et al. Ethical issues in patient safety research: a systematic review of the literature. *J Patient Saf* 2015;11:174-184.

24. Pletcher MJ, Lo B, Grady D. Informed consent in randomized quality improvement trials: a critical barrier for learning health systems. *JAMA Intern Med* 2014;174:668-670.

25. Lo B, Groman M. Oversight of quality improvement: focusing on benefits and risks. *Arch Intern Med* 2003;163:1481-1486.

26. Faden RR, Beauchamp TL, Kass NE. Informed consent for comparative effectiveness trials. *N Engl J Med* 2014;370:1959-1960.

ANNOTATED BIBLIOGRAPHY

1. Lo B, Parham L. The impact of web 2.0 on the doctor–patient relationship. *J Law Med Ethics* 2010;38:17-26. Overview of the impact of new digital communication technologies on the doctor–patient relationship.

2. Tan SS, Goonawardene N. Internet health information seeking and the patient-physician relationship: a systematic review. *J Med Internet Res* 2017;19:e9
Review of research on patients' Internet health information seeking and its influence on the patient–physician relationship.

3. Faden RR, Kass NE, Goodman SN, et al. An ethics framework for a learning health care system: a departure from traditional research ethics and clinical ethics. *Hastings Cent Rep* 2013;Spec No:S16-S27.
Thoughtful ethics framework for learning health care systems.

Ethical Issues in Genomic Medicine

INTRODUCTION

The human genome comprises 3 billion base pairs, about 25,000 genes. Ninety-eight percent of the whole genome is the noncoding portion, whose clinical significance is largely unknown (1). Whole-exome sequencing, which involves the 2% of genome that encodes proteins, is cheaper and more accurate than whole-genome sequencing (1).

With rapid advances in genomics, physicians in all specialties will increasingly be asked to advise patients about genetic testing. This chapter discusses the use cases for genomic testing in clinical practice, informed consent for genomic testing, presenting genomic test results to patients, the confidentiality of test results, and genetic enhancement and discrimination. We use the term *genomics* to refer to the DNA sequence of chromosomes; *genetics* refers simply to the science of inheritance.

WHAT IS DIFFERENT ABOUT GENOMICS?

Genetic or genomic information is commonly viewed as qualitatively different from other clinical information. On closer analysis, however, this claim is untenable in some respects.

People Overestimate the Impact of Genes

The media have characterized the human genome as a "blueprint" for life or as a "future diary," implying that a person's DNA sequence determines his or her future and that genomic information has greater predictive power than other medical information. To be sure, some severe diseases are caused by single-gene variants that have complete penetrance, such as Huntington disease. However, most genes have incomplete penetrance or variable expressivity so that their presence does not reliably predict the occurrence of disease or its severity. Furthermore, most common conditions are polygenic. For example, a person's risk of hypertension and diabetes depends on many genes, including genes that might be protective or modify the expression of other genes. Many laypeople mistakenly regard genetic influences as all-or-none, rather than as probabilistic. Furthermore, the effects of genes on clinical outcomes are modified by education, environmental, and socioeconomic factors, such as diet, exercise, and exposure to viral illness.

Genetics Provides Information About Relatives

All genetic information, whether a family history or a genomic test, provides information about relatives. Ethical dilemmas arise regarding the confidentiality of genomic information if the proband refuses to disclose information that relatives may share and would enable them to take steps to prevent or treat a serious disease.

Genomic Testing Has Significant Psychosocial Risks

Genetic and genomic information might be considered especially personal and sensitive. People commonly regard information about their heredity and future health as highly private. They might believe that genetic information reveals something essential about themselves that would not otherwise be apparent. Furthermore, genetic information might reveal family secrets, for example, about adoptions and nonpaternity. Genomic testing might also contradict a person's beliefs about parentage or ancestry.

The risks of genomic tests are psychosocial as well as than medical. Persons found to be at risk for adult-onset illness might change their self-image and might be labeled by others as abnormal even if they are asymptomatic (2). Breaches of confidentiality might cause stigma, discrimination, and distress. Generally patients receiving gnomic test results do not experience psychological distress (3). However, adults who were low in optimism or self-esteem before testing were more likely to be anxious after receiving positive results (4).

Genetic Information Might Be Stigmatizing

Scientifically flawed ideas about inheritance were used in the late 19th and early 20th centuries to support ideas of racial superiority and discriminatory social policies (5). Eugenic laws were passed, forbidding marriage or mandating sterilization of people categorized as feebleminded, insane, and criminals. In addition, miscegenation laws and restrictive immigration policies were enacted. Given this history, some people fear that genetic research today might be used to support discriminatory social policies (6).

Genomic Knowledge Might Undermine Traditional Beliefs

Critics fear that advances in genetic science might contradict moral and religious teachings about human nature or undermine human dignity (7). For example, some people oppose preimplantation genetic diagnosis as fostering a desire for the "perfect" baby, disrespecting persons with disabilities, violating the natural order, and undermining the awe of procreation. Advances in genetics might also change beliefs about individual responsibility. Identification of genes that predispose to alcoholism or drug addiction might allow persons with these conditions to escape responsibility for their behaviors because people generally are not considered responsible for inherited conditions.

INTERPRETATION OF GENOMIC SEQUENCE RESULTS

Every clinical test should meet several criteria before being accepted into clinical practice (8). *Analytic validity* means that the test is reliable and accurate: If the test is repeated, the same results will be reported. *Clinical validity* means that the test predicts the presence or absence of a clinical disease or condition. That is, the test has high positive and negative predictive values. *Clinical utility* means that testing leads to a net health benefit for the patient. The potential benefits of testing must outweigh the risks, and the balance of benefits to risks must be acceptable to the patient.

Interpreting genomic sequencing data involves many challenges. First, both false-positive and false-negative results may occur. False-positive reports may be due to several causes. Automated next-generation sequencing (NGS) methods have good reliability for detecting single base pair substitutions, which are the overwhelming majority of variants detected (1). However, these methods are less sensitive detecting other variants, including insertions, deletions, inversions, and transpositions. In addition, the vast majority of identified variants are common, observed in greater than 3% of the population and thus unlikely to be pathogenic.

False negatives may also occur. First, genomic testing methods have limitations. With targeted multigene panels for specific conditions, such as hereditary breast cancer, the proband may have a variant that was not included on the panel and thus not detected (1). NGS also has technical limitations in reconstructing the exome or genome from the fragments that were actually analyzed (1). Results of whole-exome and whole-genome sequencing need to be verified by clinical laboratory that is certified under the Clinical Laboratory Improvement Amendment before they can be used in clinical practice (1).

Second, many detected variants are categorized as "of unknown significance" because they have not been previously reported to be associated with a clinical disease. It is therefore not known whether a newly discovered variant is pathogenic or not.

Third, as with all diagnostic tests, the interpretation will depend on the prior probability of disease before the test is ordered. If testing is carried out in a population in which the prevalence of disease is low, false positives will outnumber false negatives. If the individual patient in whom a test is ordered presents a very low clinical suspicion for the condition for which testing is carried out, for example, if the patient is asymptomatic, the prior probability of disease is low, and the probability of a false-positive result increases. The prior probability of disease is also very low if an association is identified between a gene and a disease other than the one the patient is suspected of having.

Are the Results Actionable?

The case for providing the results of genomic testing to the patients and their physicians is strongest if the variant is known to be a pathogenic mechanism, and there is a prevention or treatment known to be effective, interventions are more effective if started early in the course of illness or before clinical symptoms develop, and the medical intervention would not otherwise be recommended. When these conditions are present, the test result is said to be actionable.

A test might have *personal utility*, however, even if it is not actionable. Some patients might desire screening for predisposition for a serious adult-onset illness even if there is no prevention or treatment known to be effective. Similarly, some patients may want genomic tests that predict prognosis, even if there is no treatment available. If they were found to be at risk, they might change plans regarding education, career, marriage, or childbearing. On the other hand, some persons would not want to know they are at increased risk for serious untreatable conditions such as Alzheimer disease.

For many common conditions, such as coronary artery disease and diabetes, many variants confer only a small increase in risk, and the same interventions would be recommended regardless of the results of genomic testing, namely weight loss, exercise, smoking cessation, and treatment of high blood pressure and high cholesterol. Although some believe that genomic information will help patients become more adherent to these preventive measures, the evidence does not support this belief (9).

USE CASES FOR GENOMIC TESTING

Establish a Diagnosis in Symptomatic Patients

Children who are suspected of having severe genetic disorders but remain undiagnosed after an extensive conventional workup may have a diagnosis established through genomic testing. Even if such testing does not lead to therapeutic intervention, providing a definitive diagnosis may end a long diagnostic odyssey and, in the neonatal intensive care unit, facilitate discussion about goals of care and the option of a palliative care approach (10).

Guiding Therapy in Patients with Cancer

In nonsquamous cell lung cancer, genomic tumor profiling is now the standard approach to guide therapy. Certain driver mutations indicate that molecularly targeted therapies may prolong progression-free survival compared with traditional chemotherapy.

In pediatric cancer, genetic tumor profiling is less well developed and not part of routine care. A tumor board with expertise in genetics needs to determine whether identified variants are actionable and might guide therapy or a recommendation of a clinical trial (11). In one report, the tumor board struggled with categorizing genomic variants as driving tumorigenesis, protecting, or incidental with no clinical impact.

Targeted Screening for Susceptibility to Adult-Onset Diseases

The following examples illustrate diseases for which targeted genomic testing panels are available.

BRCA

These autosomal dominant genes account for about 2% to 3% of cases of breast cancer. In families with a high incidence of breast and ovarian cancer, pathogenic variants in BRCA1 are associated with up to an 85% lifetime risk of developing breast cancer and a 40% risk of ovarian cancer (12). Women who test positive for BRCA variants should undergo more intensive mammography screening, starting at an earlier age than recommended for the general population. Moreover, they might consider preventive measures, which include chemoprevention with tamoxifen or raloxifene and prophylactic mastectomy and oophorectomy, which have medical and psychosocial ramifications (12). BRCA testing has important limitations. As with other genomic tests, false-negative tests might occur if no specific variant has been identified in the family, if the test kit used did not detect the variant present in the family, or if inheritance in the family is due to another gene than BRCA.

Hereditary Nonpolyposis Colorectal Cancer (HNPCC)

This autosomal dominant syndrome is caused by variants in mismatch-repair genes. The most common pathogenic variants, MLH1 and MSH2, occur in up to 3% of cases of newly diagnosed colorectal cancer (13). In persons with these variants, the lifetime risk of colorectal cancer is about 80%, and such cancers are more likely to be earlier onset and synchronous. Screening colonoscopy starting around age 20 to 25 cuts the risk of colorectal cancer by around 60% and improves survival (13). Thus, genomic screening is useful to identify persons who should start colonoscopy earlier than usually recommended. Negative tests, however, have low predictive value because many other variants can cause this syndrome.

Hemochromatosis

Hemochromatosis is a syndrome of cirrhosis, diabetes, and gonadal failure due to iron overload. About 1 in 200 persons of Northern European descent are homozygous for the variant C282YP. The clinical validity of population-based DNA screening is unproven because of low penetrance and variable expressivity (14).

Pharmacogenomics

Pharmacogenomic tests can identify some patients at increased risk of a serious adverse reaction or lack of effectiveness with a given medication due to genomic variations. Genomic testing is recommended to prevent hypersensitivity reactions to abacavir, life-threatening adverse reactions to carbamazepine and phenytoin, and treatment failure with clopidrogel and with combination therapy for hepatitis C (15). For several conditions, HLA serotyping is required.

With other drugs, genomic testing for drug metabolism genes can identify some patients who would benefit from dose adjustment, for example, when starting warfarin. However, it is not clear that genomic testing will reduce the time to achieve an effective dose of warfarin or improve patient outcomes (15).

Adoption of pharmacogenomics into clinical practice is challenging because treating physicians are not knowledgeable about it. Point of service decision support for prescribers will be required (15).

Screening Healthy Persons

The role of whole-genome sequencing or whole-exome sequencing in asymptomatic persons remains to be demonstrated (16). Generally a screening test is recommended in asymptomatic patients only if there is an intervention that is known to prevent or treat the disease and is more effective when started early in the disease (17). Earlier diagnosis *per se* is not considered a justification when screening for risk factors. As with any test, the positive predictive value will be low in a population with a low prevalence of disease.

The current ethical and clinical standard is to return genomic screening test results to patients only if the results are actionable, leading to specific recommendations for treatment. To determine whether a variant is actionable requires genomics experts to spend considerable time reviewing the literature on the clinical significance of an identified variant (11).

Testing Children for Adult-Onset Diseases

Testing children for susceptibility to adult-onset diseases raises special ethical concerns because testing children denies them the opportunity to make informed decisions of whether or not to be tested (18). Because many adults choose not to be tested, it cannot be assumed that children would agree with testing when they reach maturity. Thus, genomic testing is best deferred until the child reaches maturity, unless there are effective preventive measures or treatments that need to be instituted during childhood if the test is abnormal (18).

Direct-to-Consumer Genomic Testing

Genomic tests are available over the Internet (19). Patients might ask physicians about such testing, or bring in results of DNA tests obtained over the Internet. Tests might concern physical characteristics such as eye color, hair color, height, and earwax. Sometimes, such testing is combined with recommendations for skin care, anti-aging, or nutritional products. These "recreational" genomics tests currently are not regulated by the FDA. However, direct-to-consumer (DTC) tests for genetic health risk is now regulated by the FDA (20). Patients send a buccal swab or blood spot. If a state requires a physician to order the test, a physician employed by the company, who has not met the patient, does so. Consumers pay out-of-pocket for the test and receive the results directly from the Internet site.

Direct-to-consumer genetic testing raises several ethical dilemmas, including the validity of testing, the completeness of variants tested for an allele, and the quality of counseling over the telephone or the Internet (19). Concerns about adverse psychological effects from the DTC test results have not been substantiated empirically (20). Furthermore, there are confidentiality concerns because the Internet testing company may not be subject to HIPAA privacy regulations.

Ancestry Testing

Several Internet companies offer genomic testing to help people learn their continent of origin or trace their genealogy. People have many reasons for obtaining such tests, including satisfying their curiosity about their heritage or the geographical origins of their ancestors, to connect to their homeland, to identify genetic relatives, and to obtain benefits such as race-based scholarships or Native American casino profits. These tests have a number of limitations (21). Mitochondrial DNA (inherited through the maternal lineage) or Y-chromosome DNA (inherited through the paternal lineage) tests trace inheritance only through a single genetic lineage, so that contributions from many other distant ancestors is not taken into account. Moreover, these tests sample only a limited amount of the subject's DNA, classifications are derived from small, selected population samples, and there are no quality-control requirements. Given these limitations, it is not surprising that a person who sends a sample to different companies for genetic ancestry testing often receives inconsistent results. Genetic ancestry testing might have adverse psychological consequences if test results contradict clients' deeply held beliefs about their ethnic heritage (21).

These Internet genealogy websites are not confidential; indeed, one of their attractions is that after testing people can identify distant genetic relatives and contact them. Recently law enforcement officials have used these sites to identify suspects in unsolved cases of multiple murders and rapes by matching DNA found at the crime scene to relatives of the alleged perpetrator (22). Customers of ancestry testing sites probably did not realize such forensic uses of the site were possible under company policies. When law enforcement seeks to use ancestry databases, respecting the autonomy of persons who subscribed to the website needs to be balanced against the public benefit of identifying and prosecuting alleged perpetrators of repeated serious crimes.

INFORMED CONSENT FOR GENOMIC TESTING

Careful attention to informed consent can maximize the benefits of genomic testing and minimize its risks. Informed consent is particularly important for genomic testing because individuals differ on whether the benefits of testing outweigh the risks. Some people will want more information about genomic risk, even if its significance is uncertain and no proven preventive or therapeutic intervention is available. Others might decline testing because they do not want to receive information about serious genomic risks.

Genetic concepts and probabilities are complicated and difficult to comprehend. Misunderstandings about genomic testing and the interpretation of results are widespread among health professionals and laypeople alike. For example, people may not appreciate that physicians may not be able to interpret the clinical significance of many genomic variants.

PRESENTING RESULTS OF GENOMIC TESTING TO PATIENTS AND THEIR PHYSICIANS

Most clinicians lack training about genomic testing and are not well equipped to interpret the clinical significance of specific genomic variants, identify options for treatment and prevention, assess their benefits and risks of those options, and effectively communicate findings to patients.

Genetic counselors and medical geneticists, who have special training on such issues, are in very short supply and cannot be expected to see all patients who undergo genomic testing. A variety of approaches to informing patients have been proposed and tested, including consultative expert committees and decision aids (11, 23, 24).

In disclosing genomic results with patients, physicians should first make sure they understand the limitations and clinical implications of the results; consultation with genomics specialists may be useful. As with any other test results, physicians should check that patients understand the information provided and answer any questions.

Nondirective Genetic Counseling

Nondirectiveness has been an important belief in genetic counseling. People interpret this term in different ways (25). Commonly it means that the counselor presents all sides of an issue in an unbiased manner, the counselor's personal views should not influence the client's decision, and the client's or couple's decision is respected. Historically, nondirectiveness developed as a reaction to eugenicist policies and from the desire to distance prenatal genetic diagnosis from controversies over abortion.

Empirical studies, however, show that genetic counselors are often directive. In one study, 28% of genetic counselors said they would recommend testing or screening to a client (26). Another study found that genetic counselors gave advice an average of almost six times per session and that clients did not object (27). Some concerns about nondirectiveness might be resolved if counselors respond to clients' questions about what to do by suggesting issues to consider in making the decision, rather than by giving a direct recommendation (28).

The stance of nondirectiveness is ethically problematic for several reasons. First, patients commonly request advice determining which option is most consistent with their values and best interests (*see* Chapter 3). Second, nondirectiveness might violate the ethical guideline of beneficence. A strong case can be made that physicians have an ethical obligation to recommend cancer screening in BRCA and Lynch syndrome and to share genomic test results with relatives who might be at high risk for a preventable serious disease (25).

Disclosure of Genomic Results to Relatives

Genetic testing provides information about relatives as well as the individual being tested (29). Persons identified as having a predisposition to a serious adult-onset genetic illness that can be prevented or treated effectively have a moral duty to inform relatives who might also be at risk. Most probands agree to do so. An ethical dilemma can arise for physicians when the patient objects to such disclosure.

CASE 45.1   **Disclosure of pathogenic genomic results to relatives**

Mr. R, a 48-year-old man with colon cancer with a strong family history of colon cancer, is found to have an MLH1 variant for HNPCC. Relatives with this allele have an 80% lifetime risk of colon cancer, often at an early age. Mr. R refuses the physician's advice to inform his sister, with whom he had a falling out several years ago regarding his marriage. "After what she did to me and my wife, I wouldn't help her in any way."

After explaining why informing relatives that they are at risk, the physician offered to send a letter to the sister or to the sister's physician advising her that she is at risk for HNPCC and advising her to be tested so that Mr. R need not have any direct contact with his sister. About one quarter of patients with HNPCC who would not contact a relative would agree to have their physician do so (30). Mr. R continues to decline to notify his sister.

When Is Overriding Confidentiality Justified?

The guidelines in Chapter 5 on exceptions to confidentiality can be applied to genetic testing in Case 45.1. The potential harm to identifiable third parties is serious and likely if a high risk of cancer is missed. There is an effective intervention to avert the risk—annual screening colonoscopy beginning at a much earlier age than usually recommended. There is no less invasive means for warning relatives at risk if the proband declines to notify relatives. The finding of HNPCC provides much more specific prognostic information than the family history alone.

There is a presumption that physicians should respect patient confidentiality, as Chapter 5 discusses. Mr. R may feel wronged if the physician contacts his sister without his permission. State law and the federal HIPAA privacy regulations protect the confidentiality of his health information. However, there are also good reasons to override confidentiality in this case, to prevent serious harm to persons who do not know they are at risk.

The law does not give definitive guidance to physicians in this situation. Appellate rulings in such cases are not consistent and some find that physicians can fulfill their legal duties by advising the proband to disclose to relatives, as the physician did in Case 45.1 (31).

Recommendations

Physicians should consider the issue of informing relatives of actionable genomics test results a process that requires the involvement of the health care team over time. First, physicians should discuss the importance of disclosure during informed consent for testing. Second, after tests have been carried out, physicians should recommend disclosing positive results to relatives if the information would lead to a significant change in their medical care, as in Case 45.1. Third, the health care team should elicit patients' concerns about informing relatives, help them resolve them, and provide support and counseling repeatedly on how to disclose information (32). As in Case 45.1, the team can offer to contact relatives directly if the patient does not wish to do so personally. Fourth, in exceptional situations, there may be compelling ethical reasons to offer to disclose results of genetic testing to relatives over the objections of the patient. Such disclosure should be a last resort. Practically speaking, if Mr. R does not want his sister contacted he can refuse to provide contact information. Relatives at risk should be offered the information; if they do not want to know it, their refusal should be respected.

GENETIC DISCRIMINATION

Screening for genetic disorders might lead to stigmatization and discrimination. Asymptomatic persons at increased risk for adult-onset genetic conditions might regard themselves, or be regarded by others, as impaired. Although there is no evidence of widespread discrimination on the basis of genetic testing, fears about it are widespread and might prevent persons from accepting genetic testing in clinical care or participating in research (33).

Insurers

In the United States, life, disability, and long-term care insurance companies have incentives to avoid adverse selection, which occurs when patients increase coverage after they learn they are at risk for diseases but insurers do not have that information (34). Insurers who are unaware of such risk would sell coverage at relatively low rates to individuals who know they are at increased risk for claims. Insurers, therefore, want to know any pertinent medical information that the applicant knows and, if they do not have such information, seek to limit coverage for preexisting diseases, exclude the diseases from coverage, or set prohibitive premiums.

Employers

Employers also have incentives to use genetic screening. Excluding employees who are likely to become sick might increase future productivity and cut health insurance premiums. Employers might also want to identify workers at genetic risk for occupational diseases because it might be cheaper to exclude them from the workplace than to reduce occupational exposure. Genetic testing by employers, however, might be a tragedy for employees identified as at risk for adult-onset conditions. They might be unable to find employment, even if they are asymptomatic and able to work productively.

Antidiscrimination Law

In 2008, the federal Genetic Information Nondiscrimination Act (GINA) was passed. It prohibits health insurers from using a person's genetic information to set eligibility or premiums. Employers may not use a person's genetic information to make employment decisions, such as hiring, job assignments, promotions, and firing (35). Neither health insurers nor employers may request or require a person or family to provide genetic information. The law does not apply to disability, long-term care, and life insurance. The 2010 Patient Protection and Affordable Care Act extends GINA by banning insurers from determining eligibility on the basis of health status, medical condition, or receipt of health care, and from setting premiums on the basis of health status (36).

GENETIC ENHANCEMENT

In the future, gene transfer might offer the possibility of enhancing athletic or cognitive performance. This possibility raises dilemmas similar to those discussed in Chapter 14. The dilemma is sometimes framed as enhancement or "beyond therapy": a medical intervention is being used to augment and improve a person's native capacity, not to treat a serious disease. In this view, success from enhancement is less worthy of admiration and praise (7). Even if genetic enhancements were shown to be safe and effective, critics object that they would exacerbate existing health and social disparities and create pressure for competitors or other students to use them. Others object that such enhancements disrupt the connection between effort and success. From this perspective, success is praiseworthy only if it results from the fulfillment of one's natural capacities, developed through effort and discipline. In this view, success from other means is less worthy of admiration and praise (7).

In rebuttal, others argue that biomedical enhancements do not differ in kind from attending better schools and access to academic help and counseling from parents and tutors, which are also more accessible to the wealthy and do not eliminate the need for practice and training. Debates over enhancement in sports are prominent. To achieve short-term competitive advantage and glory, some athletes might use performance-enhancing drugs with long-term serious adverse effects. Some interventions to enhance performance are accepted, including better equipment, diet, and coaching. One astute commentator argues that the sole justification for banning performance-enhancing drugs or genomic interventions in athletic competition is an agreement on the rules of the game, which are based on socially constructed conventions, not on deep moral principles (37).

SUMMARY

1. In advising patients about genomic testing, physicians need to be aware of the clinical limitations of testing, the risk of discrimination, the importance of informed consent, the importance of confidentiality, and the implications for relatives.
2. Physicians should recommend genomic tests only if the results would lead to a significant change in clinical care or the patient values the likely diagnostic and prognostic information very highly, even if care would not change.

References

1. Holm IA, Yu TW, Joffe S. From sequence data to returnable results: ethical issues in variant calling and interpretation. *Genet Test Mol Biomarkers* 2017;21:178-183.
2. Harris RP, Sheridan SL, Lewis CL, et al. The harms of screening: a proposed taxonomy and application to lung cancer screening. *JAMA Intern Med* 2014;174:281-285.
3. Broadstock M, Michie S, Marteau T. Psychological consequences of predictive genetic testing: a systematic review. *Eur J Hum Genet* 2000;8:731-738.
4. Michie S, Bobrow M, Marteau TM. Predictive genetic testing in children and adults: a study of emotional impact. *J Med Genet* 2001;38:519-526.
5. Kevles DJ. *In the name of eugenics: genetics and the uses of human heredity.* New York: Knopf; 1985.
6. Nuffield Council on Bioethics. *Genetics and Human Behavior: The Ethical Concerns.* London: Nuffield Council on Bioethics; 2002.
7. The President's Council on Bioethics. *Beyond Therapy: Biotechnology and the Pursuit of Happiness.* 2003. Available at: http://bioethics.georgetown.edu/pcbe/reports/beyondtherapy/. Accessed September 12, 2012.
8. Secretary's Advisory Committee. *Enhancing the oversight of genetic tests: recommendations of the SACGT.* 2000. Available at: http://www4.od.nih.gov/oba/sacgt/gtdocuments.html. Accessed November 16, 2007.
9. Hollands GJ, French DP, Griffin SJ, et al. The impact of communicating genetic risks of disease on risk-reducing health behaviour: systematic review with meta-analysis. *BMJ* 2016;352:i1102.
10. Berg JS, Agrawal PB, Bailey DB, Jr., et al. Newborn sequencing in genomic medicine and public health. *Pediatrics* 2017;139.
11. McGraw SA, Garber J, Janne PA, et al. The fuzzy world of precision medicine: deliberations of a precision medicine tumor board. *Per Med* 2017;14:37-50.
12. Couch FJ, Nathanson KL, Offit K. Two decades after BRCA: setting paradigms in personalized cancer care and prevention. *Science* 2014;343:1466-1470.
13. Giardiello FM, Allen JI, Axilbund JE, et al. Guidelines on genetic evaluation and management of Lynch syndrome: a consensus statement by the US Multi-Society Task Force on colorectal cancer. *Gastroenterology* 2014;147:502-526.
14. Whitlock EP, Garlitz BA, Harris EL, et al. Screening for hereditary hemochromatosis: a systematic review for the U.S. Preventive Services Task Force. *Ann Intern Med* 2006;145:209-223.
15. Haga SB. Integrating pharmacogenetic testing into primary care. *Expert Review of Precision Medicine and Drug Development* 2017;2:327-336.

16. Vassy JL, Christensen KD, Schonman EF, et al. The impact of whole-genome sequencing on the primary care and outcomes of healthy adult patients: a pilot randomized trial. *Ann Intern Med* 2017.

17. Newman TB, Kohn MA. *Evidence-Based Diagnosis.* New York: Cambridge University Press; 2009.

18. McCullough LB, Brothers KB, Chung WK, et al. Professionally responsible disclosure of genomic sequencing results in pediatric practice. *Pediatrics* 2015;136:e974-e982.

19. Lu M, Lewis CM, Traylor M. Pharmacogenetic testing through the direct-to-consumer genetic testing company 23andMe. *BMC Med Genomics* 2017;10:47.

20. Allyse MA, Robinson DH, Ferber MJ, et al. Direct-to-consumer testing 2.0: emerging models of direct-to-consumer genetic testing. *Mayo Clinic Proceedings* 2018;93:113-120.

21. Royal CD, Novembre J, Fullerton SM, et al. Inferring genetic ancestry: opportunities, challenges, and implications. *Am J Hum Genet* 2010;86:661-673.

22. Ram N, Guerrini CJ, McGuire AL. Genealogy databases and the future of criminal investigation. *Science* 2018;360:1078-1079.

23. Lewis MA, Paquin RS, Roche MI, et al. Supporting parental decisions about genomic sequencing for newborn screening: the NC NEXUS decision aid. *Pediatrics* 2016;137:S16-S23.

24. Wright CF, McRae JF, Clayton S, et al. Making new genetic diagnoses with old data: iterative reanalysis and reporting from genome-wide data in 1,133 families with developmental disorders. *Genet Med* 2018.

25. Elwyn G, Gray J, Clarke A. Shared decision making and non-directiveness in genetic counselling. *J Med Genet* 2000;37:135-138.

26. Bartels DM, LeRoy BS, McCarthy P, et al. Nondirectiveness in genetic counseling: a survey of practitioners. *Am J Med Genet* 1997;72:172-179.

27. Michie S, Bron F, Bobrow M, et al. Nondirectiveness in genetic counseling: an empirical study. *Am J Hum Genet* 1997;60:40-47.

28. Kessler S. Psychological aspects of genetic counseling: nondirectiveness revisited. *Am J Med Genet* 1997;72:164-171.

29. Korngiebel DM, Thummel KE, Burke W. Implementing precision medicine: the ethical challenges. *Trends Pharmacol Sci* 2017;38:8-14.

30. Kohut K, Manno M, Gallinger S, Esplen MJ. Should healthcare providers have a duty to warn family members of individuals with an HNPCC-causing mutation? A survey of patients from the Ontario familial colon cancer registry. *J Med Genet* 2007;44:404-407.

31. Wolf SM, Branum R, Koenig BA, et al. Returning a research participant's genomic results to relatives: analysis and recommendations. *J Law Med Ethics* 2015;43:440-463.

32. Hodgson J, Metcalfe S, Gaff C, et al. Outcomes of a randomised controlled trial of a complex genetic counselling intervention to improve family communication. *Eur J Hum Genet* 2016;24:356-360.

33. Greely HT. Banning genetic discrimination. *N Engl J Med* 2005;353:865-867.

34. Dodge JH. Predictive medical information and underwriting. *J Law Med Ethics* 2007;35:36-39.

35. Rothstein MA. GINA at ten and the future of genetic nondiscrimination law. *Hastings Cent Rep* 2018;48:5-7.

36. Hudson KL. Genomics, health care, and society. *N Engl J Med* 2011;365:1033-1041.

37. Murray TH. *Good Sport: Why Our Games Matter—and How Doping Undermines Them.* New York: Oxford University Press; 2018.

ANNOTATED BIBLIOGRAPHY

1. Rothstein MA. GINA at ten and the future of genetic nondiscrimination law. *Hastings Cent Rep* 2018;48:5-7. Analysis of the antidiscrimination protections in the Genetic Information Nondiscrimination Act and the Affordable Health Care and Patient Protection Act.

2. Allyse MA, Robinson DH, Ferber MJ, et al. Direct-to-consumer testing 2.0: emerging models of direct-to-consumer genetic testing. *Mayo Clinic Proceedings* 2018;93:113-120. Recent review summarizing FDA oversight of DTC genetic testing for medical conditions.

3. Royal CD, Novembre J, Fullerton SM, et al. Inferring genetic ancestry: opportunities, challenges, and implications. *Am J Hum Genet* 2010;86:661-673. Discusses limitations of ancestry testing and the ethical issues it raises.

4. Lucassen A, Parker M. Confidentiality and sharing genetic information with relatives. *Lancet* 2010;375:1507-1509. Analyzes clinical, ethical, and legal issues regarding disclosure of genetic information to relatives.

Ethical Issues with Big Data and Artificial Intelligence

Unprecedentedly large data sets can now be combined and analyzed to improve our understanding of health and disease and to improve the care of individual patients. The first step was combining clinical data in electronic health records (EHRs) with genomic sequencing data, other "omics" findings, and biomarkers (1).

The amount and variety of "big data" are continually and rapidly expanding. The decreasing cost of next-generation genomic sequencing makes it affordable and widely available for research and clinical practice.

The next major addition to big data comes from mobile devices and wearable sensors. They can record and transmit to the cloud data about blood pressure, glucose, heart rhythm, electrocardiograms, and pulmonary function and thus allow detailed monitoring of chronic conditions in real-world settings outside the physician's office. These mobile health applications are useful both for research on and clinical management of common chronic diseases. These apps can detect unsuspected abnormal results, identify the frequency and patterns of abnormal results, and monitor response to therapy. Wearable sensors also are being developed to measure cardiopulmonary parameters to help predict exacerbations and rehospitalizations in patients with congestive heart failure and to identify nicotine cravings and stress in patients who are trying to stop smoking (2).

Mobile devices and wearable sensors also can provide information on physical activity, sleep, social interactions, diet, and geolocation. In turn, geolocation provides information on many other variables, including neighborhood income, employment rates, population density, crime rates, and the built environment (such as the presence of grocery stores, parks, sidewalks, and public transportation). These data on lifestyle and social determinants of health can be added to biomedical and clinical data.

Metadata from mobile devices and Internet application automatically track an individual's patterns of speech and voice tone, typing and scrolling, sleep, social interactions, and Internet searches. Researchers are using these data to try to diagnose depression, mania, or psychosis, monitor response to therapy, and predict relapses (3).

Even more types of digital data could be added. For example, dietary intake might be assessed through cell phone photos of meals and snacks, and payments to restaurants and food stores. This information could lead to improved counseling and management for obesity and diabetes.

PRECISION MEDICINE

Precision medicine aims to identify subgroups of patients who are more likely to benefit from an intervention and also who are unlikely to benefit or are more likely to experience significant adverse effects. Precision medicine tries to identify susceptibility to disease at a molecular level (4a). Precision medicine thus tailors treatments to small groups of patients; it does not provide personalized recommendations to individual patients (4). By targeting treatments to patients whose net benefit is greater, precision medicine seeks to reduce the number of patients who need to be treated in order to benefit on patient, as well as increase the number of patients who need to be treated in order to harm one patient.

Early use cases for precision medicine in cancer patients include individualizing therapy, reducing overtreatment, and identifying germline mutations for which increased cancer screening is recommended (5). In breast cancer, precision medicine has identified early-stage patients who have such a low probability of benefiting from adjuvant therapy, more extensive radiation therapy, and more extensive surgery that these standard treatments would likely do more harm than good (6). Another use case is pharmacogenomics, to identify people who need lower or higher doses of a medication or for whom the medicine is likely to be ineffective (7).

Precision medicine is still developing, and more clinical applications are anticipated in the future. A particular challenge is to move beyond a biomedical focus to incorporate the social determinants of health into predictive models and therapeutic algorithms.

Ethical Issues in Precision Medicine

Facilitating Precision Medicine Discoveries

The basic and translational research to develop precision medicine presents many ethical challenges, including access to specimens and data previously collected in research studies or routinely collected in clinical care, consent for access and use, privacy, and security. Precision medicine requires combining large amounts of data from multiple sources for each patient.

Before a precision medicine therapeutic algorithm can be accepted as part of clinical care, it should be carefully assessed. Clinical trials of the treatment recommended by the algorithm may need to be conducted. Identifying and enrolling the appropriate target patients will be challenging. New precision medicine therapies will have much smaller target audiences than current small molecule drugs and thus will require sufficient incentives for product development and a higher price to recoup investments in products (8).

Fair Distribution of Benefits

The benefits of precision medicine and artificial intelligence applied to medicine need to be distributed equitably across groups in the population, particularly subgroups who suffer from health disparities.

Genomic knowledge does not match the diverse ancestry backgrounds in the population. Under 5% of participants in genome-wide association studies are from African American, Hispanic, or indigenous backgrounds (9). Eighty-one percent of samples are from participants of European ancestry, and 14% from persons of Asian ancestry. Findings derived in studies of persons of predominantly European descent may not replicate in other groups. The strength of an association between a genomic variant and the risk of disease or response to a therapy may differ significantly in various populations. Lack of diversity also leads to missed opportunities to identify variants that are strongly associated with diseases and more prevalent in underrepresented populations.

Groups who already suffer from health disparities may fail to gain the benefits of genomic medicine because of a lack of research about them. Patients of African, Hispanic/Latin American, and native peoples ancestry are more likely to be told that genomic variants are ambiguous or of unknown significance (9). For the benefits of precision medicine to be equitably distributed, the diversity of populations studied in genomic research must be broadened (10). This will require overcoming skepticism in these underrepresented populations regarding biomedical research.

More broadly, some scholars question whether precision medicine will improve overall population health. Common diseases like hypertension and obesity usually have multifactorial causes in most patients, and effect sizes identified in precision medicine have been small. Moreover, precision medicine many not lead to more precise therapy in the majority of patients, for whom diet and exercise will still be recommended as first steps. Indeed a focus on biomedical factors might detract attention from ameliorating social determinants of health, such as poverty and poor education (11).

ARTIFICIAL INTELLIGENCE AND MACHINE LEARNING

Analysis of big data increasingly uses the techniques of artificial intelligence and machine learning to draw inferences and conclusions. In artificial intelligence (AI), computers perform tasks that are characteristic of human intelligence (12). Common daily examples of AI are programs to correct spelling errors, recommend consumer purchases, detect potentially fraudulent financial transactions, translate text or audio recordings from one language to another, suggest friends to whom to send a photo, and recognize individuals from facial or retinal images or speech patterns.

Machine learning is a type of AI that can improve its performance and learn from greater experience without being explicitly programmed by humans to modify the algorithm (12). Machine learning requires vast compounds of computing power, which has been feasible only recently (13).

Deep learning is a type of machine learning. It uses mathematical models that resemble neural networks in the human brain. Each layer of "neurons" takes data from the layer below it, performs a calculation, and provides its output to the layer above it. The term *deep* refers to models that have many layers of neural networks.

Applications of AI to clinical medicine will almost certainly increase in the future. The current cohort of trainees is likely to experience great increases in the proposed uses of artificial intelligence in medicine.

MEDICAL EXAMPLES OF ARTIFICIAL INTELLIGENCE

Medical recommendations based on AI can match or exceed performance of physicians in some situations.

Classification of Images

Machine learning can learn to classify images to determine whether a specific condition is present or not. The computer is trained on a large data set that has been interpreted by human experts with regard to a specified outcome or classification. With more experience the program improves its own performance in predicting the outcome of interest. The machine learning program can then be applied to new digital images. Once developed and validated, machine learning is standardized, repeatable, and scalable, and it reduces interreader variability (14).

In radiology, machine learning programs can match or exceed radiologists in detecting breast cancer and lung and liver nodules (15). Moreover, machine learning can measure the size of lesions and compare them to previous imaging studies. In some clinical situations, diagnostic radiology findings are needed as soon as possible, for example, to detect stroke within the time window for thrombolytic therapy to be instituted or to prioritize interventions in patients with multiple injuries after severe trauma. AI readings of radiology studies might provide results more rapidly than a system that relies on human readers, particularly real-time readings by treating physicians who are not trained in radiology.

In ophthalmology, machine learning has been used to detect diabetic retinopathy and may be useful in screening for and following glaucoma (16). Because ophthalmology already makes wide use of digital images, the specialty may be ripe for advances in machine learning.

In dermatology, machine learning can distinguish skin cancers from benign lesions with comparable accuracy as dermatologists (17). In conjunction with photos of skin lesions taken by mobile devices, such AI-based algorithms might provide universal access to skilled dermatology diagnosis.

In pathology, AI might be useful in predicting prognosis in patients diagnosed with Stage 1 adenocarcinoma of the lung and in identifying metastatic breast cancer in sentinel lymph node biopsies (18). However, because pathology data are stored on slides and not routinely as digital images, applying AI to clinical care would require considerable additional investments in equipment, processing, data storage, and personnel.

In classifying images, AI could compensate for known problems with human reading and interpretation (15). Computer programs do not develop fatigue or have lapses of attention, unlike humans.

Predictions of Prognosis and Adverse Effects

AI can predict which patients are at risk for adverse events or complications, such as a high risk of needing intensive care, requiring rehospitalization, or developing surgical site infections (19). These predications, which could be made in real time, allow physicians to intervene in a timely manner to prevent the adverse outcome. Because of reimbursement incentives to reduce adverse clinical outcomes, health care organizations are eager to implement these uses of AI.

Treatment Recommendations

In some patients, the genomic sequence of a patient's cancer cells reveals alleles that may be responsive to targeted therapies. These therapies would not be recommended by expert physicians following the usual classification of cancer by site of primary cancer, histology, and stage. These cases led to the hypothesis that classifying diseases according to molecular markers that identify pathogenic mechanisms would be a more useful classification of disease than current clinical classifications. Furthermore, because these precision medicine recommendations could not have been made by expert clinicians, the idea that computers might provide better recommendations than expert physicians was credible.

LIMITATIONS OF AI

Quality of Data

AI recommendations are only as good as the data fed into algorithm development (20). Good machine learning programs require a very large number of detailed real cases, with accurate human judgments regarding outcomes. The accuracy of machine learning predictive algorithms depends more on the amount of data used to train the algorithm rather than on the type of machine learning program (13). Moreover, an AI algorithm may not generalize to situations that were not included in the data set used to derive it. The derivation population of patients may differ in important ways from the patient population to whom the algorithm is applied in practice because of differences in patients' severity of illness, comorbid conditions, age, and social determinants of health. In addition, the treating health care provider may differ from the providers in the derivation set in terms of staffing, workflow, and resources.

There can be marked temporal changes in disease presentation and treatment. For instance, during outbreaks of emerging infections such as AIDS, Lyme disease, or pandemic influenza, machine learning diagnostic and predictive algorithms based on older datasets would be inaccurate. A current major, rapid change in clinical medicine is the rise in opioid abuse, more potent street drugs, and drug overdoses. Serious mistakes might occur if an AI algorithm faces situations that were not included in the derivation and training databases. If singularities or "black swan" events occur, predictions based on older data would be erroneous. Treatment options and recommendations in the derivation dataset may also become obsolete. For example, the new targeted cancer treatments based on genomic variants and biomarkers are not included in older cancer datasets. Thus, AI recommendations may be useful in a setting at one time but not in other situations.

Important data may be missing from derivation datasets. For example, EHRs and administrative data, which are readily fed into an AI dataset, may not contain information on patient-centered outcomes, such as functional status and quality of life. Yet these outcomes may be crucial for patients.

Reasoning for Recommendations Is Not Transparent

Machine learning algorithms cannot explain the reasons for their diagnosis or recommendation. Thus, recommendations will be a "black box" to physicians and patients. Physicians may find it difficult to answer questions from patients regarding their diagnosis or treatment recommendations made by AI. If the recommendations from AI are clinically counterintuitive, physicians will be challenged to exercise critical thinking and determine whether the recommendation is a brilliant insight or a serious error.

ETHICAL ISSUES INTEGRATING AI INTO CLINICAL PRACTICE

CASE 46.1	AI algorithm recommending cancer treatment

IBM's Watson Cancer, which was intended to deliver precision treatment recommendations, floundered after its recommendations were noted to be inconsistent with treatment guidelines and standard practice by oncologists whose hospitals had purchased the system (21). One problem was that Watson Cancer was trained on a small number of hypothetical cases, not on a large number of real cases in which the outcome was known. Another problem was that Watson could not keep up with rapidly changing information on new drugs and combinations. Serious errors have also occurred with AI applications in other fields, for example, traffic fatalities due to AI limitations in self-driving cars.

Several ethical issues regarding how an AI algorithm can be integrated into clinical practice should be discussed as part of comprehensive planning for a specific AI project.

Multiple Goals and Priorities for AI Algorithms

Different stakeholders may prioritize different outcomes or goals for AI algorithms in addition to biomedical outcomes, such as levels of blood pressure or glucose, or disease-free survival in cancer (19). Patients and surrogates might also be concerned about their ability to carry out daily activities or their quality of life. Physicians might also be interested in workflow and income. Leaders of health care organizations might be interested in reducing expenses, maximizing reimbursement, or enhancing reputation. AI algorithms themselves cannot set priorities among different outcomes of interest; these issues need to be determined by human stakeholders. In contrast, successful applications of AI to other areas of life do not have multiple conflicting outcomes. In language translation, accuracy is the key outcome. In business, increased sales and profits are the goal.

Benefits and Risks of AI

The clinical utility of an AI algorithm should be evaluated critically. Standards for validation should depend on the stakes for patients. If the outcome of an algorithm is to offer additional supportive services to patients to prevent serious adverse clinical outcomes, false positives have little risk other than cost and perceived intrusiveness by the patient. Nonrandomized trial designs would be adequate to evaluate clinical utility. But more rigorous evaluation of benefits and risks should be carried out if an AI is making treatment recommendations, particularly if the recommendation is markedly different from the current standard of care. In high-stakes situations, it may be appropriate to conduct a pragmatic clinical trial comparing recommendations based on AI to the current standard of care (19).

Incorporating AI Algorithms into Patient-Centered Care

AI is being used to identify patients who are at risk of needing critical care or rehospitalization. The question of whether and how to intervene with such patients to decrease adverse outcomes is outside the scope of AI projects themselves. The AI algorithm can identify patients in whom an intervention might be useful to prevent poor clinical outcomes, and perhaps suggest what interventions might be useful. However, the AI algorithm is unlikely to provide insights into how physicians or health care institutions should interact with patients identified as being at risk. A common response to patients at risk for needing critical care is to mobilize a rapid response team to provide aggressive medical interventions to improve the patient's condition. However, some patients at risk for needing critical care may not want it, and for others a discussion of goals of care is desirable to reach goal-concordant care. In one study of cancer patients at risk for critical care that did not involve AI predictions, goals of care discussions commonly led to a choice for palliative care and a decreased use of critical care

(22). Similarly, for patients at high risk for readmission to an acute care hospital, the usual response is to put in place home-based chronic disease management. However, for some such patients, it might be more appropriate to discuss goals of care; some patients might choose palliative care as the goal and implement a "do not hospitalize" order.

Impact on Health Disparities

AI might fail to improve health disparities or even exacerbate them (23). First, bias in data used to derive an AI algorithm will be carried over into the algorithm. For example, there is a lack of next-generation sequencing data on patients not from Caucasian or Asian continents of origin. Also, datasets used to derive AI algorithms may include clinical decisions that reflect discrimination, such as lower use of pain medication for African American patients with fractures and less evaluation for coronary artery disease in women with chest pain. Algorithms based on such discriminatory decisions will perpetuate disparities in health outcomes. Second, safety net hospitals and clinics that disproportionately care for vulnerable and uninsured patients may not be able to benefit from AI. These institutions have few resources to invest in personnel and information technology needed to capture, curate, and store data for AI applications. As a result, health disparities may widen. Third, individual patients who lack access to good health insurance may be identified as being at high risk for poor outcomes without having the root causes of the problem identified. Information on insurance coverage in the data set may not discern that the co-payments and coverage limits make it impossible for some patients with limited income to afford medications for multiple chronic conditions. The data feeding into the AI algorithm may not routinely include information on whether patients have difficulty paying for medicines and what they do when that occurs. Although it is possible for AI algorithms to incorporate geocoding and other proxies for social determinants of poor health at the community level, they may not be able to address these issues on the individual patient level or give a thick description of the impact of social factors. Finally, the AI algorithm, by focusing on individual patients at risk for poor outcomes, may not give due attention to addressing organizational or system-wide issues that may be a root cause of patients' poor outcomes.

Impact of AI on Health Care Workers

Like workers in many other fields, physicians are concerned that they will be replaced by AI or lose less prestige and income. As noted, above AI programs already are as good as physicians in some tasks.

A common response to such concerns about the impact of AI on jobs is that AI will be most fruitful when it collaborates with human workers rather than replacing them (24). In this view, humans and computers can contribute complementary skills and strengths to a task. Although this is true in the abstract, how to do this for a specific medical task remains to be specified.

Physician's Role in Assessing Machine Learning Algorithms

AI algorithms in medicine may be wrong, as in Case 46.1. In applications of AI to other areas, such as self-driving cars, algorithm errors have caused fatalities. Thus, prudent physicians would ask whether an AI algorithm improves patient outcomes and whether overall the benefits outweigh the risks, just as they do with other clinical innovations. Such prudence and critical thinking, which are key aspects of physician professionalism, are particularly important in fields like oncology, where new drugs and combinations are rapidly introduced.

However, there are cognitive and organizational challenges in expecting physicians to critically assess AI algorithms. First, machine learning algorithms are "black boxes." These algorithms cannot explain the variables that were used to calculate the algorithm or the reasoning that led to recommendations in a specific case. Nor can the computer scientists who developed the machine learning project provide such explanations. Thus, when a machine learning recommendation diverges from practice guidelines or expert recommendations or seems implausible or counterintuitive, treating physicians cannot obtain an explanation of the reasoning behind the recommendation, as they can from human consultants.

Second, it might become increasingly difficult for physicians to identify wrong recommendations as machine learning algorithms become more widely used. As physicians become more dependent on machine learning, there are fewer incentives for them to stay up to date on the most recent clinical literature and guidelines. It will be easy to assume that a computer knows them, when in fact the program may not have been updated recently to include new diagnostic categories or therapies. Physicians might wait for the machine learning recommendation and then ask whether it seems reasonable, rather than thinking through the case independently. If this occurs, physician expertise and judgment might atrophy. Moreover, if review of machine learning recommendations becomes routine because errors are expected to be infrequent, physicians will be more prone to lapses of attention and concentration when reviewing AI recommendations.

Physician Role in Implementing AI Recommendations

After an AI algorithm is judged to be appropriate to introduce into clinical practice, physicians will have an important role in integrating them into clinical workflows. Choice architecture or behavioral economics can suggest how to do so (19), taking into account the clinical issue, the stakes for the patient, the practice setting, physician workflow, and other tasks and issues competing for the physician's attention.

Current attempts to incorporate computer-generated reminders and suggestions for patients have often floundered because they do not fit well into the physician's priorities, needs, workflow, and constraints. Physician information overload and attention fatigue are common if many computer-generated recommendations are generated during the limited time of an outpatient visit. Currently, reminders of drug interactions are exhaustive rather than prioritized to those having clinical significance.

Implementation requires multiple steps to be worked out. In the hospital setting, an AI algorithm might identify a patient at high risk of sepsis. Who should be notified: the treating physician or an interdisciplinary rapid response team? After the initial evaluation confirms impending sepsis, how should standardized orders be carried out for laboratory evaluation, monitoring, and transfer to a higher level of care: as prewritten suggestions for the physician to sign or default orders that are implemented after initial clinical evaluation unless the physician overrides them? The best choices will likely depend on the hospital organization and culture.

Physician Role in Interacting with the Patient

If AI generates a valid clinical recommendation for a patient, for example, a diagnosis of skin cancer or clinically significant lung nodule, physicians will have to accomplish several important tasks, such as disclosing the diagnosis, discussing options for further evaluation and treatment, addressing the patient's concerns and needs, discussing the patient's goals, values, and preferences, and reaching agreement on a plan for care. In these discussions, physicians need to be attentive to the patient's needs, concerns, emotional reactions, and preferred decision-making style.

For the foreseeable future, machine learning is unlikely to replace humans at these complex interactions with patients. First, there is no agreement on how to measure success in doctor–patient discussions about different problems in patients from diverse backgrounds. Because these discussions have multiple goals, they may be successful at some but unsuccessful at others. Second, there are no large datasets of actual doctor–patient conversations in many clinical situations that could be used to train machine learning systems to carry out such conversations. Even if there were such training databases, without some annotation of desirable and undesirable outcomes, a machine learning algorithm could reproduce the shortcomings of current discussions.

Improving AI Algorithms Through Feedback from Stakeholders

In a major cultural shift, physicians and health care institutions now acknowledge that errors occur and can harm patients. Increasingly the accepted approach to medical errors is to disclose them to patients, apologize, carry out a root cause analysis, implement a quality-improvement plan to prevent similar errors in the future, and explain to the patient or family the plan to prevent future errors (see Chapter 34). Moreover, near misses are not to be dismissed, but valued as opportunities for improvement before a patient is actually harmed. The leaders of the health care organization need to support this approach.

Errors by machine learning algorithms in patient care should follow these standards for responding to errors and unintended adverse patient outcomes. However, there are several challenges when responding to errors by machine learning algorithms. First, who is the responsible human actor (19): The computer scientist who developed the algorithm? The head of the technology company that developed the algorithm? The leader of the health care organization that implemented the algorithm into clinical practice? The treating physician who did not override the erroneous recommendation? Second, how can the patient or family be told what caused a machine learning error if the algorithm cannot provide an explanation for its recommendations? Third, what should be the standards for correcting errors in machine learning systems? How can the algorithm be modified to prevent similar errors in the future? How often should programs be updated? How can the ethical responsibilities and legal duties of treating physicians and health care organizations be harmonized with the business model of the for-profit organization selling the algorithm? A for-profit artificial intelligence company may not be willing to disclose errors, analyze root causes, or implement timely corrective steps.

SUMMARY

Applications of AI to medicine will continue to increase in the future. Physicians have a crucial role in assuring AI is introduced into clinical medicine in a manner that patients will benefit, the risks are acceptable, and that the benefits and burdens are distributed fairly across society.

References

1. Kulynych J, Greely HT. Clinical genomics, big data, and electronic medical records: reconciling patient rights with research when privacy and science collide. *J Law Biosci* 2017;4:94-132.
2. Kumar S, Abowd G, Abraham WT, et al. Center of excellence for mobile sensor data-to-knowledge (MD2K). *IEEE Pervasive Comput* 2017;16:18-22.
3. Insel TR. Digital phenotyping: technology for a new science of behavior. *JAMA* 2017;318:1215-1216.
4. Juengst E, McGowan ML. Why does the shift from "personalized medicine" to "precision health" and "wellness genomics" matter? *AMA Journal of Ethics* 2018;20:E881-E890.
4a. National Academy of Sciences. *Toward Precision Medicine: Building a Knowledge Network for Biomedical Research and a New Taxonomy of Disease.* Washington, DC: National Academies Press; 2011. https://www.ncbi.nlm.nih.gov/books/NBK91503/.
5. McGraw SA, Garber J, Janne PA, et al. The fuzzy world of precision medicine: deliberations of a precision medicine tumor board. *Per Med* 2017;14:37-50.
6. Katz SJ, Jagsi R, Morrow M. Reducing overtreatment of cancer with precision medicine: just what the doctor ordered. *JAMA* 2018;319:1091-1092.
7. Korngiebel DM, Thummel KE, Burke W. Implementing precision medicine: the ethical challenges. *Trends Pharmacol Sci* 2017;38:8-14.
8. Dzau VJ, Ginsburg GS. Realizing the full potential of precision medicine in health and health care. *JAMA* 2016;316:1659-1660.
9. Popejoy AB, Fullerton SM. Genomics is failing on diversity. *Nature* 2016;538:161-164.
10. Feero WG, Wicklund CA, Veenstra D. Precision medicine, genome sequencing, and improved population health. *JAMA* 2018;319:1979-1980.
11. Khoury MJ, Galea S. Will precision medicine improve population health? *JAMA* 2016;316:1357-1358.
12. Bell L. *Machine learning versus AI: what's the difference.* 2016. Available at: http://www.wired.co.uk/article/machine-learning-ai-explained. Accessed July 17, 2018.
13. Buchanon B, Miller T. *Machine Learning for Policymakers*: Harvard Kennedy School Belfer Center for Science and International Affairs; 2017. https://www.belfercenter.org/publication/machine-learning-policymakers.
14. Beam AL, Kohane IS. Big data and machine learning in health care. *JAMA* 2018;319:1317-1318.

15. Thrall JH, Li X, Li Q, et al. Artificial intelligence and machine learning in radiology: opportunities, challenges, pitfalls, and criteria for success. *J Am Coll Radiol* 2018;15:504-508.

16. Lee A, Taylor P, Kalpathy-Cramer J, et al. Machine learning has arrived! *Ophthalmology* 2017;124:1726-1728.

17. Esteva A, Kuprel B, Novoa RA, et al. Dermatologist-level classification of skin cancer with deep neural networks. *Nature* 2017;542:115-118.

18. Golden JA. Deep learning algorithms for detection of lymph node metastases from breast cancer: helping artificial intelligence be seen. *JAMA* 2017;318:2184-2186.

19. Cohen IG, Amarasingham R, Shah A, et al. The legal and ethical concerns that arise from using complex predictive analytics in health care. *Health Aff (Millwood)* 2014;33:1139-1147.

20. Chen JH, Asch SM. Machine learning and prediction in medicine—beyond the peak of inflated expectations. *N Engl J Med* 2017;376:2507-2509.

21. Ross C. IBM's Watson supercomputer recommended "unsafe and incorrect" cancer treatments, internal documents show. *STAT News* July 25, 2018. https://www.statnews.com/2018/07/25/ibm-watson-recommended-unsafe-incorrect-treatments/.

22. Apostol CC, Waldfogel JM, Pfoh ER, et al. Association of goals of care meetings for hospitalized cancer patients at risk for critical care with patient outcomes. *Palliat Med* 2015;29:386-390.

23. Gianfrancesco MA, Tamang S, Yazdany J, et al. Potential biases in machine learning algorithms using electronic health record data. *JAMA Intern Med* 2018.

24. Verghese A, Shah NH, Harrington RA. What this computer needs is a physician: humanism and artificial intelligence. *JAMA* 2018;319:19-20.

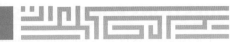
INFORMED CONSENT

CASE 1	Choosing among therapeutic options for breast cancer

An asymptomatic 52-year-old computer programmer is diagnosed with stage T1 localized breast cancer. Options for treatment include total mastectomy or lumpectomy plus radiation therapy. Suppose that you are the attending surgeon.

QUESTIONS FOR DISCUSSION

1. You are hosting a visiting physician from China, who says he does not understand why Americans regard informed consent as so important: "I can understand that in your country, you tell patients they have cancer. But why don't you then just do what is the best treatment for them, rather than going through what you call informed consent?" How would you explain (a) the purposes of informed consent and (b) the ethical reasons for informed consent?
2. An intern asks you how to determine what information about surgery he needs to discuss with the patient. "I just read a chapter in a surgery textbook, and I'm not sure how much information I should tell her before asking her to sign the consent form," he says. "There's no way I can tell her everything! What do I need to discuss with her?" How would you answer the intern's question?
3. Suppose, on the basis of your critical reading of the published evidence, you believe that breast-conserving surgery plus radiation therapy offers the best outcome for this patient. How do you incorporate this judgment in your discussions with the patient?
4. One resident has read articles reporting that patients do not understand basic information that physicians discuss with them and says, "Why do we bother with the informed consent? Patients don't understand what we tell them and don't remember any of it." How do you respond to the resident's objections?
5. A student asks if patients need to be told of the role that students and residents play during surgery and in postoperative care. One of the residents says, "We don't need to tell the patient about that. They have given implied consent to have residents and students participate in their care by choosing to come to a teaching hospital." Do you agree or disagree? Give the ethical considerations for your position. How have the courts used the term *implied consent*?

REFUSAL OF CARE

CASE 2	Refusal of treatment by a patient with inoperable cancer

A 64-year-old man has inoperable pancreatic cancer and obstructive jaundice. He had an internal drainage tube placed in the common duct in an attempt to decompress his biliary tree. However, he developed cholangitis, which was treated with antibiotics. He entered hospice care, and over the next 2 weeks he developed progressive jaundice, abdominal pain, nausea, pruritis, anorexia, and weight loss. He understands that he is unlikely to live more than a few weeks. His drainage tube obstructs and he is admitted with another episode of biliary sepsis. As his physician, you discuss with him plans for care. He is lucid and shows no sign of mental impairment during your conversation.

QUESTIONS FOR DISCUSSION

1. The patient says he does not want cardiopulmonary resuscitation (CPR) attempted if he suffers a cardiac arrest. Would you write a Do Not Attempt Resuscitation (DNAR) order? What are the ethical reasons for your decision?
2. What would you do if his wife or family disagrees with his refusal of CPR? What is the ethical rationale for your response?
3. The patient also refuses antibiotics for biliary sepsis, saying, "There isn't any point in going through this again only to have another infection next week or the week after." The intern exclaims, "How can we not give him antibiotics? He'll die without them, and we have an ethical duty to save lives." Do you agree to withhold antibiotics? What is the ethical rationale for your position?

CASE 3	**Refusal of blood transfusions by a Jehovah's Witness**

A 34-year-old grade school teacher is hospitalized after an automobile accident that ruptures his spleen. A devout Jehovah's Witness, he refuses a blood transfusion. He does agree to a splenectomy and states emphatically, "I wish to live, but with no blood transfusions." He also refuses blood components and court-ordered transfusions. He declares, "It is between me and God, not the courts. I'm willing to take my chances. My faith is that strong." He is lucid throughout the conversation.

QUESTIONS FOR DISCUSSION

1. His hematocrit drops to 14.1%. One of the residents says, "How can we just stand by and let him bleed to death when we could bring him back to full health with transfusions? Aren't doctors supposed to act for the good of the patient? How can it be good for a young, healthy man to die needlessly?" Do you agree with the resident? What is the ethical rationale for your position?
2. The patient's wife was a Jehovah's Witness but left the faith. "I know that he says he doesn't want a blood transfusion, but I also know he loves his children and his work," she says. "He could never agree to a transfusion, but he couldn't bear to leave us either. Can't you just give him blood without telling him when he's in surgery? Then he would get the care he needs." How do you respond to the wife? Explain the ethical rationale for your approach.
3. The surgeon is reluctant to operate without transfusion support. "What's the point of taking someone to the operating room to have him die on the table?" he says. "If he wants to refuse transfusions and die in the emergency room, then that's his right. But he can't force me to operate and be responsible for his death." Do you agree or disagree with the surgeon? What is the ethical rationale for your position?

CASE 4	**No clear reason for refusal of medically effective treatment**

A 45-year-old sales clerk has a 1/2-cm breast mass that is found to be malignant on needle aspiration. With either mastectomy or lumpectomy plus radiation, she has an excellent chance of being cured of her cancer. She refuses any form of therapy, saying that she wants to try natural healing through herbal remedies, megavitamin therapy, spiritual healing, and relaxation techniques.

QUESTIONS FOR DISCUSSION

1. One resident objects, "How do we just stand by when she would most likely be cured of her cancer with surgery? Aren't we supposed to act in the patient's best interests? How can it be in the patient's best interests to lose the chance to cure her cancer?" Another resident says, "Wait a minute, we're supposed to respect patient autonomy. It's her body and her life, and it's her decision." How do you respond to these viewpoints? What is the ethical rationale for your position? How would you carry out your views in practice?

CONFIDENTIALITY

CASE 5	Reporting a patient with syncope to the Department of Motor Vehicles

A 76-year-old retired teacher with a history of coronary artery disease is hospitalized after a syncopal episode. He is found to have ventricular tachycardia. He had two previous syncopal episodes during the past 3 years. An automatic implantable cardioverter defibrillator (AICD) is implanted. During the first year after implantation, about 10% of patients experience syncope or near-syncope because of defibrillation.

QUESTIONS FOR DISCUSSION

1. A nurse in a clinic asks if the patient needs to be reported to the Department of Motor Vehicles. How do you respond? What ethical considerations support your position?
2. Suppose that your patient is a 47-year-old bus driver instead of a retiree. The patient tells you that he is willing to try anything, even take temporary leave from work, as long as you don't report him to the Department of Motor Vehicles. "Doc, if you take my license away, I can't support my family," he pleads. "I need this job." How do you respond? What ethical considerations support your position?

CASE 6	Use of anabolic steroids by an athlete

A colleague asks your advice on a difficult case. A 19-year-old college swimmer reveals that she has started to take anabolic steroids, which she obtains through friends at the gym where she lifts weights. She says that she is aware of the long-term side effects but plans to use the drugs only while she is competing in intercollegiate athletics. She doesn't want to lose her athletic scholarship. Because many of her opponents are using steroids, she believes there is no other way for her to be competitive.

QUESTIONS FOR DISCUSSION

1. Your colleague asks whether she should tell the swim coach about the patient's steroid use, saying, "Maybe the coach can discourage her from taking these drugs. It's so dangerous for her, and her health can't be worth winning a few races. We need to act in her best interests." How do you respond? What ethical considerations support your position?
2. Another colleague, joining your discussion, suggests, "She should be reported to the intercollegiate athletic officials. It isn't fair to other swimmers for her to have an advantage. If she wants to risk her health, then that's her business, but let's keep the pool lanes fair." How would you respond? What ethical considerations support your position?
3. A third colleague says, "If you tell anyone, it should be her parents. If I were her mother, I'd certainly want to know." What is your view on talking to her parents? What ethical considerations support your position?

CASE 7	Disclosure of genetic illness to relatives

A 40-year-old auto mechanic is found to have localized breast cancer, which is treated with lumpectomy and radiation. Because of a family history of both ovarian and breast cancer in several first-degree relatives, she is tested for BRCA-1 and is found to be positive for a variant that confers a greatly increased risk for these cancers. As her physician, you discuss the implications of this

(continued)

CASE 7	Disclosure of genetic illness to relatives (*continued*)

autosomal recessive condition for her 34-year-old and 36-year-old sisters and urge her to disclose her test results to them so they can be tested for BRCA-1. A relative who has the same mutation has a lifetime 85% risk of breast cancer and a 50% risk of ovarian cancer. An affected relative will probably want to begin screening mammography earlier than is usually recommended and also may want to consider interventions such as bilateral mastectomy, tamoxifen, and experimental therapies. Your patient refuses to disclose her results to her sisters or to allow you to do so. "We had a major falling out when mom died," she tells you. "They did some things that I don't think I can ever forgive. I just don't want to get involved with them at this point in my life."

QUESTIONS FOR DISCUSSION

1. A nurse is outraged at the patient's refusal to inform her sisters that they might be at high risk for cancer. "We should pick up the phone and call them," she says. "This is more serious than tuberculosis, and we notify contacts of TB patients. What if her sisters years later present with inoperable cancer?" How do you respond to the nurse? What ethical considerations support your position?

DECISION-MAKING CAPACITY

CASE 8	Refusal of colonoscopy

A 72-year-old retired lawyer comes into the hospital with lower abdominal pain. He is found to have guaiac positive stools and anemia. You plan to do a colonoscopy, but the patient refuses. During your conversation, you learn that the patient spends all day inside his house where the electricity has been turned off because of outstanding bills.

One intern says that it is appropriate to seek a court order, saying, "This guy can't even pay his bills, how can we expect him to make decisions about his health care?" Another intern responds, "Look, I have trouble paying my bills on time. I hope that no court would override my medical decisions."

The patient's only relative is a niece who lives in a distant state. She says that he is somewhat cantankerous and has always been independent and stubborn. She is unable to persuade him over the phone to have the colonoscopy. She tells the doctors, "If you believe that he's not able to make decisions for himself, then I would certainly give permission for you to do the tests and treatments he needs. I want the best care for him."

QUESTIONS FOR DISCUSSION

1. What will happen if it is determined that the patient is competent to make medical decisions? What if he is determined to lack decision-making capacity?
2. What questions would you ask this patient to better evaluate whether he is competent to make decisions about his care?
3. The intern says, "I was told that we have to get a psychiatry consultation to declare a patient incompetent." Do you agree or disagree? What ethical considerations support your position?

DECISIONS FOR INCOMPETENT PATIENTS

CASE 9	Mechanical ventilation in end-stage lung disease

Mrs. O, a 64-year-old retired grocery store owner with end-stage interstitial lung disease, presents to the emergency department for shortness of breath that began several days ago. On room air, she is breathing at a rate of 36 and has an O2 saturation of 54%. She is cyanotic and using her accessory muscles. On examination, she is afebrile and has no signs of consolidation. She is unable to have a coherent conversation. Her chest x-ray shows no acute infiltrates. At baseline, her FEV1 is 0.8 L, and her room air blood gas is PH 7.38, PO2 46 mm Hg, PCO2 55 mm Hg. She has shortness of breath walking around her house. She lives with her daughter and two grandchildren, her closest relatives. Mrs. O pulls off both nasal cannulae and a mask delivering oxygen. Her daughter is unable to get her to keep the supplemental O2 on.

Mrs. O has never completed a durable power of attorney for health care, and has no Do Not Intubate (DNI) order in the computerized record system. You are unable to get the primary care physician's records, and the on-call physician does not know the patient.

QUESTIONS FOR DISCUSSION

1. The daughter says that her mother knows that she has end-stage lung disease and has told her primary physician several times that she does not want to be intubated. The patient has also told the daughter that she would not want intubation. Her daughter reports, "She knows what intubation is. She had it several years ago when she had pneumonia. But she knows that her lungs have just gotten worse and worse. She's ready to die when the time comes, but she wants to die with dignity, without machines or tubes." Your resident says doctors must provide treatment for potentially reversible conditions, saying, "This may be aspiration pneumonia, from which she could recover. Without a written advance directive or DNI order, we have to intubate her." Do you agree? What are the ethical justifications for your position?

2. One intern says, "We have to intubate her. All we know is what the daughter is telling us. How can we be sure that she is saying what her mother wants? You can't always trust family members; maybe she is trying to get an inheritance. Whenever there is any doubt, we have to err on the side of preserving life." The other intern responds, "But that means we would never trust a family to make decisions for an incompetent patient, except when patients complete a health care proxy. That doesn't seem right." Do you agree with either intern? What are the ethical justifications for your position? How might the first intern's concerns be addressed in emergency situations?

CASE 10	Stroke and aspiration pneumonia

Mr. S, a 74-year-old retired gas station owner with Alzheimer disease and coronary artery disease, is admitted with a stroke. An ECG also shows an acute myocardial infarction with many premature ventricular contractions. He develops an aspiration pneumonia that is treated with antibiotics. Three days after admission, he has a dense hemiplegia, is unable to speak coherently, and has difficulty swallowing. At his baseline, he often does not recognize family members and needs help with all activities of daily living. He has not given any written advance directives.

QUESTIONS FOR DISCUSSION

1. According to his wife and daughter, he had said many times that becoming demented and living in a nursing home would be a fate worse than death. He had helped care for an uncle with Alzheimer disease and had said that not being able to recognize people and take care of himself would be intolerable. The wife and daughter request that he be transferred out of the intensive care unit (ICU) and allowed to die. They want a DNAR order, no intubation, no feeding tube, and no antibiotics for infections. "Just keep him comfortable and let him die in peace," they say. In the emergency room, they agreed to active treatments because they were told that his stroke might be reversible and that he might return home. However, he has not improved after 3 days. They are unable to care for him at home because of his wife's medical problems and his daughter's job. They cannot afford to hire full-time help. The nurses comment that his family seem devoted to him. Do you agree with the DNAR and DNI orders? What are the ethical justifications for your position?
2. How would the ethical and legal analysis be different if the patient had completed an advance directive appointing his wife as proxy?

CASE 11	Stroke and aspiration pneumonia

Assume the same medical facts as in Case 10, but Mr. S has made no statements about his preferences for care. His wife and daughter believe that he would not want to receive continued intensive care after failing to improve from his stroke. "He never really talked about what he would want in this situation for himself," his wife explains. "But he was a man who prided himself on his independence and dignity. He never wanted anyone to help him when he was injured or sick. He was always immaculately dressed. He would never even go out to pick up the newspaper in the morning before getting dressed because he didn't want anyone to see him in his robe or pajamas. It's hard enough for him to have us help him. He would be mortified to have strangers help him with his bathing and dressing. We've been married over 50 years, and I know in my heart he wouldn't want to live like this."

QUESTIONS FOR DISCUSSION

1. The intern says that without some indication of the patient's own preferences, either written or oral, it is inappropriate to discontinue antibiotics or write DNAR and DNI orders. "What the family is saying is pure speculation," the intern points out. "Also he may still improve from his stroke." Do you agree with the intern? What are the ethical justifications for your position?

CASE 12	Stroke and aspiration pneumonia

Assume the same medical facts as in Case 10, but Mr. S has made no statements about his preferences for care and has no family members. He has lived in a nursing home for several years and has no friends who visit him regularly. The nurses did not know him before he became demented.

QUESTIONS FOR DISCUSSION

1. One of the interns says, "We have to continue ICU care because we don't know what the patient would want in this situation. Without any surrogate, we have to give maximal treatment. How can we say that it's better for him to be dead than to live like this, when we don't know him?" Do you agree with the intern? What are the ethical justifications for your position?

CONFUSING ETHICAL DISTINCTIONS

CASE 13	Withdrawal of mechanical ventilation

Assume that Mrs. O, the 64-year-old retired grocery store owner with end-stage interstitial lung disease from Case 9, was intubated in the ED. The next morning you obtain old records, which document extensive discussions with her primary physician that she does not want to be intubated or have resuscitation attempted. You also speak with the primary physician, who confirms that the patient did not want to be intubated and says, "This is exactly what she most feared—being on a ventilator with nothing readily reversible."

QUESTIONS FOR DISCUSSION

1. An ICU nurse says, "I would have no problem if we hadn't intubated her in the first place. But we can't just turn off the ventilator or extubate her. She would die in a couple of minutes. That would be killing her, pure and simple, just as if we injected potassium." Do you agree with the nurse? What are the ethical justifications for your position?
2. Because the patient will be dyspneic, you want to administer morphine and also provide sedation. An intern objects, saying that it could reduce her respirations or lower her blood pressure, which would kill her: "That would be active euthanasia, and that's wrong." Do you agree? What are the ethical justifications for your position?

CASE 14	Withdrawal of antibiotics and withholding tube feedings

Assume that Mrs. O, the 64-year-old retired grocery store owner with end-stage interstitial lung disease from Case 9, is transferred out of the ICU with DNAR and DNI orders, based on the family reports of her previous statements. The family requests that no tube feedings be given.

QUESTIONS FOR DISCUSSION

1. The neurology consultant exclaims, "I have no problem with the DNAR and DNI orders. But feeding her and giving her antibiotics are basic, ordinary care. It would be inhumane to withhold them." Do you agree? What are the ethical justifications for your position?

DNAR ORDERS

CASE 15	DNAR orders during endoscopy

A 58-year-old woman with dysphagia is found to have inoperable carcinoma of the esophagus. She realizes her poor prognosis and opts for palliation. With the concurrence of her family, she agrees to DNAR and DNI orders. Because she has difficulty maintaining adequate oral intake, she agrees to endoscopic placement of an intraluminal esophageal stent.

QUESTIONS FOR DISCUSSION

1. The gastroenterologist who performs the procedure insists that the DNAR order be lifted during the procedure, saying, "I understand that she has chosen palliative care, and I respect that. But if she has a cardiac arrest during the endoscopy, it is due to the medications that we give for

conscious sedation. Our ability to resuscitate patients in this situation, even those with inoperable cancer, is close to 100%. The situation is completely different from a cardiopulmonary arrest that occurs spontaneously in the course of illness." Do you agree with the gastroenterologist that the DNAR order should be suspended during the procedure? What are the ethical justifications for your position?

CASE 16	**Pneumonia and Alzheimer disease**

A 74-year-old man with severe Alzheimer disease is transferred from a nursing home for treatment for pneumonia. Except for mild hypercholesterolemia and osteoarthritis of the knees and hips, he has no active medical problems and takes no medications regularly. He has no living relatives or friends, and before becoming demented he had not indicated what he would want done in such a situation. His baseline state in the nursing home is that he requires assistance with all activities of daily living, including eating. He usually does not recognize nursing home staff, but he does smile when watching television. The nursing home physician says that he does not know what the patient would want, but that it seems reasonable to administer antibiotics but not to provide more intensive interventions, such as mechanical ventilation.

QUESTIONS FOR DISCUSSION

1. The resident on the team says, "He should be DNAR. It doesn't make any sense to resuscitate someone with such a terrible quality of life. It would be futile." Do you agree with the resident's view? What are the ethical justifications for your position?

FUTILE INTERVENTIONS

CASE 17	**Multiorgan failure**

Mr. D is a 72-year-old homebound man with multisystem failure admitted to a hospital for pneumonia, a myeloproliferative disorder, and failure to thrive. He develops stupor and adult respiratory distress syndrome (ARDS), for which he requires mechanical ventilation. He then develops renal failure requiring dialysis and recurrent episodes of hypotension and sepsis. No primary site of infection has been identified.

His major problem now is abdominal pain and distention, which requires opioids. A CT scan shows dilated extrahepatic bile ducts but no intrahepatic dilatation or other abnormalities. His liver function tests are only mildly and occasionally elevated. The patient's daughter believes that an operation on his biliary tract would cure his abdominal problem and that relief of his abdominal distention would allow him to be weaned off the ventilator. The surgeon believes that there is no abdominal problem that surgery would improve and that general anesthesia would be an extremely high risk. Two attempts at endoscopic retrograde cholangio-pancreatography (ERCP) were unable to visualize the ampulla of Vater. Interventional radiology is unwilling to attempt percutaneous biliary drainage because there is no intrahepatic duct dilatation.

Mr. D has given no advance directives. The patient's wife tends to defer to the daughter in discussions and agrees with her. His family believes that if he had widespread cancer or were in a permanent coma, he would not want life-prolonging treatment, but they point out that this is not currently the case. They refuse to agree to a DNAR order or limitation of medical interventions.

QUESTIONS FOR DISCUSSION

1. The surgical chief resident says that it would be "crazy" to operate on Mr. D and remarks, "He's not a surgical candidate. There is no reason to operate. It would be futile. We won't take him to the operating room, no matter what the family wants." Do you believe that exploratory laparotomy would be futile and that the surgery team may refuse to do the procedure? What are the ethical justifications for your position?
2. The gastrointestinal (GI) service declines to make another attempt at ERCP. The GI fellow says, "We've already tried the procedure twice. There's no point in trying again. The family can't force us to do something that's futile." Do you believe that ERCP would be futile and that the GI team may refuse to do the procedure? What are the ethical justifications for your position?
3. The nephrology service believes that continuing dialysis is futile, saying, "What's the point of dialyzing him? That's not going to allow him to leave the ICU." Do you believe that continued dialysis would be futile and that the nephrology team may refuse to do the procedure? What are the ethical justifications for your position?
4. When you sign out the patient to the night float resident, she notes that the last time she covered, the patient suffered an episode of hypotension, which she treated with fluids, vasopressors, and antibiotics. "What if that happens again, but he doesn't respond and develops progressive hypotension despite maximal therapy?" she asks. "Do you still want me to do CPR if he suffers a cardiac arrest? Why don't you write a medical DNAR order? CPR would be futile." In that situation, would it be appropriate to withhold CPR despite the family's wishes? What are the ethical justifications for your position?

PHYSICIAN-ASSISTED SUICIDE AND ACTIVE EUTHANASIA

CASE 18	Head and neck cancer

Mrs. M is 57-year-old machinist who has recurrent head and neck cancer that has progressed despite radiation and chemotherapy. She cannot swallow foods and secretions and has to sit upright at night to spit out her secretions. She asks her physician for a prescription for a lethal dose of sleeping pills and says, "It's barbaric that the medical system does not allow me to retain the last shreds of my dignity. Why can't I have the same humane, compassionate treatment that we give our pets at the end of their lives? I do not want to wait for pneumonia or starvation to deliver me. I want to end my life freely and rationally. I am not depressed, but it is inhumane to ask me to live this way. Don't force me to shoot myself to get relief." Her husband and children agree with her decision.

QUESTIONS FOR DISCUSSION

1. What actions should a physician who supports physician-assisted suicide take before deciding that it is appropriate to write a prescription for a lethal dose of medication in this case?
2. What actions should a physician who opposes physician-assisted suicide take in addition to refusing the patient's request?
3. Does the moral responsibility of the physician differ when writing a lethal prescription compared with injecting a lethal dose of medication, such as potassium?

CASE 19	Failed suicide attempt

Mrs. M, the patient with head and neck cancer in Case 18, is found at home by her husband after a suicide attempt. She has ingested a combination of tricyclic antidepressants, benzodiazepines, and alcohol and has left a long explanatory note. She had held a good-bye party for her friends and then ingested the medications while her husband played her favorite music. As they agreed, she was left alone for 3 hours. When Mr. M returned with a friend, they found her unconscious and grunting for breath. Horrified that she was suffering, Mr. M called 911.

   Paramedics found that her O2 saturation was 70% and intubated her. In the ED, she is placed on mechanical ventilation and given intravenous fluids and vasopressors. The patient's primary physician confirms her progressive cancer, her recent deterioration, and the absence of depression or other psychiatric illness, saying, "She didn't want to be a burden on her family or spend her last days waiting for a medical complication. I personally wouldn't do what she did, but I respect her choice. There is no question that she thought about this long and hard."

QUESTIONS FOR DISCUSSION

1. Would you continue mechanical ventilation, fluids, and vasopressors? One ED resident says, "If we withdraw support, we'll be abetting a suicide. That's illegal and morally wrong. My conscience won't let me do that. What message does it send to other patients if the ED helps people kill themselves?" Do you agree with this position? What are the ethical justifications for your position?
2. While the medical and nursing staff are discussing the case, the patient begins to awaken. She is weaned off vasopressors, and 2 hours later she is extubated. As per ED protocol, a psychiatrist talks with her. She says, "Of course, I'll do this again as soon as I get home and can figure out how to do it right. We'll have to get on the Internet and find out. Don't you understand that waiting for some medical catastrophe is an inhumane way to die? Wouldn't you do the same thing? Do you expect me to lie about my intentions just to make you all feel better?" As the psychiatrist, do you place her on an involuntary hold because she is actively suicidal? What are the ethical justifications for your position?

CASE 20	Withdrawal of mechanical ventilation

Mrs. O, the 64-year-old retired grocery store owner with end-stage interstitial lung disease from Case 9, has mechanical ventilation withdrawn based on evidence that she would not want such treatment. She is placed on oxygen via nasal cannulae and morphine and diazepam drips to palliate her dyspnea and anxiety. On 10 mg morphine per hour and 2 mg diazepam per hour, the patient appears comfortable, without any tachypnea, use of accessory muscles, tachycardia, or restlessness. Her respiratory rate is 12 per minute. She does not respond when called or when an intravenous line is restarted.

QUESTIONS FOR DISCUSSION

1. The patient's family requests that you increase the dose of medications: "She said many times she didn't want to linger or to have a prolonged death." Do you agree with the family's request? What are the ethical justifications for your position?

REFUSAL TO CARE FOR PATIENTS

CASE 21	Caring for a patient with AIDS

A 34-year-old unemployed homeless man with AIDS (CD4 level 47) is admitted to your service with *Pneumocystis carinii* pneumonia. His IV has infiltrated, and you are asked to restart it.

QUESTIONS FOR DISCUSSION

1. How would you feel if you suffered a needle-stick injury while caring for an HIV-infected patient?
2. One of the interns on the admitting team refuses to take care of this patient. What are the ethical considerations if each of the following holds true?
2a. The intern says he is inexperienced at starting IVs and thinks that a more experienced physician should care for the patient.
2b. The intern is a deeply religious person who believes that homosexuality is a sin. Because the patient is gay, the intern does not want to care for him. The intern says, "I couldn't live with myself if I helped him live in sin."
2c. The patient is an injection drug user. An injection drug user at the hospital had earlier in the year mugged the intern. The intern is still experiencing flashbacks about that earlier incident and does not want to be subjected to more stress.

ETHICAL DILEMMAS FACING STUDENTS AND HOUSE STAFF: LEARNING ON PATIENTS

CASE 22   Outcomes of coronary artery bypass and graft

Suppose your favorite uncle, who lives in New York, has been recommended to have coronary artery bypass and graft (CABAG) for angina that is poorly controlled with medical management and that interferes with his usual activities. From your clinical epidemiology course you recall that the mortality rates for this operation vary from less than 1% to more than 8% and that New York State publishes mortality rates for hospitals and for individual surgeons.

QUESTION FOR DISCUSSION

1. Do you want to know the outcomes experience for the hospital or for the surgeon who would operate on your uncle? What are your reasons?
2. Would you feel comfortable having surgery residents carry out part of the operation under supervision?

CASE 23   Carrying out an invasive procedure

Recall the first time you did a lumbar puncture (LP) (or central line, or other similar procedure).

QUESTIONS FOR DISCUSSION

1. How did you feel before doing your first invasive procedure?
2. One of your classmates says that by coming to a teaching hospital, patients have given implied consent to having students and residents do procedures. Thus, there is no need to tell the patient that a student will be performing a procedure. Do you agree, and why?
3. What would you do if before your first LP, the resident calls to say go ahead and do it yourself because he and the interns are in the ED with critically ill new patients? The LP needs to be done today. How would you respond?

| CASE 24 | Unethical behavior of an attending physician |

On a clerkship, you observe what you consider unethical behavior by one of your attending physicians. On several occasions, his speech is slurred and you smell alcohol on his breath. He also fails to round on his patients for days at a time, without having anyone cover for him, and does not return your pages or those of your resident.

QUESTIONS FOR DISCUSSION

1. What are the ethical reasons for reporting the situation to an appropriate senior physician?
2. What are some of the risks to you if you report the situation?
3. In practical terms, how might you proceed?

DISCLOSING ERRORS

| CASE 25 | Muscle weakness due to inadequate potassium replacement |

A 42-year-old man is admitted to your team with diabetic ketoacidosis. After treatment with intravenous fluids and an insulin drip, the patient's glucose declines from 745 to 289 mg per dL after 4 hours. However, the patient develops progressive weakness and difficulty breathing and requires transfer to the ICU for mechanical ventilation. In reviewing the case, you check the computer for lab results and realize that the patient had a potassium of 2.3 mmol per L. No potassium replacement had been given during the treatment of the ketoacidosis.

The patient's family asks what happened and whether he had a stroke. They say that the patient has been hospitalized several times for ketoacidosis but has never required mechanical ventilation.

QUESTIONS FOR DISCUSSION

1. If you were the subintern on the case who did not order potassium replacement, what would your feelings be?
2. In your experience, how have colleagues reacted to serious mistakes?
3. What would your concerns be about telling the attending physician about this mistake?
4. Would you tell the attending physician about the episode?
5. A nurse asks you what she should tell the patient and family, saying that they are very concerned about what happened. How do you respond? What are the ethical reasons for your response?

ETHICAL ISSUES IN PEDIATRICS

| CASE 26 | Treating adolescents without parental consent |

A 15-year-old high school student comes to the physician because of dysuria and a discharge from his penis after intercourse without a condom. He wants to be tested and treated but does not want his parents to know about his problems. "They would completely freak out if they knew I was having sex," he says.

QUESTIONS FOR DISCUSSION

1. You ask a colleague whether you can treat the patient without his parents' authorization. She says that you may do so, provided that he is capable of giving informed consent to treatment. Do you agree with her advice? What are the ethical justifications for your position?
2. The patient is so concerned about his parents' finding out that he asks you to write on the encounter form that the visit is for shoulder pain. "I don't want them getting a bill that tells them why I came in." How do you respond to his request? Give the ethical considerations for your decision.

CASE 27	Treating children despite refusals

A 10-year-old boy is taken to the ED with vomiting and right lower quadrant abdominal pain and is found to have appendicitis.

QUESTIONS FOR DISCUSSION

1. The patient says that he does not want surgery, saying that the pain is getting better and he does not want to have a scar the rest of his life. His parents are willing to authorize surgery for him. The resident on the team says, "We're not going to operate on a patient who is screaming that he doesn't want surgery. That's assaulting the patient." Do you agree with the resident? What are the ethical reasons supporting your position?
2. Suppose instead that the parents refuse surgery after an aunt who was baby-sitting brought the child to the ED. The parents are devout Christian Scientists who believe that their child will recover with prayer therapy. The intern says that parents are not permitted to make irrational decisions, so the surgery should proceed as recommended. Do you agree with the intern? What are the ethical reasons supporting your position?

Index

Note: Page numbers followed by *f* indicate figures; those followed by *t* indicate tables respectively.